Wearable Sensors Applied in Movement Analysis

Wearable Sensors Applied in Movement Analysis

Editors

Fabien Buisseret
Frédéric Dierick
Liesbet Van der Perre

MDPI • Basel • Beijing • Wuhan • Barcelona • Belgrade • Manchester • Tokyo • Cluj • Tianjin

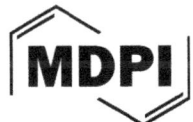

Editors

Fabien Buisseret
CeREF-Technique
Mons
Belgium

Frédéric Dierick
LAMP
Rehazenter
Luxembourg
Luxembourg

Liesbet Van der Perre
DRAMCO Lab
KU Leuven
Gent
Belgium

Editorial Office
MDPI
St. Alban-Anlage 66
4052 Basel, Switzerland

This is a reprint of articles from the Special Issue published online in the open access journal *Sensors* (ISSN 1424-8220) (available at: www.mdpi.com/journal/sensors/special_issues/Wearable_Sensors_Applied_in_Movement_Analysis).

For citation purposes, cite each article independently as indicated on the article page online and as indicated below:

LastName, A.A.; LastName, B.B.; LastName, C.C. Article Title. *Journal Name* **Year**, *Volume Number*, Page Range.

ISBN 978-3-0365-5860-8 (Hbk)
ISBN 978-3-0365-5859-2 (PDF)

© 2022 by the authors. Articles in this book are Open Access and distributed under the Creative Commons Attribution (CC BY) license, which allows users to download, copy and build upon published articles, as long as the author and publisher are properly credited, which ensures maximum dissemination and a wider impact of our publications.

The book as a whole is distributed by MDPI under the terms and conditions of the Creative Commons license CC BY-NC-ND.

Contents

About the Editors vii

Fabien Buisseret, Frédéric Dierick and Liesbet Van der Perre
Wearable Sensors Applied in Movement Analysis
Reprinted from: *Sensors* **2022**, *22*, 8239, doi:10.3390/s22218239 1

Trung C. Phan, Adrian Pranata, Joshua Farragher, Adam Bryant, Hung T. Nguyen and Rifai Chai
Machine Learning Derived Lifting Techniques and Pain Self-Efficacy in People with Chronic Low Back Pain
Reprinted from: *Sensors* **2022**, *22*, 6694, doi:10.3390/s22176694 5

Paul Thiry, Martin Houry, Laurent Philippe, Olivier Nocent, Fabien Buisseret and Frédéric Dierick et al.
Machine Learning Identifies Chronic Low Back Pain Patients from an Instrumented Trunk Bending and Return Test
Reprinted from: *Sensors* **2022**, *22*, 5027, doi:10.3390/s22135027 23

Woosoon Jung and Hyung Gyu Lee
Energy–Accuracy Aware Finger Gesture Recognition for Wearable IoT Devices
Reprinted from: *Sensors* **2022**, *22*, 4801, doi:10.3390/s22134801 37

Dylan den Hartog, Marjolein M. van der Krogt, Sven van der Burg, Ignazio Aleo, Johannes Gijsbers and Laura A. Bonouvrié et al.
Home-Based Measurements of Dystonia in Cerebral Palsy Using Smartphone-Coupled Inertial Sensor Technology and Machine Learning: A Proof-of-Concept Study
Reprinted from: *Sensors* **2022**, *22*, 4386, doi:10.3390/s22124386 55

Renaud Hage, Fabien Buisseret, Martin Houry and Frédéric Dierick
Head Pitch Angular Velocity Discriminates (Sub-)Acute Neck Pain Patients and Controls Assessed with the DidRen Laser Test
Reprinted from: *Sensors* **2022**, *22*, 2805, doi:10.3390/s22072805 69

Frédéric Dierick, Pierre-Loup Stoffel, Gaston Schütz and Fabien Buisseret
High Specificity of Single Inertial Sensor-Supplemented Timed Up and Go Test for Assessing Fall Risk in Elderly Nursing Home Residents
Reprinted from: *Sensors* **2022**, *22*, 2339, doi:10.3390/s22062339 81

Stefano Lanzi, Joël Boichat, Luca Calanca, Lucia Mazzolai and Davide Malatesta
Supervised Exercise Training Improves 6 min Walking Distance and Modifies Gait Pattern during Pain-Free Walking Condition in Patients with Symptomatic Lower Extremity Peripheral Artery Disease
Reprinted from: *Sensors* **2021**, *21*, 7989, doi:10.3390/s21237989 91

Yeon-Wook Kim, Kyung-Lim Joa, Han-Young Jeong and Sangmin Lee
Wearable IMU-Based Human Activity Recognition Algorithm for Clinical Balance Assessment Using 1D-CNN and GRU Ensemble Model
Reprinted from: *Sensors* **2021**, *21*, 7628, doi:10.3390/s21227628 105

Cory Snyder, Aaron Martínez, Rüdiger Jahnel, Jason Roe and Thomas Stöggl
Connected Skiing: Motion Quality Quantification in Alpine Skiing
Reprinted from: *Sensors* **2021**, *21*, 3779, doi:10.3390/s21113779 121

Yosuke Tomita, Tomoki Iizuka, Koichi Irisawa and Shigeyuki Imura
Detection of Movement Events of Long-Track Speed Skating Using Wearable Inertial Sensors
Reprinted from: *Sensors* **2021**, *21*, 3649, doi:10.3390/s21113649 . . . . **135**

About the Editors

Fabien Buisseret

Dr Fabien Buisseret has a degree in Physics and a PhD in Science (University of Mons –UMONS, Belgium). After pursuing research in hadronic Physics as a post-doctoral fellow at UMONS, he is currently a teacher at Haute Ecole Louvain en Hainaut, a researcher at CeREF (HELHa's research center) and a scientific collaborator at UMONS. His research interests are human motion analysis through mechanical, nonlinear and sensor-based approaches, as well as theoretical and hadronic Physics. He also takes part in the creation and management of interdisciplinary projects for CeREF. Currently, he is part of the leading operator team of the Interreg FWVl NOMADe project.

Frédéric Dierick

Dr Frédéric Dierick holds a PhD in Physiotherapy and Rehabilitation (Université catholique de Louvain - UCLouvain, Belgium, 2006). From 2003 to 2019, he worked at the Haute Ecole Louvain in Hainaut as a teacher-researcher and developed the "Forme & Fonctionnement Humain"laboratory (Physiotherapy department, Charleroi, Belgium). In 2020, he joined the CNRFR - Rehazenter (Luxembourg, Luxembourg) as a senior researcher and manager of national and international research projects. His research are devoted to human motion analysis in healthy and pathological states, especially the development of multidisciplinary methods involving low-cost sensors, medical imaging or nonlinear time series analysis. Currently, he is the leader of the Interreg FWVl NOMADe project.

Liesbet Van der Perre

Liesbet Van der Perre received the MSc and PhD degree in Electrical Engineering from the KU Leuven, Belgium, in 1992 and 1997 respectively. The research for her thesis was completed at the Ecole Nationale Superieure de Telecommunications in Paris. She was appointed honorary doctor at Lund University, Sweden, in 2015. Dr. Van der Perre joined imec's wireless group in 1997 in the wireless group and took up responsibilities as senior researcher, system architect, project leader and program director, until 2015.

Liesbet Van der Perre was appointed Professor in the DRAMCO lab of the Electrical Engineering Department of the KU Leuven in 2016. She's an author and co-author of over 300 scientific publications. Prof. L. Van der Perre was the scientific leader for the FP7-MAMMOET and is the technological lead of the EU H2020 project REINDEER and supervisor of the wireless sensors team in the Interreg FWVl NOMADe project. Liesbet Van der Perre served on the Board of Directors of Zenitel (2015–2021) and Crescent (2019–2021). She is a guest Professor at the University of Lund since 2017.

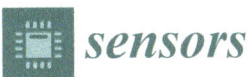

Editorial

Wearable Sensors Applied in Movement Analysis

Fabien Buisseret [1,2,*], Frédéric Dierick [1,3,4] and Liesbet Van der Perre [5]

1. Centre de Recherche, d'Étude et de Formation Continue de la Haute École Louvain en Hainaut (CeREF Technique), Chaussée de Binche 159, 7000 Mons, Belgium
2. Service de Physique Nucléaire et Subnucléaire, Research Institute for Complex Systems, UMONS Université de Mons, Place du Parc 20, 7000 Mons, Belgium
3. Centre National de Rééducation Fonctionnelle et de Réadaptation–Rehazenter, Laboratoire d'Analyse du Mouvement et de la Posture (LAMP), Rue André Vésale 1, 2674 Luxembourg, Luxembourg
4. Faculté des Sciences de la Motricité, UCLouvain, Place Pierre de Coubertin 1-2, 1348 Ottignies-Louvain-la-Neuve, Belgium
5. DraMCo Lab of the Electrical Engineering Department, KU Leuven, 9000 Ghent, Belgium
* Correspondence: buisseretf@helha.be or fabien.buisseret@umons.ac.be

Citation: Buisseret, F.; Dierick, F.; Van der Perre, L. Wearable Sensors Applied in Movement Analysis. *Sensors* **2022**, *22*, 8239. https://doi.org/10.3390/s22218239

Received: 30 September 2022
Accepted: 20 October 2022
Published: 27 October 2022

Publisher's Note: MDPI stays neutral with regard to jurisdictional claims in published maps and institutional affiliations.

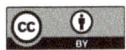

Copyright: © 2022 by the authors. Licensee MDPI, Basel, Switzerland. This article is an open access article distributed under the terms and conditions of the Creative Commons Attribution (CC BY) license (https://creativecommons.org/licenses/by/4.0/).

Recent advances in the miniaturization of electronics have resulted in sensors whose sizes and weights are such that they can be attached to living systems without interfering with their natural movements and behaviors. They may be worn on the body as accessories or as part of clothing, enabling personalized mobile information processing. Wearable sensors enable unobtrusive and continuous monitoring of body orientation, movements, and various physiological parameters during real-life activities. Thus, they may become crucial tools not only for researchers but also for clinicians, as they have the potential to improve diagnosis, better monitor disease progression, and thus individualize treatment. We also expect that after the SARS-CoV-2 crisis, interest in devices that promote telemedicine, such as low-cost wearable sensors, will increase significantly.

To be used in real-life situations, wearable sensors should meet the following three criteria: (1) *Be imperceptible to the wearer*. They should have wireless connectivity and consume little power. An example of algorithm development that optimizes both gesture recognition and energy consumption is presented in [1]. There, a finger gesture recognition system was developed using a lightweight multi-layer perceptron implemented on a low-end micro-controller unit with a two-axis flex sensor. The final prototype achieves up to 95.5% recognition accuracy while consuming less than 2.74 mJ of energy per gesture on a low-end embedded wearable device, which is 10% better than previous algorithms. (2) *Be intuitive to install*. The developed systems should provide high-performance body fixation solutions that are easily accepted by the user. Moreover, the electronic system should be self-calibrating and operating. An interesting way to increase the acceptance in domestic applications may be to use smartphones—very broadly accepted electronic devices—as control devices for the developed sensors. In [2], it is shown that dystonia assessment using smartphone-coupled inertial sensors and machine learning is a promising way to detect dystonia in real-life applications. (3) *Provide accurate and easy-to-interpret information*. Cross-platform interfaces that enable secure data storage and easy data analysis and visualization are needed. As an illustration, using Inertial Measurement Units (IMUs) to assess gait pattern evolutions during a 6-min walk test before and after a supervised exercise training program, the authors of [3] obtained such easy-to-interpret information in patients with symptomatic peripheral artery disease of the lower extremities. Two results can be quoted: a significant increase in walking speed after supervised exercise training and a significant positive correlation between the change in stride length and the change in 6-min walking distance. Therefore, the use of IMUs with the aim to investigate gait pattern during physical examination has potential applications for optimizing exercise prescription in patients with peripheral artery disease. Beyond the above examples, the papers published in this Special Issue show that several domains may benefit from wearable sensors when these three criteria are considered.

Sport is a clear example of a domain where imperceptible sensors are needed so as not to interfere with movement. The information from the sensors may help to improve the efficiency of training through accurate biofeedback. The authors of [4] have shown that a system of eight IMUs was able to identify the different phases (stance times) in a 1000 m speed skating trial for 12 competitive athletes. The IMUs results compare well with a foot pressure detector, which is considered the gold standard: between 90.1% and 96.1% for the average stance time. In [5], it is shown that two IMUs attached to the ski boots of nineteen experienced alpine skiers allow researchers to distinguish between an experienced skier and a beginner by comparing the recorded time series with those of a group of reference skiers. More generally, wearable sensors offer accurate methods of monitoring real-time movement parameters during sport, with an expected high relevance in optimizing training programs and performance or in minimizing risk of injury [6,7]. Note that wearable sensors also offer non-invasive and portable techniques to monitor the sports practices of persons with disability, especially in wheelchair sports [8].

Wearable sensors may also provide clinicians with additional quantitative information when assessing musculoskeletal conditions, such as neck pain and low-back pain. Regarding neck pain, the authors of [9] used a single IMU placed on a participant's forehead while performing a test to assess sensorimotor performance of the neck through repeated head rotations. A Linear Support Vector Machine can discriminate acute and subacute non-specific neck pain patients from healthy control participants with 82% accuracy by analyzing time series of angular speed and acceleration. The study was conducted with 38 acute and subacute non-specific neck pain patients and 42 healthy control participants and demonstrates that machine-learning methods can provide relevant information from relatively small datasets. The same observation is made in [10], where the kinematics of 20 patients with chronic low-back pain (CLBP) and 20 healthy participants without CLBP were recorded from three IMUs attached to the participants while they performed 1-min repetitive bending (flexion) and return (extension) trunk movements. It was found that Gaussian Naive Bayes machine learning achieved 79% accuracy in identifying CLBP patients. Moreover, machine learning identified that simple kinematic indicators were sensitive to low-back pain and therefore could gradually be used by clinicians in the assessment of CLBP patients. Machine learning can even go beyond binary classification in CLBP patients, as shown in [11]. From the video analysis of 115 CLBP participants lifting an 8 kg weight, Ward clustering suggests that there are four different lifting techniques in people with CLBP. One of the clusters, moving the trunk the least and the knee the most, demonstrates the least pain self-efficacy. Again, these results may help clinicians determine the best motor strategies to relieve pain in their patients.

A final topic explored in this Special Issue is gait analysis and its relationship to fall risk in the elderly. One challenge in this population is the implementation of automated gait assessment for continuous monitoring, either at home or in care institutions and hospitals. In [12], an IMU was used to assess patients with automated assessment based on the Berg balance scale. Optimal agreement (98.4%) with the therapist's scoring can be achieved using a one-dimensional convolutional neural network and a gated recurrent unit in a population of 53 hospitalized patients with brain diseases aged 50 to 80 years. Finally, it was shown in [13] that additional information from a single IMU, placed on the lower back of 73 care institute residents who performed a Timed-Up and Go (TUG) test considerably improved fall risk prediction. Kinematic observations and TUG time were included in a multiple logistic regression. The proposed new test, called i+TUG, achieved an accuracy of 74.0%, with a specificity of 95.9% and a sensitivity of 29.2% in classifying residents into fallers and non-fallers.

Beyond applications in elderly aiming at favoring an autonomous, active, and healthy ageing [14], wearable sensors may bring important improvement in monitoring patients with neurological diseases. As shown in the review [15], e-health approaches, including wearable sensors, may be beneficial for self-management and disease understanding of patients suffering from multiple sclerosis. Wearable motion sensors can be helpful in measuring physical activity of patients suffering from multiple sclerosis [16]. Another case of interest is the application of motion sensors to detect freezing of gait (FOG) in Parkinsons's disease, i.e., a gait disturbance typical of the mid- and late-stages of the disease. As discussed in the review [17], many challenges are still to be addressed in FOG detection, such as building large enough datasets allowing a more accurate detection via machine-learning techniques. In addition, wearable sensors may be used to estimate the metabolic energy expenditure and physical activity levels of different intensities in stroke patients with hemiparesis [18].

Wearable sensors can clearly bring great value in the analysis of movement, in sports as well as medical contexts, and not in the least for patients suffering from chronic diseases. While the potential is shown in the papers presented here and many others, we are confident that with further development of hardware and signal processing, many new opportunities will follow.

Acknowledgments: The Guest Editors thank all the authors, reviewers, and members of MDPI's editorial team whose work has led to the publication of this Special Issue. Financial support from the European Regional Development Fund (Interreg FWVl NOMADe) is acknowledged.

Conflicts of Interest: The authors declare no conflict of interest.

References

1. Jung, W.; Lee, H.G. Energy–Accuracy Aware Finger Gesture Recognition for Wearable IoT Devices. *Sensors* **2022**, *22*, 4801. [CrossRef] [PubMed]
2. Den Hartog, D.; van der Krogt, M.M.; van der Burg, S.; Aleo, I.; Gijsbers, J.; Bonouvrié, L.A.; Harlaar, J.; Buizer, A.I.; Haberfehlner, H. Home-Based Measurements of Dystonia in Cerebral Palsy Using Smartphone-Coupled Inertial Sensor Technology and Machine Learning: A Proof-of-Concept Study. *Sensors* **2022**, *22*, 4386. [CrossRef] [PubMed]
3. Lanzi, S.; Boichat, J.; Calanca, L.; Mazzolai, L.; Malatesta, D. Supervised Exercise Training Improves 6 min Walking Distance and Modifies Gait Pattern during Pain-Free Walking Condition in Patients with Symptomatic Lower Extremity Peripheral Artery Disease. *Sensors* **2021**, *21*, 7989. [CrossRef] [PubMed]
4. Tomita, Y.; Iizuka, T.; Irisawa, K.; Imura, S. Detection of Movement Events of Long-Track Speed Skating Using Wearable Inertial Sensors. *Sensors* **2021**, *21*, 3649. [CrossRef] [PubMed]
5. Snyder, C.; Martínez, A.; Jahnel, R.; Roe, J.; Stöggl, T. Connected Skiing: Motion Quality Quantification in Alpine Skiing. *Sensors* **2021**, *21*, 3779. [CrossRef] [PubMed]
6. Li, R.T.; Kling, S.R.; Salata, M.J.; Cupp, S.A.; Sheehan, J.; Voos, J.E. Wearable Performance Devices in Sports Medicine. *Sports Health* **2016**, *8*, 74–78. [CrossRef] [PubMed]
7. Seshadri, D.R.; Li, R.T.; Voos, J.E.; Rowbottom, J.R.; Alfes, C.M.; Zorman, C.A.; Drummond, C.K. Wearable sensors for monitoring the physiological and biochemical profile of the athlete. *NPJ Digit. Med.* **2019**, *22*, 72. [CrossRef] [PubMed]
8. Rum, L.; Sten, O.; Vendrame, E.; Belluscio, V.; Camomilla, V.; Vannozzi, G.; Truppa, L.; Notarantonio, M.; Sciarra, T.; Lazich, A.; et al. Wearable Sensors in Sports for Persons with Disability: A Systematic Review. *Sensors* **2021**, *21*, 1858. [CrossRef] [PubMed]
9. Hage, R.; Buisseret, F.; Houry, M.; Dierick, F. Head Pitch Angular Velocity Discriminates (Sub-)Acute Neck Pain Patients and Controls Assessed with the DidRen Laser Test. *Sensors* **2022**, *22*, 2805. [CrossRef] [PubMed]
10. Thiry, P.; Houry, M.; Philippe, L.; Nocent, O.; Buisseret, F.; Dierick, F.; Slama, R.; Bertucci, W.; Thévenon, A.; Simoneau-Buessinger, E. Machine Learning Identifies Chronic Low Back Pain Patients from an Instrumented Trunk Bending and Return Test. *Sensors* **2022**, *22*, 5027. [CrossRef]
11. Phan, T.C.; Pranata, A.; Farragher, J.; Bryant, A.; Nguyen, H.T.; Chai, R. Machine Learning Derived Lifting Techniques and Pain Self-Efficacy in People with Chronic Low Back Pain. *Sensors* **2022**, *22*, 6694. [CrossRef]
12. Kim, Y.-W.; Joa, K.-L.; Jeong, H.-Y.; Lee, S. Wearable IMU-Based Human Activity Recognition Algorithm for Clinical Balance Assessment Using 1D-CNN and GRU Ensemble Model. *Sensors* **2021**, *21*, 7628. [CrossRef]
13. Dierick, F.; Stoffel, P.-L.; Schütz, G.; Buisseret, F. High Specificity of Single Inertial Sensor-Supplemented Timed Up and Go Test for Assessing Fall Risk in Elderly Nursing Home Residents. *Sensors* **2022**, *22*, 2339. [CrossRef] [PubMed]
14. Stavropoulos, T.G.; Papastergiou, A.; Mpaltadoros, L.; Nikolopoulos, S.; Kompatsiaris, I. IoT Wearable Sensors and Devices in Elderly Care: A Literature Review. *Sensors* **2020**, *20*, 2826. [CrossRef] [PubMed]
15. Matthews, P.M.; Block, V.J.; Leocani, L. E-health and multiple sclerosis. *Curr. Opin. Neurol.* **2020**, *33*, 271–276. [CrossRef] [PubMed]
16. Sasaki, J.E.; Sandroff, B.; Bamman, M.; Motl, R.W. Motion sensors in multiple sclerosis: Narrative review and update of applications. *Expert. Rev. Med. Devices* **2017**, *14*, 891–900. [CrossRef] [PubMed]

17. Pardoel, S.; Kofman, J.; Nantel, J.; Lemaire, E.D. Wearable-Sensor-Based Detection and Prediction of Freezing of Gait in Parkinson's Disease: A Review. *Sensors* **2019**, *19*, 5141. [CrossRef] [PubMed]
18. Fonte, G.; Schreiber, C.; Areno, G.; Masson, X.; Chantraine, F.; Schütz, G.; Dierick, F. Metabolic Energy Expenditure and Accelerometer-Determined Physical Activity Levels in Post-Stroke Hemiparetic Patients. *J. Stroke Cerebrovasc. Dis.* **2022**, *31*, 106397. [CrossRef] [PubMed]

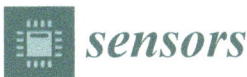

Article

Machine Learning Derived Lifting Techniques and Pain Self-Efficacy in People with Chronic Low Back Pain

Trung C. Phan [1], Adrian Pranata [2,3], Joshua Farragher [2,4], Adam Bryant [4], Hung T. Nguyen [1] and Rifai Chai [1,*]

[1] School of Science, Computing and Engineering Technologies, Swinburne University of Technology, Hawthorn, VIC 3122, Australia
[2] School of Health Sciences, Swinburne University of Technology, Hawthorn, VIC 3122, Australia
[3] School of Kinesiology, Shanghai University of Sports, Shanghai 200438, China
[4] Centre for Health, Exercise and Sports Medicine, Department of Physiotherapy, The University of Melbourne, Melbourne, VIC 3010, Australia
* Correspondence: rchai@swin.edu.au

Citation: Phan, T.C.; Pranata, A.; Farragher, J.; Bryant, A.; Nguyen, H.T.; Chai, R. Machine Learning Derived Lifting Techniques and Pain Self-Efficacy in People with Chronic Low Back Pain. *Sensors* 2022, 22, 6694. https://doi.org/10.3390/s22176694

Academic Editors: Fabien Buisseret, Frédéric Dierick and Liesbet Van der Perre

Received: 21 July 2022
Accepted: 31 August 2022
Published: 4 September 2022

Publisher's Note: MDPI stays neutral with regard to jurisdictional claims in published maps and institutional affiliations.

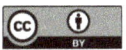

Copyright: © 2022 by the authors. Licensee MDPI, Basel, Switzerland. This article is an open access article distributed under the terms and conditions of the Creative Commons Attribution (CC BY) license (https://creativecommons.org/licenses/by/4.0/).

Abstract: This paper proposes an innovative methodology for finding how many lifting techniques people with chronic low back pain (CLBP) can demonstrate with camera data collected from 115 participants. The system employs a feature extraction algorithm to calculate the knee, trunk and hip range of motion in the sagittal plane, Ward's method, a combination of K-means and Ensemble clustering method for classification algorithm, and Bayesian neural network to validate the result of Ward's method and the combination of K-means and Ensemble clustering method. The classification results and effect size show that Ward clustering is the optimal method where precision and recall percentages of all clusters are above 90, and the overall accuracy of the Bayesian Neural Network is 97.9%. The statistical analysis reported a significant difference in the range of motion of the knee, hip and trunk between each cluster, $F (9, 1136) = 195.67$, $p < 0.0001$. The results of this study suggest that there are four different lifting techniques in people with CLBP. Additionally, the results show that even though the clusters demonstrated similar pain levels, one of the clusters, which uses the least amount of trunk and the most knee movement, demonstrates the lowest pain self-efficacy.

Keywords: low back pain; lifting technique; camera system; ward clustering method; K-means clustering method; ensemble clustering method; Bayesian neural network; pain self-efficacy questionnaire

1. Introduction

Chronic low back pain (CLBP) is a multifactorial condition that is the leading cause of activity limitations and work absenteeism, affecting 540 million people worldwide [1]. Adaptation in trunk muscle control is commonly observed in people with CLBP, which is associated with changes in trunk muscle properties [2] and delayed reaction time in response to external perturbations [3]. These adaptations could be reflected in trunk and lower limb movement variability, especially during lifting [4].

Lifting is a complex activity that requires coordination of the lower limbs (e.g., hip and knee) and the trunk [4]. In simplistic terms, lifting techniques could be classified as a stoop lift (i.e., lifting with flexed back) or leg lift (i.e., lifting with hips and knees bent and back straight). Although lifting with the legs was traditionally considered to be a safer lifting technique, this has been disputed in several studies [5,6]. Lifting movements can vary considerably between individuals depending on factors such as hamstring tightness and movement speed—both of which have been demonstrated in people with CLBP or in risk factors for CLBP [7–9]. Therefore, dichotomous classification of lifting techniques may not be appropriate in people with CLBP. It is currently unknown how many different lifting techniques people with CLBP would demonstrate. This information may guide clinicians in identifying and individualizing target areas for rehabilitation for people with CLBP.

Moreover, it is well established that CLBP is associated with changes in psychosocial domain such as pain self-efficacy [10]. Pain self-efficacy is defined as the belief in one's ability to perform painful or perceived painful tasks or movements to achieve a desirable outcome. Pain self-efficacy is typically measured using a Pain Self-Efficacy Questionnaire (PSEQ) [11]. In people with CLBP, low pain self-efficacy is associated with higher pain intensity, disability, and fear-avoidance beliefs [12–14]. Therefore, pain self-efficacy is an important attribute to be assessed in people with CLBP.

Recent technology using the computational intelligence technique for classification [15] may assist with the identification of different lifting techniques in people with CLBP. In principle, there are three main steps for activity recognition: (i) data capture by appropriate sensor; (ii) segmentation of the captured data and feature extraction; (iii) recognition of the activity using appropriate classification/identification techniques.

In classification, machine learning is known as one of the categories of artificial intelligence. In general, there are two types of machine learning: supervised and unsupervised. In supervised machine learning, once the data set has been labelled with each input, a pre-set correct output is assigned [16]. By contrast, unsupervised machine learning techniques utilize unlabelled data sets to identify patterns which will then be clustered into different groups [16]. In different medical and health applications, clustering algorithms have been applied to cluster patient records to identify a trend in health care [17,18], detect a set of co-expressed genes [19], categorize patients from medical records [20], and from the symptoms, find out patient subgroups [21]. It is unknown whether different movement patterns could be identified using unsupervised machine learning techniques or clustering algorithms in people with CLBP.

Thus, this study aims to present an innovative methodology for identifying different lifting movement patterns in people with CLBP using unsupervised machine learning techniques and range of motion. Therefore, the main contribution of this paper is the novel application of unsupervised machine learning techniques for lifting movement pattern classification in the CLBP participants. We hypothesized that people with CLBP will lift utilizing various techniques when clustered using the trunk, hip and knee movement integration.

2. Materials and Methods

The components for the camera-based cluster classification system introduced in this paper are presented in Figure 1.

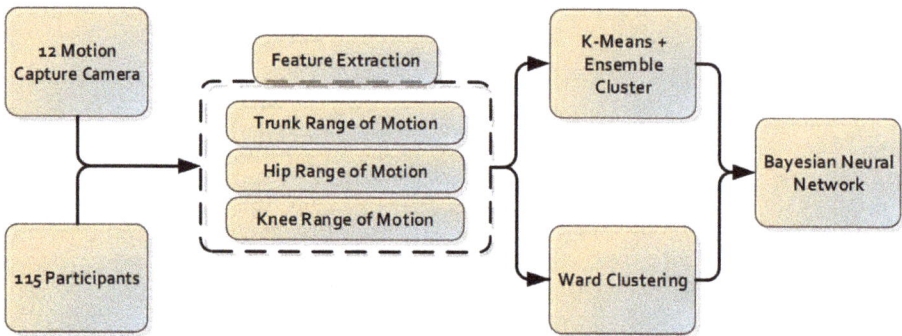

Figure 1. The components for the camera-based cluster classification system.

2.1. Participants

One-hundred and fifteen males and females ($n_{females}$ = 57) with CLBP aged 25 to 60 years old with CLBP were recruited from a large physiotherapy clinic in Melbourne (VIC, Australia). This study was approved by the University of Melbourne Behavioural and Social Sciences Human Ethics Sub-Committee. Participants were included in the study if they had reported pain between the gluteal fold and the twelfth thoracic vertebra (T12) level, with or without leg pain that had persisted for >3 months. Participants were excluded from the study if they demonstrated overt neurological signs, such as muscle weakness and loss of lower limb reflexes, had had spine and lower limb surgery, had been diagnosed with active inflammatory conditions such as rheumatoid arthritis, had been diagnosed with cancer or did not comprehend written or verbal English. The participants in this study had not received any physiotherapy intervention during their assessment of lifting technique. All participants completed assessments of pain self-efficacy using the PSEQ [10].

2.2. Data Collection

The lifting task protocol has been published previously [4,22]. In summary, participants began the test standing upright, barefooted, with their arms by their sides. Participants were instructed to bend down and lift an 8 kg weight (i.e., an average weight of groceries [23]) placed between their feet with both hands from the ground up to the level of their abdomen. Participants were instructed to utilize a lifting technique of their choosing. Eight lifting trials were performed, with the first 2 trials serving as practice trials, hence excluded from data analysis. The sequence of consecutive actions during the lifting task is summarized and presented in Figure 2.

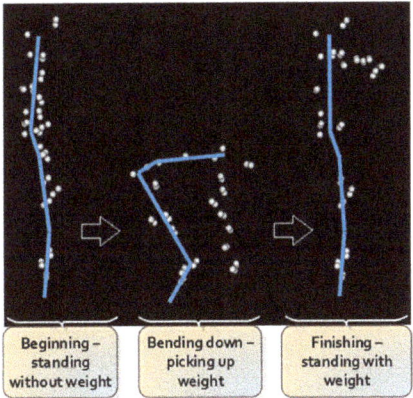

Figure 2. Sequence of consecutive actions during lifting.

Kinematic data were collected using non-reflective markers placed on the participants' skin to mark the head, trunk, pelvis, upper and lower limbs [22]. A 12-camera motion analysis system (Optitrack Flex 13, NaturalPoint, Corvallis, OR, USA) with 120 Hz sampling rate was utilized to provide the three-dimensional recording of anatomical landmarks. Kinematic data were grouped, named, cleaned and gap-filled using Optitrack Motive software (NaturalPoint, Corvallis, OR, USA). The data were then passed through to a custom-written analysis pipeline of Visual3D v5.01.6 (C-Motion, Inc., Germantown, MD, USA). Angular displacement and velocity data of different joints in all planes were derived using custom-written software (LabVIEW 2009, National Instruments).

2.3. Pre-Processing and Features Extraction

The angular displacement of the trunk, hip and knee joints during lifting were used for analysis and were inputted into the machine learning algorithm.

A joint range of motion is chosen to simplify the complex data into efficient features. The joint range is calculated by taking the difference between maximum and minimum values of that joint's angular displacement.

$$Range\ of\ motion\ (ROM) = Max(\theta) - Min(\theta) \tag{1}$$

where $Max(\theta)$ is the maximum value of joint's angular displacement, and $Min(\theta)$ is the minimum value of the joint's angular displacement.

One perspective of inter-joint coordination in manual lifting is a distal-to-proximal pattern of extension of the knee, hip, and lumbar vertebral joints [24]. In addition, the movement of the knee, the hip and the lumbar take an important role in achieving the lifting task and generating different types of lifting techniques. From the provided data, the range of motion of the trunk, hip and knee in the sagittal plane are extracted for further analysis. A between-side average value was used for the knee and hip, as there was no statistically significant ROM differences between the left and right sides.

2.4. Partitional Clustering

Clustering is known as one of the common techniques which is used to generate homogeneous groups of objects [25]. From the provided data points, all the data points that are similar and closely resemble each other will be placed into the same cluster [26]. Partitional clustering is known as one of the most popular algorithm in clustering [27–29]. In partitional clustering, data points are separated into a predetermined number of clusters without a hierarchical structure.

The K-means clustering algorithm is most commonly used as a partitional clustering [30]. In K-means clustering algorithm, h clusters are generated so that the distance between the points within its own clusters and centroids is less than the distance to centroids of other clusters. The algorithm's operation begins with the selection of h points as the centroid. Following the selection of the h points, all points are allocated to the closest centroid, resulting in the formation of t clusters. The average of each cluster's points will then be used to generate a centroid. These centroids make up the mean vector, with each field of the vector equalling each cluster centroid. A new centroid generates the new cluster as a result of this process. In the situation where the centroids remain unchanged, K-means clustering algorithm will be completed. K-means clustering has certain advantages such as less space and time complexity or optimal results accomplished for equal-sized globular and separated clusters [30]. However, K-means clustering algorithm shows sensitivity to outliers and noises. Moreover, a poor initial choice of centroid in partitioning process might produce increasingly poor result. In this study, K-means clustering algorithm was implemented using kmean function from Matlab.

2.5. Ensemble Clustering

In recent years, clustering ensemble has widely been used to improve the robustness and quality of results from clustering algorithms [31–34]. In ensemble clustering, multiple results from different clustering algorithms are combined into final clusters without retrieving features or base algorithm information. In ensemble clustering, the only requirement is obtaining the base clustering information instead of the data itself. This is useful for dealing with privacy concerns and knowledge reuse [35].

The ensemble clustering algorithm consists of two main stages: diversity and consensus function. The data set is processed in the diversity stage with a single clustering algorithm with several initializations or multiple standard clustering algorithms. The results of this process are recorded-based clustering. Afterwards, the consensus function is implemented to combine the based clustering result and produce the final consensus solution. Currently, there is a different approach for consensus function, such as conducting co-association matrix or hypergraph partitioning. With a co-association matrix, a key advantage is the specification of a number of clusters in consensus partition is not required [30]. However, hypergraph partitioning requires this specification information [30]. However, in this research, the cluster number will be investigated and is used as input of hypergraph partitioning. As a result, a co-association matric will be unsuitable in this case. Thus, hypergraph partitioning is chosen for the consensus function in this research.

In the hypergraph, there are two main components: hyperedges present clusters, and vertices present equivalent samples or points. A clustering is presented as a label vector ϑ^t. Label vector ϑ with mixture of r label vector $\vartheta^1, \vartheta^2, \ldots, \vartheta^r$, where r is known as number of clustering, is the procedure by consensus function. The objective function is described by function $T : V^{v*r} \to V^v$ mapping a set of clustering to an integrated clustering $T : \{\vartheta^t \,|\, t \in \{1, 2, \ldots, r\} \to \vartheta\,\}$. Labelled vector of ϑ^t is demonstrated by binary matrix L^t where each cluster is specified with a column. In situation where the row is relating to an object with a known label, and all entries of the row in the binary membership indicator matrix L^t are considered equal to 1. In contrast, in the situation where the row is relating to an unknown label, objects are considered equal to 0. Matrix $L = (L^1 L^2 \ldots L^r)$ as a hypergraph adjacency matrix is explained with v vertices and $a = \sum_{e=1}^{r} g^e$ hyperedges.

There are three algorithms in hypergraph methods: Cluster-based Similarity Partitioning Algorithm (CSPA), HyperGraph Partitioning Algorithm (HGPA) and Meta-Clustering Algorithm (MCLA).

In the Cluster-based Similarity Partitioning Algorithm, clustering can be used to generate a measure of pair-wise similarity because it illustrates the relationships among the objects that reside within the same cluster. The fraction of the clustering, where two objects occur within the same cluster and can be calculated in one sparse matrix multiplication $\frac{1}{r} L L^c$ where L is indicator matrix and L^c is matrix transposition, it is indicated by the entries of B [35]. The purpose of the similarity matrix is to re-cluster the items using any suitable similarity-based clustering technique.

HyperGraph Partitioning Algorithm (HGPA) partitions the hypergraph by cutting the smallest number of hyperedges possible. All hyperedges are weighed to ensure that they are all of the same weight. Furthermore, all vertices have the same weight. The partitions are created using the minimal cut technique, which divides the data into J unconnected components of roughly equal size. For these partitions, Han et al. (1997) employed the HMETIS hypergraph partitioning package [36]. In contrast to CSPA, which considers local piecewise similarity, HGPA solely considers the comparatively global links between items across partitions. Furthermore, HMETIS has a proclivity for obtaining a final partition in which all clusters are nearly the same size.

Cluster correspondence is dealt with in MCLA integration. MCLA finds and consolidates cluster groups, transforming them into meta-clusters. Constructing the meta-graph, computing meta-clusters, and computing clusters of the objects are the three key aspects of this method for finding the final clusters of items. The hyperedges J^e, $e = 1, 2, \ldots, a$ are the meta-vertices, and the graph and edge weights are proportional to the similarity between vertices. Matching labels can be identified by partitioning the meta-graph into o balanced meta-clusters. Each vertex is appropriately weighted to the size of the cluster to which it belongs. Balancing ensures that the sum of vertex-weights is generally equal within each meta-cluster. To achieve clustering of the J vectors, the graph partitioning package METIS is used in this stage. Each vertex in the meta-graph represents a distinct cluster label; as a result, a meta-cluster denotes a collection of corresponding labels. The hyperedges are crushed into a single meta-hyperedge for each of the o meta-clusters. An object is assigned to the meta-cluster with the highest entry in the association vector. Ties are broken in an ad hoc manner using this approach.

For this research, ensemble clustering is used to improve the robustness and quality of results from the K-means clustering algorithm. At the diversity stage, the K-means clustering algorithm with various initial choices of a centroid is applied to the data set to create base clustering. Following base clustering, in the consensus function stage, CSPA, HGPA, and MCLA algorithms are used separately to conduct the final results. Following base clustering, in the consensus function stage, the CSPA, HGPA, and MCLA algorithms are used separately to conduct the final results. The ROM of trunk, hip and knee as features were passed through K-means with squared Euclidean distance and random initial choice of centroid using Matlab multiple times (50 times) to form-based clustering for ensemble cluster. Before passing these results to ensemble clustering, duplicated results from K-means were removed to increase the quality and diversity of based clustering. From obtained-based clustering, ensemble clustering uses CSPA, HGPA, and MCLA as consensus functions processed to finalize the final result using the python ClusterEnsembles package.

2.6. Clustering—Wards

Besides partitioning clusters, the other widely utilized clustering algorithm is Hierarchical Clustering. The Hierarchical Clustering algorithm produces clusters in a hierarchical tree-like structure or a dendrogram [26,37].

In the beginning, each data point is assigned as a single unique cluster. By combining two data sets, allocating the data to an existing cluster, or merging two clusters after each loop, a new cluster can be formed [38]. The condition to create a new cluster is when the similarity or dissimilarity between every pair of objects (data or cluster) is found. Currently, there are four common kinds of linkage techniques, but research has shown that Ward's linkage is the most effective technique for dealing with noisy data compared to the other three [26,38,39].

The linkage technique developed by Ward in 1963 uses the incremental sum of squares, which means the growth in the total within-cluster sum of squares as a consequence of merging two clusters [26]. The sum of squares of the distance between entire objects in the cluster and the cluster's centroid is explained as the within-cluster sum of squares [38]. The sum of squares metric is equal to the distance metric d_{AB}, which is shown below:

$$d^2{}_{EF} = \frac{2n_E n_F}{n_E + n_F} \|\overline{y_E} + \overline{y_F}\|^2 \qquad (2)$$

where the Euclidean distance is represented by $\| \ \|$, the centroid of cluster E and F is represented by y_E and y_F respectively, and the number of elements in cluster E and F is represented by n_E and n_F. In some research studies as references, Ward's linkage does not contain the factor of 2 in Equation (2) when n_E is multiplied by n_F. This factor's main purpose is to ensure that the distance between two singleton clusters will be the same as the Euclidean distance.

To calculate the distance from cluster D to a new cluster C, cluster C is formed by merging clusters E and F, and the updated equation is shown as follows:

$$d^2{}_{DC} = \frac{n_E + n_D}{n_C + n_D} d^2{}_{DE} + \frac{n_F + n_D}{n_C + n_D} d^2{}_{DF} - \frac{n_D}{n_C + n_D} d^2{}_{EF} \qquad (3)$$

where the distance between cluster D and cluster E is represented by d_{DE}, the distance between cluster D and cluster F is represented by d_{DF}, the distance between cluster F and cluster E is represented by d_{EF}, the number of elements in clusters E, F, C and D are represented by n_E, n_F, n_C and n_D.

After the hierarchical cluster is formed, a cut point is determined which can be at any position in the tree so that a full description of the clusters (final output) can be extracted [26]. In this study, the ROM of the trunk, hip and knee were passed through Ward clustering with Euclidean distance using the linkage and cluster function in Matlab.

2.7. Determining Optimal Number of Cluster

In partitioning clustering, for example, K-means clustering, the number of cluster h to be formed is defined and given, and choosing the correct optimal number of clusters for a single data set is challenging. This question, unfortunately, has no definitive answer. The method for determining similarity and the partitioning parameters define the ideal number of clusters, which is highly subjective. A basic and popular strategy is to examine the dendrogram produced by hierarchical clustering to see if it offers a specified number of clusters. Unfortunately, this strategy is as subjective. Direct technique and statistical testing method are two of these methods. Optimizing a criterion, such as the sum of squares within a cluster or the average silhouette, is a direct strategy. The equivalent procedures are known as the elbow and silhouette methods. The silhouette method analyses the average distance between clusters while the elbow method analyses the total within-cluster sum of square (WSS) for different clusters. In this research, both elbow and silhouette methods are used to determine optimal number of cluster for K-means cluster and Ward clustering using evalclusters function from Matlab and KElbowVisualizer function from Yellowbrick.

2.8. Machine Learning—Classification

A Bayesian neural network [15,40] construction operates a feed-forward structure with three layers, and it is formed by:

$$z_k(x,w) = f\left(b_k + \sum_{i=1}^{l} w_{ki} f\left(b_i + \sum_{j=1}^{m} w_{ij} x_j\right)\right) \quad (4)$$

where the transfer function is represented by $f(.)$, and in this paper, the hyperbolic tangent function is applied, the number of input nodes is represented by m (j starts from 1 to m), the number of hidden nodes is represented by l (i starts from 1 to l), the quantity of output is represented by q (k starts from 1 to q), the weight from input unit x_j to the hidden unit y_i is represented by w_{ij}, the weight from hidden unit y_i to the output z_k is represented by w_{ki}, and biases are represented by b_i and b_k.

Bayesian regularization structure is suggested to improve the generalization capabilities of the neural network irrespective of whether the presented data are noisy and/or finite [41]. In Bayesian learning, the probability distribution of network factors will be observed; thus, the trained network's greatest generalization can be delivered. Particularly, all of the obtainable data can be compatible and used in this kind of neural network to train. Consequently, the application with a small data set is appropriate.

The best possible model in the Bayesian framework, which the training data S corresponded to, is acquired automatically. Founded on Gaussian probability distribution on weight values, applying Bayes' theorem can compute the posterior distribution of the weights w in the network H and this is presented below:

$$p(w \mid S, H) = \frac{p(S \mid w, H) p(w \mid H)}{p(S \mid H)} \quad (5)$$

where $p(S \mid w, H)$ represents the probability that knowledge about the weight from observation is included, the knowledge about background weight set is contained in the prior distribution $p(w \mid H)$, and lastly, the $p(S \mid H)$ represents the network H evidence.

For a MLP neural network described in Figure 3, the cost function $G(w)$ can be minimized to achieve the most possible value for the neural network weight w^{MP}, and the cost function is shown below:

$$G(w) = \beta K_S(w) + \alpha K_W(w) \quad (6)$$

where hyper-parameters are symbolized by α and β, and the effective difficulty of network structure is operated by the ratio α/β, the error function is symbolized by $K_S(w)$ and the total square of weight function is symbolized by $K_W(w)$; this function can be calculated using the below equation:

$$K_W(w) = \frac{1}{2} \|w\|^2 \quad (7)$$

Updating the cost function with hyper-parameters, the neural network with a too large weight can lead to poor generalization when new test cases are used and can be avoided. Consequently, during a neural network training process, a set of validation is not compulsory.

To update hyper-parameters, the Bayesian regularization algorithm is used, and it is shown below:

$$\alpha^{MP} = \frac{\gamma}{2 K_W(w^{MP})}; \quad \beta^{MP} = \frac{N - \gamma}{2 K_S(w^{MP})} \quad (8)$$

where the effective number of parameters is represented by $\gamma = c - 2\alpha^{MP} tr(H^{MP})^{-1}$, the total number of parameters in the network is represented by c, the total number of errors is represented by N, and the Hessian matrix of $G(w)$ at the smallest, minimum point of w^{MP} is represented by H.

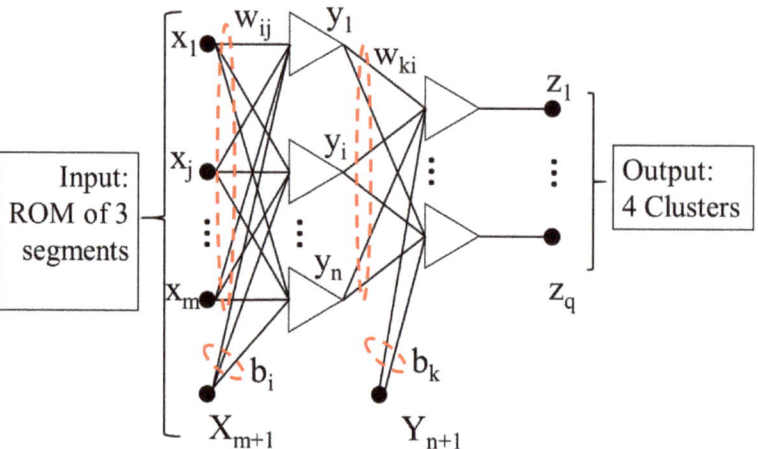

Figure 3. Artificial neural network (ANN) structure (weights and biases are highlighted in red dotted circle).

The Bayesian framework can estimate and evaluate the log evidence of model H_i, and it is shown below:

$$\ln p(S|H_i) = -\alpha_{MP} K_W^{MP} - \beta_{MP} K_W^{MP} - \frac{1}{2}\ln|A| + \frac{W}{2}\ln \alpha_{MP} + \frac{N}{2}\ln \beta_{MP} + \ln M + 2\ln M + \frac{1}{2}\ln\frac{2}{\gamma} + \frac{1}{2}\ln\frac{2}{N-\gamma} \quad (9)$$

where the number of network parameters is represented by W, the number of hidden nodes is represented by M, and the cost function Hessian matrix is represented by A. The best optimal structure will be found out based on the log evidence value; a structure which has the highest value will be chosen.

To measure multi-class classification performance, the familiar performance metric can be considered and used: precision, recall and accuracy. These indicators are shown as follows:

$$Recall = \frac{TP_O}{TP_O + FN_O} \quad (10)$$

$$Precision = \frac{TP_O}{TP_O + FP_O} \quad (11)$$

$$Accuracy = \frac{Total\ of\ correctly\ classified\ data}{Total\ number\ of\ data} \quad (12)$$

where the number of the data inputs, which is denoted as O and is classified correctly, is represented as TP_O (true positive of O), and O denotes one of the classes in multi-class. The number of the data inputs, which does not denote as O and is classified as O, is represented as FP_O (false positive of O), and the number of the data inputs, which denotes as O and is classified as not O, is represented as FN_O (false negative of O).

The clustering algorithm's output is combined with the original input data set to create a new Bayesian neural network classification data set. For the Bayesian neural network classification, the data set is separated into two sets: the first set contains 50% of the overall sets used for training purposes and the second sets has the remaining sets for testing purposes. In addition, to train this neural network classifier, the Levenberg–

Marquardt with Bayesian regularization algorithm is implemented, and the mean squared error function is selected as the error function $K_D(w)$ [41]. In this study, cluster result (Wards Clustering, combination of K-means and CPSA, HGPA and MCLA) and features of the clustering algorithm's data (ROM of trunk, hip and knee) were passed to the Bayesian neural network with maximum number of epochs of 600 and maximum mu of 1×10^{100}. Minimum performance gradient is 1×10^{-20} using Matlab script. Fifty percent of the data set (239 trials) was used for training purposes, and the other half (234 trials) was used for testing purposes.

2.9. Statistical Analysis

Besides using the Bayesian neural network to choose the better unsupervised machine learning algorithm for classifying the lifting technique, the Partial η^2 (partial eta squared) is used to measure the effect size of different algorithms from the statistical point of view.

A one-way multivariate analysis of variance (MANOVA) was used to examine the trunk, hip, and knee ROM differences between each cluster. Tukey's Honestly Significant Difference test was conducted to analyse significant group differences. The statistical analysis methods (least significant difference) were performed with patient-reported outcome measures such as the pain self-efficacy questionnaire (PSEQ). All analyses were conducted with a significance level set at 0.05 using IBM SPSS software version 28.0.1 (SPSS Inc., Chicago, IL, USA).

3. Results

Four-hundred and seventy-three lifting trials were included in this study. The participants' demographic information is summarized in Table 1.

Table 1. Descriptive participants' demographic information.

Variables (Units)	Mean (SD)
Age (years)	45.4 (11.6)
Height (cm)	173.4 (11.1)
Weight (kg)	79.6 (17.6)
BMI (m/kg^2)	26.3 (5.4)
Pain Level (VAS out of 100)	45.8 (19.9)
Duration of Pain (months)	89.2 (113.3)
ODI (%)	31.5 (14.4)
PSEQ (out of 60)	45.2 (9.9)

BMI, body mass index; ODI, Oswestry Disability Index; PSEQ, Pain self-efficacy questionnaire; VAS, Visual Analogue Scale; SD, standard deviation.

The results of elbow and silhouette methods for the Ward clustering algorithm are shown in Figures 4 and 5. The results of the elbow and silhouette methods for the K-means clustering algorithm are shown in Figures 6 and 7. The elbow method for both Ward and K-means suggests the optimal number of clusters is two, while the silhouette method suggests that four is the optimal number of clusters. In this study, the cluster result represents the lifting technique that people with CLBP uses. Currently, lifting techniques can be classified as two techniques: a stoop lift or leg lift. The main object of this research is to identify how many possible lifting techniques people with CLBP can perform besides the two lifting techniques. As a result, the optimal number of clusters for both K-means and Ward clustering is four.

The descriptive statistics pertaining to the range of motion of the trunk, hip and knee for each cluster between different unsupervised machine learning methods are summarized in Table 2.

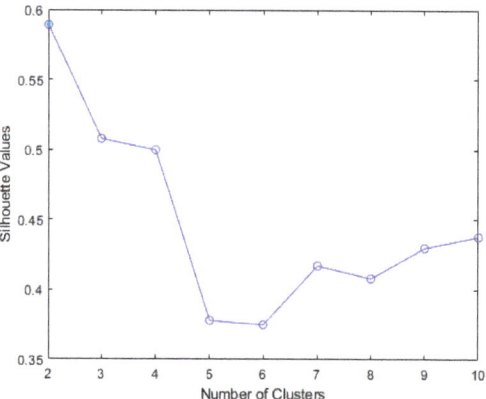

Figure 4. Silhouette score results for Ward clustering algorithm.

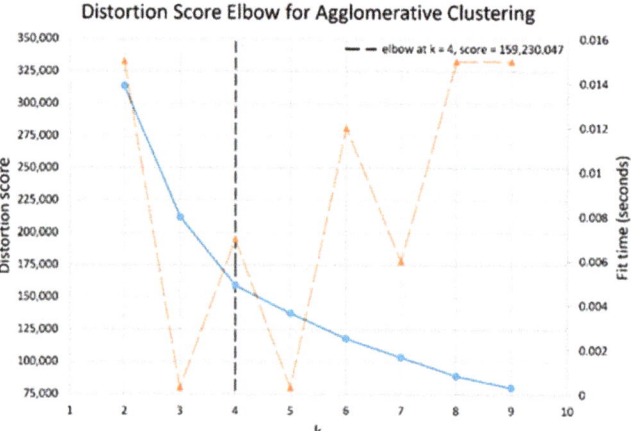

Figure 5. Elbow method results for Ward clustering algorithm (blue line indicates distortion score, and orange dashed line indicates the time to train the clustering model).

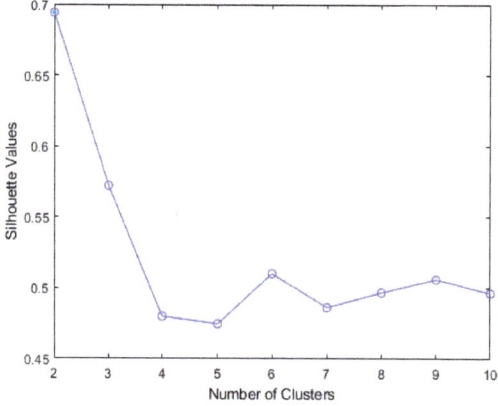

Figure 6. Silhouette score results for K-means clustering algorithm.

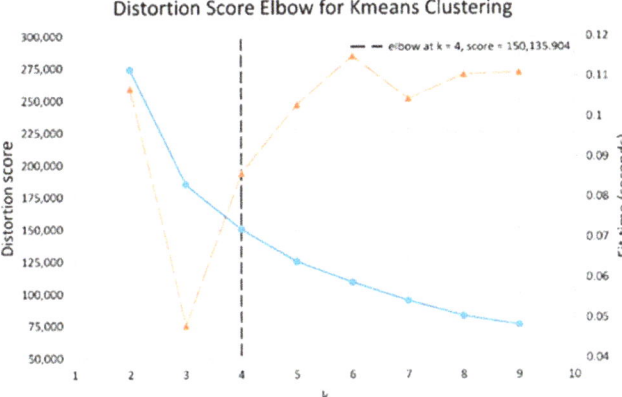

Figure 7. Elbow method results for K-means clustering algorithm (blue line indicates distortion score, and orange dashed line indicates the time to train the clustering model).

Table 2. Descriptive statistics (mean (SD)) of trunk, hip and knee range of motion for each cluster between methods.

		Mean (Standard Deviation)		
		Trunk	Hip	Knee
Ward Clustering	Cluster 1	34.19 (6.84)	114.58 (9.74)	136.24 (12.35)
	Cluster 2	41.88 (7.84)	107.37 (9.27)	96.39 (12.66)
	Cluster 3	54.00 (9.26)	83.92 (13.02)	26.70 (10.36)
	Cluster 4	48.04 (9.73)	93.54 (9.61)	67.29 (13.72)
K-means + CSPA	Cluster 1	34.19 (6.84)	105.20 (9.67)	88.75 (7.46)
	Cluster 2	33.01 (7.35)	108.60 (11.55)	115.13 (15.31)
	Cluster 3	53.17 (9.09)	86.44 (13.84)	31.72 (16.95)
	Cluster 4	47.28 (9.82)	93.91 (10.35)	64.57 (10.53)
K-means + HGPA	Cluster 1	52.80 (9.89)	84.26 (13.06)	30.92 (14.99)
	Cluster 2	47.65 (9.24)	96.07 (9.26)	65.36 (10.90)
	Cluster 3	44.92 (8.93)	105.23 (9.61)	89.02 (7.81)
	Cluster 4	38.11 (7.38)	108.59 (11.62)	115.08 (15.45)
K-means + MCLA	Cluster 1	47.52 (9.52)	95.24 (10.68)	65.59 (11.18)
	Cluster 2	42.58 (8.59)	105.79 (10.47)	95.49 (10.07)
	Cluster 3	53.90 (9.16)	84.23 (12.98)	27.18 (10.60)
	Cluster 4	36.09 (7.05)	111.80 (9.95)	129.71 (13.84)

Classification of four clusters by applying the Bayesian neural network as a classifier on the test set of different methods is summarized in Table 3. Additionally, the effect sizes of different unsupervised machine learning are shown in Table 4. For trunk, hip and knee features, Ward clustering provided the highest effect compared to the combination of K-means and ensemble clustering. The Bayesian neural network and effect size calculation result suggests that Ward clustering is the optimal algorithm for this study.

The optimum number of hidden nodes of the Bayesian neural network training versus log evidence is plotted and represented in Figure 8. Based on the plot, the training model with nine hidden nodes is determined as the best classification indication.

Cluster 2 was the most common, which constituted 40.80% of all self-selected techniques. The least chosen was Cluster 1 (6.76% of all data analysed). The descriptive statistics pertaining to PSEQ and pain level for each cluster are summarized in Table 5.

Table 3. Classification results (recall, precision and accuracy) of Bayesian neural network between each cluster on test set.

Method	Cluster	Recall	Precision	Accuracy
Ward Clustering	Cluster 1	93.8%	93.8%	97.9%
	Cluster 2	99.0%	96.9%	
	Cluster 3	98.0%	100%	
	Cluster 4	97.2%	98.6%	
K-means + CSPA	Cluster 1	93.1%	88.5%	93.6%
	Cluster 2	88.1%	94.5%	
	Cluster 3	94.9%	98.2%	
	Cluster 4	98.3%	93.5%	
K-means + HGPA	Cluster 1	98.3%	96.7%	94.9%
	Cluster 2	89.8%	98.1%	
	Cluster 3	96.6%	89.1%	
	Cluster 4	94.9%	96.6%	
K-means + MCLA	Cluster 1	94.2%	98.5%	97.0%
	Cluster 2	100%	94.8%	
	Cluster 3	98.1%	98.1%	
	Cluster 4	91.7%	100%	

Table 4. Partial eta squared effect size result between different methods.

Method	Trunk	Hip	Knee
Ward Clustering	0.015	0.078	0.122
K-means + CSPA	0.002	0.013	0.029
K-means + HGPA	0.007	0.010	0.043
K-means + MCLA	0.001	0.003	0.058

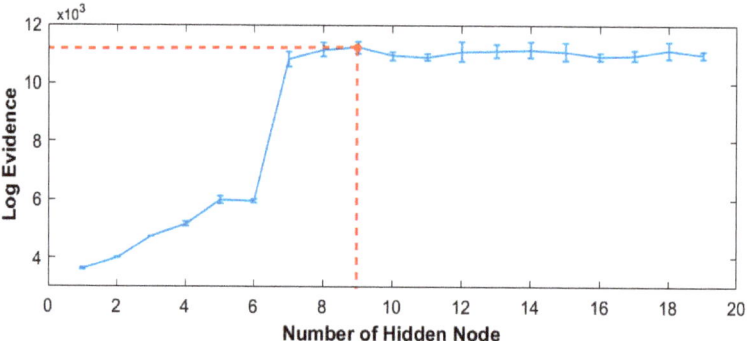

Figure 8. Evidence framework of Bayesian inference (optimum number of hidden node of 9, indicated by red dashed line).

Table 5. Descriptive statistics (mean (SD)) of PSEQ, and pain level for each cluster.

		Cluster 1	Cluster 2	Cluster 3	Cluster 4
PSEQ	Mean	35.56	43.89	46.13	45.57
	(SD)	(8.45)	(9.95)	(10.53)	(9.5)
Pain	Mean	51.03	50.33	47.73	48.17
	(SD)	(10.22)	(20.40)	(21.21)	(19.27)

SD, standard deviation.

The result of the hierarchical tree is represented using a dendrogram shown in Figure 9. Four clusters were created. A 3D scatter plot was generated to visualize the clustering algorithm's output in three-dimensional space, and it is shown in Figure 10.

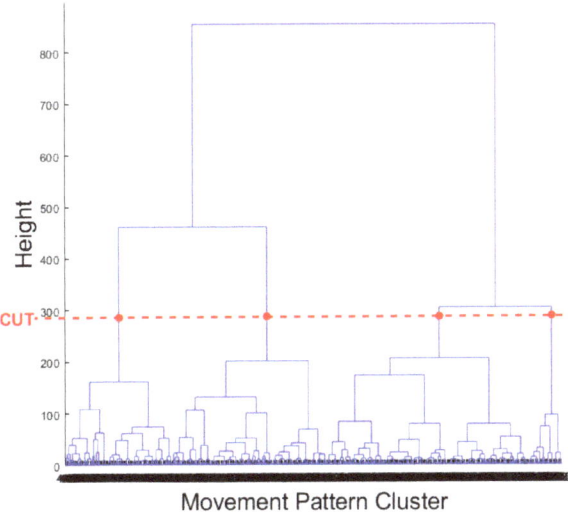

Figure 9. Dendrogram of output hierarchical tree (red dashed line indicates a cut point to form four clusters).

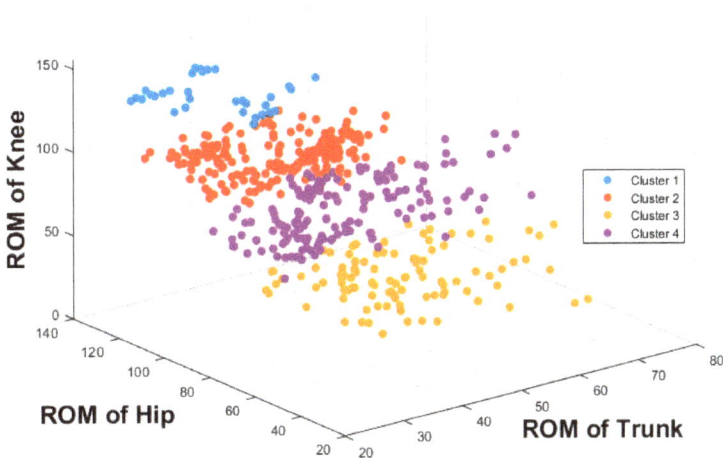

Figure 10. Three-dimensional scatter plot of output of cluster algorithm.

There were significant differences between all clusters and body regions ($F\,(9,1136)$ = 195.67, $p < 0.0001$). The post hoc test revealed different features between the clusters summarized in Figure 11. Post hoc test results show that there were significant differences between all clusters for trunk, hip and knee ROM. This shows that the four cluster results are completely distinctive from a statistical point of view.

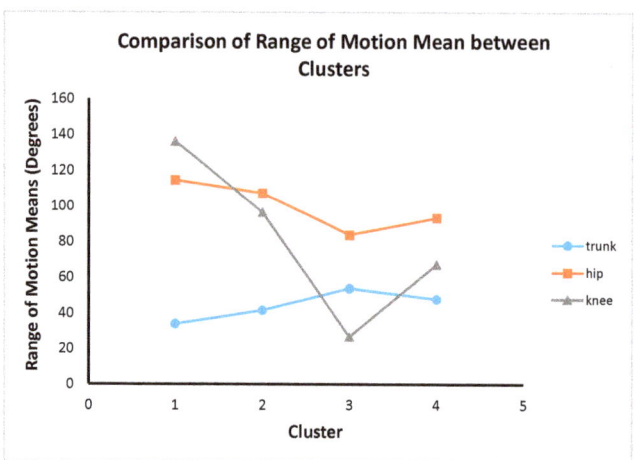

Figure 11. Estimated marginal means of trunk, hip and knee ROM between clusters.

Clusters 2 and 4 are hip dominance with more knee movement than the trunk. Cluster 3 is hip dominance with more trunk movement compared to the knee. Cluster 1 is knee dominance with more hip movement than the trunk.

Post hoc test revealed PSEQ between the clusters, summarized in Figure 12. The PSEQ mean scores of cluster 1 is statistically significantly different from other clusters ($p < 0.05$). The PSEQ mean scores are not statistically significantly different between clusters 2, 3, and 4 ($p > 0.05$ for each pair of clusters). From a clinical point of view, if the PSEQ is greater than 40, there is minimal impairment, and the patient is very confident. If the PSEQ value is less than 40, it means there is an impairment, and the patient is not too confident. As a result, it makes only cluster 1 (PSEQ mean score is 36.56) different from the other clusters.

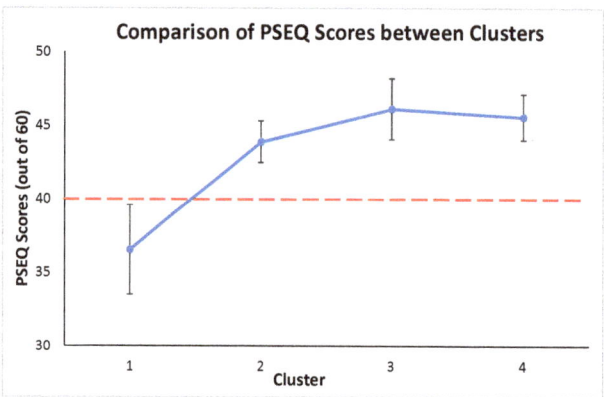

Figure 12. Estimated marginal means of PSEQ between clusters (red dashed line indicates threshold value for PSEQ; below red line suggests clinically significant finding or low pain self-efficacy).

4. Discussion

To the best of our knowledge, this is the first study to utilize unsupervised and supervised machine learning algorithms to classify different movement strategies during a dynamic task using motion capture camera. Besides stoop lift (represent as cluster 3) and leg lift (represent as cluster 1), the study found two additional lifting techniques in people with CLBP, which is in agreement with our study hypothesis. In clusters 2 and 4, people with CLBP tend to use the hip mainly with additional support from knee to lift. Although the Ward clustering method is different from the combination of K-means and ensemble clustering method, descriptive statistics of the trunk, hip and knee ROM results for each cluster between methods are similar. Both the Ward clustering method and the combination of K-means and ensemble clustering method suggest that there would be four different lifting techniques: hip dominance with more trunk movement (cluster 3—ward clustering, cluster 3—K-means and CSPA, cluster 1—K-means and HGPA, and cluster 3—K-means and MCLA); knee dominance with more hip movement (cluster 1—ward clustering, cluster 2—K-means and CSPA, cluster 4—K-means and HGPA, and cluster 4—K-means and MCLA); hip dominance with more knee movement than the trunk (cluster 4—ward clustering, cluster 4—K-means and CSPA, cluster 2—K-means and HGPA, and cluster 1—K-means and MCLA); and hip dominance with much more knee movement than the trunk (cluster 2—ward clustering, cluster 1—K-means and CSPA, cluster 3—K-means and HGPA, and cluster 2—K-means and MCLA). Additionally, the study suggested that Ward clustering was the optimal clustering method for the current data set.

The algorithm in this study resulted in high recall and precision values for all lifting clusters. These indicate that most of the data have been classified correctly, and the model performs well. There is potential to classify any new data using this result. In previous research, hierarchical clustering techniques have been applied in psychiatry. Paykel and Rassaby [42] applied hierarchical clustering to classify suicide attempters. The result has helped to investigate the causes and to guide some improvement for the method of therapy. Additionally, Kurz et al. [43] used Ward's hierarchical agglomerative method to classify suicidal behaviour. This study's accuracy is 95.7% (Ward's method had classified 96% of all cases) [43]. Their clusters were found to have implications for clinical interpretation, therapy and prognostication. This demonstrates that hierarchical clustering can successfully provide some valuable information for further application.

In this study, there are a few variables and aspects that might impact lifting technique in people with CLBP such as height, weight, age, duration of pain and lumbar muscle strength. However, multivariant analysis of covariance (MANCOVA) was conducted as further analysis to determine whether trunk, hip and knee ROM performances differed between each cluster whilst controlling for these variables. MANCOVA results indicated that there is a statistically significant difference between clusters in terms of combined trunk, hip and knee ROM, after controlling for height, weight, age, duration of pain and lumbar muscle strength. Therefore, the results from MANCOVA suggested that there was no significant differences in our initial MANOVA analysis.

Lifting is an important risk factor associated with work-related CLBP [44]. People with CLBP utilized different lifting techniques compared to people without CLBP, particularly, less trunk ROM and increased knee ROM, which are identified as one of many phenotypes of lifting techniques in this study [45]. Identification of lifting techniques in people with CLBP is potentially important in rehabilitation. Physiotherapists and manual handling advisors often encourage CLBP patients to lift with a straight back, which is already the most common lifting technique identified in this study [46]. It is unclear whether the straight-back lifting technique is the cause or the result of the motor adaptation of CLBP. Therefore, it is perhaps unsurprising that the general advice to keep the back straight during lifting did not prevent future low back pain [46]. Identifying lifting techniques and their impact on the lumbar spine can help clinicians to guide LBP patients in adopting a lifting technique that imposes the least amount of force on the lumbar spine. This information can help clinicians in directing effective ergonomic interventions in people with occupational LBP. Additionally, identifying lifting techniques in people with CLBP may help physiotherapists direct and prioritize rehabilitation towards appropriate areas of the body that may be associated with a painful lifting technique (e.g., trunk, hip, and knee). This may result in positive changes in pain and CLBP-related disability (i.e., precision medicine).

An important finding of this study is that despite the majority of the clusters demonstrating similar pain levels, cluster 1 demonstrated the lowest pain self-efficacy, which was associated with the least amount of trunk movement and the most knee movement during lifting (i.e., lifting with a 'straight' back). This finding is consistent with the previous literature that pain self-efficacy is positively correlated with lifting lumbar ROM in people with CLBP [47]. The lower self-efficacy in this group may manifest as reluctance to bend the lumbar spine during lifting, which in a past study has been associated with higher lumbar extension load [48]. This in turn, may sensitize lumbar tissues resulting in pain perpetuation. Thus, observation of a patient's lifting technique and pain self-efficacy may be key clinical assessments to define this group and develop appropriate multicomponent interventions, such as education and exercise [49].

One should interpret these study results with caution. One limitation of this study is the small sample size. The reader needs to be cautious when applying the result to a larger sample size. However, in previous studies with an even smaller sample size (n = 236 [42] and 486 [43]), this method could still cluster participants accurately. Another limitation of this study is the clustering performed on the repetitions instead of mean joint angles for each participant, as this study aims to identify and capture as many different lifting techniques that people with CLBP could demonstrate. This means that we could not account for within-participant lifting technique variability (i.e., variation between each lifting repetition performed by a single participant). Pain alters movement variability within and between participants due to differences in muscle recruitment strategies, psychological features (e.g., fear-avoidant behaviour) and muscle function (e.g., strength, flexibility) to name a few [50,51]. As a result, a small number of CLBP participants in this study (n = 17 or 15% of total participants) demonstrated employed >1 lifting technique (i.e., belonged to >1 lifting clusters). The clinical implication of this limitation is currently unclear and should be evaluated in future studies. Third, the experiment only focused on the sagittal plane's trunk, hip and knee ROM. As such, we were unable to capture movement of the trunk, hip and knee in the other coronal and axial planes. However, the symmetrical lifting task involves mainly movements of the lumbar spine, hip and knee in the sagittal plane. Future studies should explore clustering techniques involving movements in all planes.

It is currently unknown if lifting technique clusters in healthy people are different from those with CLBP. Future studies should aim to compare different lifting techniques in healthy people and people with CLBP. This information will guide the assessment and rehabilitation of movement in people with CLBP. A validation of this novel methodology from a clinic point of view can be conducted in future studies. Authors should discuss the results and how they can be interpreted from the perspective of previous studies and of the working hypotheses. The findings and their implications should be discussed in the broadest context possible. Future research directions may also be highlighted.

5. Conclusions

To the best of our knowledge, this research is the first study introducing an innovative methodology for classifying different movement strategies during lifting tasks in people with CLBP using unsupervised and supervised machine learning techniques. The optimal unsupervised machine learning technique based on Ward's clustering accurately differentiated four distinct movement groups in people with CLBP instead of two lifting techniques, as in current state-of-the-art research studies. The output of the clustering (four clusters) has been validated by the supervised machine learning using Bayesian Neural Network with an accuracy of 97.9%. This promising technique could aid in more precise assessment and rehabilitation of people with CLBP.

Author Contributions: Conceptualization, T.C.P., A.P. and R.C.; methodology, T.C.P., A.P. and R.C.; software, T.C.P. and R.C.; validation, T.C.P., A.P. and R.C.; formal analysis, T.C.P.; investigation, T.C.P., A.P., J.F., A.B., H.T.N. and R.C.; resources, A.P., J.F., A.B., H.T.N. and R.C.; data curation, A.P., J.F. and A.B.; writing—original draft preparation, T.C.P., A.P., J.F. and R.C.; writing—review and editing, T.C.P., A.P., J.F., A.B., H.T.N. and R.C.; visualization, A.P. and R.C.; supervision, A.P., H.T.N. and R.C.; project administration, T.C.P., A.P., H.T.N. and R.C. All authors have read and agreed to the published version of the manuscript.

Funding: This research received no external funding.

Institutional Review Board Statement: The study was approved by the University of Melbourne Behavioural and Social Sciences Human Ethics Sub-Committee (reference number 1749 845 and 8 August 2017).

Informed Consent Statement: Informed consent was obtained from all subjects involved in the study.

Data Availability Statement: For third-party data, restrictions apply to the availability of these data. Data were obtained from the University of Melbourne and are available from Pranata, A. et al. or at https://www.sciencedirect.com/science/article/pii/S0021929018301131 (accessed on 26 July 2020) with the permission of the University of Melbourne.

Conflicts of Interest: The authors declare no conflict of interest.

References

1. Wu, A.; March, L.; Zheng, X.; Huang, J.; Wang, X.; Zhao, J.; Blyth, F.M.; Smith, E.; Buchbinder, R.; Hoy, D. Global low back pain prevalence and years lived with disability from 1990 to 2017: Estimates from the Global Burden of Disease Study 2017. *Ann. Transl. Med.* **2020**, *8*, 299. [CrossRef]
2. van Dieën, J.H.; Reeves, N.P.; Kawchuk, G.; van Dillen, L.R.; Hodges, P.W. Motor Control Changes in Low Back Pain: Divergence in Presentations and Mechanisms. *J. Orthop. Sports Phys. Ther.* **2019**, *49*, 370–379. [CrossRef] [PubMed]
3. Prins, M.; Griffioen, M.; Veeger, T.T.J.; Kiers, H.; Meijer, O.G.; van der Wurff, P.; Bruijn, S.M.; van Dieën, J.H. Evidence of splinting in low back pain?: A systematic review of perturbation studies. *Eur. Spine J.* **2018**, *27*, 40–59. [CrossRef] [PubMed]
4. Pranata, A.; Perraton, L.; El-Ansary, D.; Clark, R.; Mentiplay, B.; Fortin, K.; Long, B.; Brandham, R.; Bryant, A. Trunk and lower limb coordination during lifting in people with and without chronic low back pain. *J. Biomech.* **2018**, *71*, 257–263. [CrossRef] [PubMed]
5. Bazrgari, B.; Shirazi-Adl, A.; Arjmand, N. Analysis of squat and stoop dynamic liftings: Muscle forces and internal spinal loads. *Eur. Spine J.* **2007**, *16*, 687–699. [CrossRef] [PubMed]
6. van Dieën, J.H.; Hoozemans, M.J.; Toussaint, H.M. Stoop or squat: A review of biomechanical studies on lifting technique. *Clin. Biomech.* **1999**, *14*, 685–696. [CrossRef]
7. Zawadka, M.; Skublewska-Paszkowska, M.; Gawda, P.; Lukasik, E.; Smolka, J.; Jablonski, M. What factors can affect lumbopelvic flexion-extension motion in the sagittal plane?: A literature review. *Hum. Mov. Sci.* **2018**, *58*, 205–218. [CrossRef]
8. Laird, R.A.; Gilbert, J.; Kent, P.; Keating, J.L. Comparing lumbo-pelvic kinematics in people with and without back pain: A systematic review and meta-analysis. *BMC Musculoskelet. Disord.* **2014**, *15*, 229. [CrossRef]
9. Sadler, S.G.; Spink, M.J.; Ho, A.; de Jonge, X.J.; Chuter, V.H. Restriction in lateral bending range of motion, lumbar lordosis, and hamstring flexibility predicts the development of low back pain: A systematic review of prospective cohort studies. *BMC Musculoskelet. Disord.* **2017**, *18*, 179. [CrossRef]
10. Nicholas, M.K. The pain self-efficacy questionnaire: Taking pain into account. *Eur. J. Pain* **2005**, *11*, 153–163. [CrossRef]
11. Ferrari, S.; Vanti, C.; Pellizzer, M.; Dozza, L.; Monticone, M.; Pillastrini, P. Is there a relationship between self-efficacy, disability, pain and sociodemographic characteristics in chronic low back pain? A multicenter retrospective analysis. *Arch. Physiother.* **2019**, *9*, 9. [CrossRef]
12. Levin, J.B.; Lofland, K.R.; Cassisi, J.E.; Poreh, A.M.; Blonsky, E.R. The relationship between self-efficacy and disability in chronic low back pain patients. *Int. J. Rehabil. Health* **1996**, *2*, 19–28. [CrossRef]
13. Karasawa, Y.; Yamada, K.; Iseki, M.; Yamaguchi, M.; Murakami, Y.; Tamagawa, T.; Kadowaki, F.; Hamaoka, S.; Ishii, T.; Kawai, A.; et al. Association between change in self-efficacy and reduction in disability among patients with chronic pain. *PLoS ONE* **2019**, *14*, e0215404. [CrossRef]
14. de Moraes Vieira, É.B.; de Góes Salvetti, M.; Damiani, L.P.; de Mattos Pimenta, C.A. Self-Efficacy and Fear Avoidance Beliefs in Chronic Low Back Pain Patients: Coexistence and Associated Factors. *Pain Manag. Nurs.* **2014**, *15*, 593–602. [CrossRef] [PubMed]
15. Rifai, C.; Naik, G.R.; Tuan Nghia, N.; Sai Ho, L.; Tran, Y.; Craig, A.; Nguyen, H.T. Driver Fatigue Classification with Independent Component by Entropy Rate Bound Minimization Analysis in an EEG-Based System. *IEEE J. Biomed. Health Inform.* **2017**, *21*, 715–724.
16. Bell, J. *Machine Learning: Hands-On for Developers and Technical Professionals*; Wiley: Hoboken, NJ, USA, 2014.
17. McCallum, A.; Nigam, K.; Ungar, L. Efficient clustering of high-dimensional data sets with application to reference matching. In *Proceedings of the International Conference on Knowledge Discovery and Data Mining, Boston, MA, USA, 20–23 August 2000*; ACM: New York, NY, USA, 2000; pp. 169–178.
18. Fiorini, L.; Cavallo, F.; Dario, P.; Eavis, A.; Caleb-Solly, P. Unsupervised Machine Learning for Developing Personalised Behaviour Models Using Activity Data. *Sensors* **2017**, *17*, 1034. [CrossRef] [PubMed]
19. Pagnuco, I.A.; Pastore, J.I.; Abras, G.; Brun, M.; Ballarin, V.L. Analysis of genetic association using hierarchical clustering and cluster validation indices. *Genomics* **2017**, *109*, 438–445. [CrossRef]
20. Kuizhi, M.; Jinye, P.; Ling, G.; Zheng, N.; Jianping, F. Hierarchical classification of large-scale patient records for automatic treatment stratification. *IEEE J. Biomed. Health Inform.* **2015**, *19*, 1234–1245.

21. Hamid, J.S.; Meaney, C.; Crowcroft, N.S.; Granerod, J.; Beyene, J. Cluster analysis for identifying sub-groups and selecting potential discriminatory variables in human encephalitis. *BMC Infect. Dis.* **2010**, *10*, 364. [CrossRef]
22. Farragher, J.B.; Pranata, A.; Williams, G.; El-Ansary, D.; Parry, S.M.; Kasza, J.; Bryant, A. Effects of lumbar extensor muscle strengthening and neuromuscular control retraining on disability in patients with chronic low back pain: A protocol for a randomised controlled trial. *BMJ Open* **2019**, *9*, e028259. [CrossRef]
23. Silvetti, A.; Mari, S.; Ranavolo, A.; Forzano, F.; Iavicoli, S.; Conte, C.; Draicchio, F. Kinematic and electromyographic assessment of manual handling on a supermarket green- grocery shelf. *Work* **2015**, *51*, 261–271. [CrossRef]
24. Burgess-Limerick, R.; Abernethy, B.; Neal, R.J.; Kippers, V. Self-Selected Manual Lifting Technique: Functional Consequences of the Interjoint Coordination. *Hum. Factors* **1995**, *37*, 395–411. [CrossRef] [PubMed]
25. Aggarwal, C.C. An Introduction to Cluster Analysis. In *Data Clustering*; Chapman and Hall: London, UK, 2014; pp. 1–27.
26. Xu, R.; Wunsch, D. *Clustering*; IEEE Press: Piscataway, NJ, USA, 2015.
27. Everitt, B.S.; Landau, S.; Leese, M.; Stahl, D. An Introduction to Classification and Clustering. In *Cluster Analysis*; John Wiley & Sons, Ltd.: Chichester, UK, 2011; pp. 1–13.
28. Hansen, P.; Jaumard, B. Cluster analysis and mathematical programming. *Math. Program.* **1997**, *79*, 191–215. [CrossRef]
29. Omran, M.G.; Engelbrecht, A.P.; Salman, A. An overview of clustering methods. *Intell. Data Anal.* **2007**, *11*, 583–605. [CrossRef]
30. Golalipour, K.; Akbari, E.; Hamidi, S.S.; Lee, M.; Enayatifar, R. From clustering to clustering ensemble selection: A review. *Eng. Appl. Artif. Intell.* **2021**, *104*, 104388. [CrossRef]
31. Fred, A.L.N.; Jain, A.K. Combining multiple clusterings using evidence accumulation. *IEEE Trans. Pattern Anal. Mach. Intell.* **2005**, *27*, 835–850. [CrossRef]
32. Berikov, V. Weighted ensemble of algorithms for complex data clustering. *Pattern Recognit. Lett.* **2014**, *38*, 99–106. [CrossRef]
33. Li, F.; Qian, Y.; Wang, J.; Dang, C.; Jing, L. Clustering ensemble based on sample's stability. *Artif. Intell.* **2019**, *273*, 37–55. [CrossRef]
34. Zhou, P.; Du, L.; Liu, X.; Shen, Y.-D.; Fan, M.; Li, X. Self-Paced Clustering Ensemble. *IEEE Trans. Neural Netw. Learn. Syst.* **2021**, *32*, 1497–1511. [CrossRef]
35. Strehl, A.; Ghosh, J. Cluster ensembles—A knowledge reuse framework for combining multiple partitions. *J. Mach. Learn. Res.* **2003**, *3*, 583–617.
36. Han, E.; Karypis, G.; Kumar, V.; Mobasher, B. *Clustering Based on Association Rule Hypergraphs*; University of Minnesota Digital Conservancy: Minneapolis, MN, USA, 1997.
37. Rajendran, S. What Is Hierarchical Clustering? An Introduction to Hierarchical Clustering. Available online: https://www.mygreatlearning.com/blog/hierarchical-clustering/ (accessed on 16 January 2021).
38. Anselin, L. Cluster Analysis Hierarchical Clustering Methods. Available online: https://geodacenter.github.io/workbook/7bh_clusters_2a/lab7bh.html (accessed on 15 January 2021).
39. Hubert, L.; Arabie, P. Comparing partitions. *J. Classif.* **1985**, *2*, 193–218. [CrossRef]
40. Mezzetti, M.; Borzelli, D.; D'Avella, A. A Bayesian approach to model individual differences and to partition individuals: Case studies in growth and learning curves. *Stat. Methods Appl.* **2022**, 1–27. [CrossRef]
41. Bishop, C.M. *Neural Networks for Pattern Recognition*; Oxford University Press: Oxford, UK, 1995.
42. Paykel, E.S.; Rassaby, E. Classification of Suicide Attempters by Cluster Analysis. *Br. J. Psychiatry* **1978**, *133*, 45–52. [CrossRef]
43. Kurz, A.; Möller, H.J.; Baindl, G.; Bürk, F.; Torhorst, A.; Wächtler, C.; Lauter, H. Classification of parasuicide by cluster analysis. Types of suicidal behaviour, therapeutic and prognostic implications. *Br. J. Psychiatry* **1987**, *150*, 520–525. [CrossRef] [PubMed]
44. Coenen, P.; Gouttebarge, V.; van der Burght, A.S.A.M.; van Dieën, J.H.; Frings-Dresen, M.H.W.; van der Beek, A.J.; Burdorf, A. The effect of lifting during work on low back pain: A health impact assessment based on a meta-analysis. *Occup. Environ. Med.* **2014**, *71*, 871–877. [CrossRef] [PubMed]
45. Nolan, D.; O'Sullivan, K.; Newton, C.; Singh, G.; Smith, B. Are there differences in lifting technique between those with and without low back pain? A systematic review. *Physiotherapy* **2020**, *107*, e76. [CrossRef]
46. Nolan, D.; O'Sullivan, K.; Stephenson, J.; O'Sullivan, P.; Lucock, M. What do physiotherapists and manual handling advisors consider the safest lifting posture, and do back beliefs influence their choice? *Musculoskelet. Sci. Pract.* **2018**, *33*, 35–40. [CrossRef]
47. La Touche, R.; Grande-Alonso, M.; Arnes-Prieto, P.; Paris-Alemany, A. How Does Self-Efficacy Influence Pain Perception, Postural Stability and Range of Motion in Individuals with Chronic Low Back Pain? *Pain Physician* **2019**, *22*, E1–E13. [CrossRef]
48. Kingma, I.; Faber, G.S.; Bakker, A.J.; van Dieen, J.H. Can Low Back Loading During Lifting Be Reduced by Placing One Leg Beside the Object to Be Lifted? *Phys. Ther.* **2006**, *86*, 1091–1105. [CrossRef]
49. Martinez-Calderon, J.; Flores-Cortes, M.; Morales-Asencio, J.M.; Fernandez-Sanchez, M.; Luque-Suarez, A. Which interventions enhance pain self-efficacy in people with chronic musculoskeletal pain? A systematic review with meta-analysis of randomized controlled trials, including over 12,000 participants. *J. Orthop. Sports Phys. Ther.* **2020**, *50*, 418–430. [CrossRef]
50. Hodges, P.W.; Smeets, R.J. Interaction between pain, movement, and physical activity: Short-term benefits, long-term consequences, and targets for treatment. *Clin. J. Pain* **2015**, *31*, 97–107. [CrossRef] [PubMed]
51. Hodges, P.W.; Tucker, K. Moving differently in pain: A new theory to explain the adaptation to pain. *Pain* **2011**, *152* (Suppl. 3), S90–S98. [CrossRef] [PubMed]

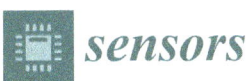

Article

Machine Learning Identifies Chronic Low Back Pain Patients from an Instrumented Trunk Bending and Return Test

Paul Thiry [1,2,3,*], Martin Houry [4], Laurent Philippe [4], Olivier Nocent [5], Fabien Buisseret [3,6], Frédéric Dierick [3,7,8], Rim Slama [9], William Bertucci [5], André Thévenon [2] and Emilie Simoneau-Buessinger [1]

1. LAMIH, CNRS, UMR 8201, Université Polytechnique Hauts-de-France, 59313 Valenciennes, France; emilie.simoneau@uphf.fr
2. CHU Lille, Université de Lille, 59000 Lille, France; andre.thevenon@univ-lille.fr
3. CeREF Technique, Chaussée de Binche 159, 7000 Mons, Belgium; buisseretf@helha.be (F.B.); frederic.dierick@rehazenter.lu (F.D.)
4. Centre de Recherche FoRS, Haute-Ecole de Namur-Liège-Luxembourg (Henallux), Rue Victor Libert 36H, 6900 Marche-en-Famenne, Belgium; martin.houry@henallux.be (M.H.); laurent.philippe@henallux.be (L.P.)
5. PSMS, Université de Reims Champagne Ardenne, 51867 Reims, France; olivier.nocent@univ-reims.fr (O.N.); william.bertucci@univ-reims.fr (W.B.)
6. Service de Physique Nucléaire et Subnucléaire, UMONS Research Institute for Complex Systems, Université de Mons, Place du Parc 20, 7000 Mons, Belgium
7. Centre National de Rééducation Fonctionnelle et de Réadaptation–Rehazenter, Laboratoire d'Analyse du Mouvement et de la Posture (LAMP), Rue André Vésale 1, 2674 Luxembourg, Luxembourg
8. Faculté des Sciences de la Motricité, UCLouvain, Place Pierre de Coubertin 1, 1348 Ottignies-Louvain-la-Neuve, Belgium
9. LINEACT Laboratory, CESI Lyon, 69100 Villeurbanne, France; rsalmi@cesi.fr
* Correspondence: thiryp@helha.be

Citation: Thiry, P.; Houry, M.; Philippe, L.; Nocent, O.; Buisseret, F.; Dierick, F.; Slama, R.; Bertucci, W.; Thévenon, A.; Simoneau-Buessinger, E. Machine Learning Identifies Chronic Low Back Pain Patients from an Instrumented Trunk Bending and Return Test. *Sensors* **2022**, *22*, 5027. https://doi.org/10.3390/s22135027

Academic Editor: Ki H. Chon

Received: 9 June 2022
Accepted: 30 June 2022
Published: 3 July 2022

Publisher's Note: MDPI stays neutral with regard to jurisdictional claims in published maps and institutional affiliations.

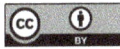

Copyright: © 2022 by the authors. Licensee MDPI, Basel, Switzerland. This article is an open access article distributed under the terms and conditions of the Creative Commons Attribution (CC BY) license (https://creativecommons.org/licenses/by/4.0/).

Abstract: Nowadays, the better assessment of low back pain (LBP) is an important challenge, as it is the leading musculoskeletal condition worldwide in terms of years of disability. The objective of this study was to evaluate the relevance of various machine learning (ML) algorithms and Sample Entropy (SampEn), which assesses the complexity of motion variability in identifying the condition of low back pain. Twenty chronic low-back pain (CLBP) patients and 20 healthy non-LBP participants performed 1-min repetitive bending (flexion) and return (extension) trunk movements. Analysis was performed using the time series recorded by three inertial sensors attached to the participants. It was found that SampEn was significantly lower in CLBP patients, indicating a loss of movement complexity due to LBP. Gaussian Naive Bayes ML proved to be the best of the various tested algorithms, achieving 79% accuracy in identifying CLBP patients. Angular velocity of flexion movement was the most discriminative feature in the ML analysis. This study demonstrated that: supervised ML and a complexity assessment of trunk movement variability are useful in the identification of CLBP condition, and that simple kinematic indicators are sensitive to this condition. Therefore, ML could be progressively adopted by clinicians in the assessment of CLBP patients.

Keywords: artificial intelligence; machine learning; inertial measurement unit—IMU; movement complexity; sample entropy; trunk flexion

1. Introduction

Low back pain (LBP) is the leading cause of a high number of years lived with disability worldwide. In both 10–24 and 50–74-year-old age groups, LBP is typically responsible for the loss of an entire year of full health [1]. A better understanding of this musculoskeletal condition and its complexity is therefore essential for clinicians involved in the care of patients with LBP.

LBP, especially chronic LBP (CLBP), leads to a fear of movement and causes patients to limit their activities of daily living and social participation to avoid pain [2,3]. The sedentary lifestyle of LBP patients is an exacerbating factor and leads to chronicity [4,5]. A better understanding of the relationship between the kinematics of the lumbo–pelvic–hip complex and LBP is currently of high importance. The evaluation of these movements can potentially be performed easily and inexpensively with one or more low-complexity devices [6], such as inertial sensors, also called inertial measurement units (IMUs) [7–11]. Low complexity can be understood as ready-to-use, which is a necessary feature in clinical practice. Information from the IMU time series can be obtained using various methods, including machine learning (ML) algorithms [12–18]. Our study focused on IMU-based testing of lumbo–pelvic–hip complex movements and ML-based algorithm analysis of CLBP patients and non-LBP (NLBP) subjects. The power of current computers and commercially available equipment allows ML to be increasingly affordable; hence it seemed logical to include it in the development of a clinical test to assess LBP.

An example of interest for the present study is the ability of a single IMU to measure the variability of repetitive trunk bending and return (b&r) movements by computing the sample entropy (SampEn) [19] from the different time series recorded in healthy subjects [20]. In the latter study [20], it was shown that 50 repetitions of trunk b&r movements could provide kinematic data that allow for the accurate computation of SampEn from the six time series recorded by a single IMU and, therefore, may be used to assess movement complexity [21]. We hypothesize that such a b&r test can be used to investigate LBP and, if possible, discriminate between the presence and absence of LBP in individuals. In the present study, we extended the results of [20] in several directions: (1) increasing the number of IMU from one to three; (2) using SampEn measurements in combination with ML methods to analyze the recorded time series; (3) including patients with CLBP in the population of NLBP subjects previously included in [20]. We will now address these three points.

1. The use of a set of three IMUs should provide more information about the b&r test and allows the whole lumbopelvic–hip complex to be examined. Some authors placed the IMUs at L2 and S2 vertebrae to measure low lumbar flexion–extension movements [22], while others chose T10-12 and S2 to be able to measure the local dynamic stability, coordination, and variability of the lumbar spine in repeated flexion–extension movements [23]. We chose T12 and S2 so to consider the entire lumbar spine for a given movement. Differences between the time series of different sensors can provide information about the relative angular velocity and acceleration between two anatomical landmarks. Typically, for sagittal plane angular velocities, the difference between the data from a sensor placed at the twelfth thoracic vertebra and a sensor placed at the second sacral vertebra should provide an estimate of the lumbar angular velocity. From a clinical perspective, the use of three IMUs placed at different points may help to identify the most relevant location for a single IMU, which may be useful when time constraints apply.

2. Two main techniques were used in this study. The first is a standard statistical analysis, which consists of computing the SampEn from the IMUs time series in two groups—NLBP subjects and CLBP patients—and comparing them. The second technique is ML, which has been used for about 40 years in the study of LBP [13], especially in the field of medical imaging and clinical data analysis for diagnostic and decision-making purposes [14,15]. Note that SampEn will be part of the data used by ML to identify CLBP patients.

3. We believe that a first step toward integrating the clinical interpretation of a test, such as the b&r test, into a biopsychosocial model must be to examine its ability to discriminate between CLBP patients and NLBP subjects. A recent study using a particular supervised ML algorithm (Support Vector Machine, SVM) to analyze IMU data has already shown that a kinematic test of the lumbar spine is able to discriminate NLBP subjects from LBP patients and classify them according to their risk of chronicity, i.e., between high risk and medium to low risk, with an accuracy of >75% [12]. Moreover, it has been shown in [24] that SVM can detect neck pain from

rotational head movements with an accuracy of 82%. These last two studies show that a diagnostic analysis using ML algorithms supplied with kinematic parameters is a promising way to investigate these spinal conditions further. Our work focuses on the kinematic signature of patients suffering from CLBP and, more specifically, on the complexity of their variability during repetitive movements of the trunk along the lines of [20].

The main question addressed by this study is: "Can an instrumented b&r test identify CLBP patients by resorting to ML algorithms?" Our hypothesis is that algorithms such as SVM can accurately discriminate CLBP patients from NLBP subjects using raw data from three IMUs and SampEn values.

2. Materials and Methods

2.1. Population

Data were collected from a group of CLBP patients and from a matched group of healthy NLBP subjects. The study protocol was approved by the Intercommunale de Santé Publique du Pays de Charleroi Ethics Committee (ISPPC/OM008) under the number B325-2020-43666 and complied with the Helsinki Declaration on the Ethical Principles for Medical Research Involving Human Beings. All of the patients and subjects received an information sheet explaining the purpose of the study and gave informed consent before participation.

Twenty CLBP patients were recruited on a voluntary basis between the 3 November and the 1 December 2020 from the pool of patients treated for CLBP at the University Hospital of Charleroi (CHUC) in the "Sport Santé" department in Monceau-sur-Sambre, Belgium. The inclusion criteria were: the presence of LBP diagnosed by a physician and lasting longer than three months, ability to perform three trunk flexions with the lower limbs extended, aged between 18 and 65 years, body mass index (BMI) between 18 and 35 $kg \cdot m^{-2}$, and a pain score of less than 8/10 on a verbal Numerical Rating Scale (NRS) the day of the test. The exclusion criteria were: the presence of tumor, fracture, neurological signs (loss of strength and/or sensitivity), decrease or abolition of reflexes, and presence of pain of neuropathic origin evaluated by a positive DN4 ("diagnostic de Douleur Neuropathique", i.e., neuropathic pain diagnostic) questionnaire [25], recent trauma, surgery at the spinal level, vertigo and balance disorders due to positional changes, musculoskeletal disorders in another region that could interfere with the b&r test, or systemic and metabolic disorders.

Twenty healthy NLBP subjects were recruited on a voluntary basis between 1 December and 15 December 2020 from CHUC staff or their personal acquaintances. They were matched with the CLBP patients using the following criteria: age, BMI, and physical activity level. For these subjects, the exclusion criteria were: the presence of LBP in the past year, history of spinal surgery, musculoskeletal disorders in another region that could interfere with the b&r test, systemic and metabolic disorders, and the use of analgesics.

2.2. Protocol, Data Collection and Preprocessing

The general characteristics were collected from all participants: gender, age, BMI, and physical activity level were collected through the Global Physical Activity Questionnaire (GPAQ) [26]. Two experienced examiners (physiotherapists) were involved in the protocol. A first examiner (examiner #1) gave standardized instructions to each participant and showed a video demonstrating how to perform the b&r test. The same examiner (#1) cleaned the skin with cotton wool and ether at the sites where the three IMUs were taped. These were attached with hypoallergenic double-sided adhesive tape (Figure 1): Sensor #1 (SENS1) on the opposite to the spinous process of the twelfth thoracic vertebra (T12); Sensor #2 (SENS2) opposite to the second sacral vertebra (S2) on a horizontal line connecting the posterior-superior iliac spines; and Sensor #3 (SENS3) on the lateral side of the thigh, 10 cm below the greater trochanter.

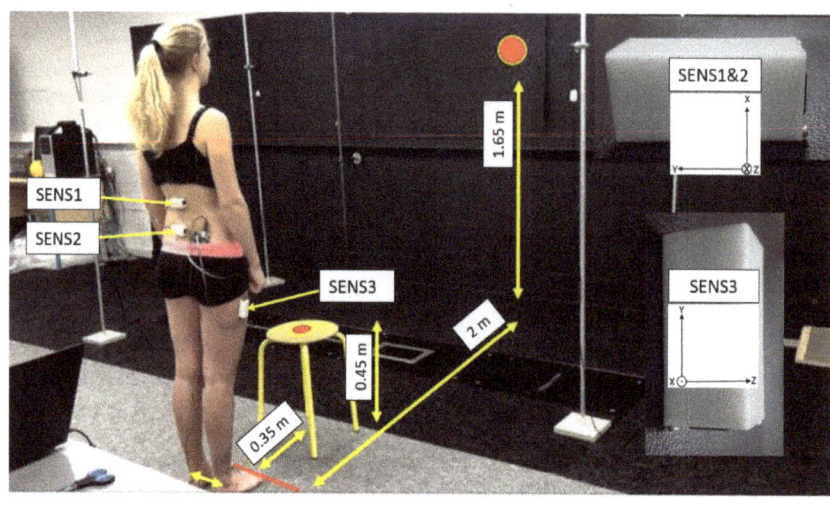

Figure 1. NLBP subject in starting position for the b&r test. The targets on the stool and on the wall in front of the subject are shown (red points). A zoom on the sensors is shown in the inset of the figure (on the right). The respective coordinate system (X, Y, Z) used is shown for SENS1&2 and for SENS3.

Each participant was then placed in a standing position with their arms by their sides, as shown in Figure 1. To perform the b&r test, the participants were instructed to bend the trunk forward (flexion) without flexing their lower limbs and to touch a target in the center of a stool with the fingertips of both hands, followed by an immediate trunk extension to return to the starting position while focusing on a target in front of them (Figure 1). This movement was repeated continuously, as quickly and comfortably as possible. The test was performed once and lasted 70 s. The participants were allowed to stop the test before the end of the 70 s if they felt unable to continue; however, in this case, they were then excluded from the study. The examiner was present near the participant during the test but gave no verbal instructions.

A second examiner (examiner #2) recorded the data from the IMUs on a computer located less than 3 m from the patient or subject, with the IMUs connected to the computer via a cable [27]. Examiner #2 informed the participant of the time remaining every 10 s. The computer screen was visible to neither examiner #1 nor the participant. The data were stored on the computer's hard disk drive for later analysis.

The IMUs used are part of a homemade system called DYSKIMOT (for Motor Dyskinesia), which has been presented in detail previously in [27]. The DYSKIMOT system software (v. 3.1) recorded the data from the three IMUs with a sampling frequency of 100 Hz. The system is based on commercial IMUs (LSM9DS1, SparkFun Electronics, Niwot, CO, USA) equipped with a triaxial accelerometer, gyroscope, magnetometer, and thermometer. Time series of accelerations (Acc X, Y, Z) along each of the 3 axes of each sensor and angular velocities (Gyr X, Y, Z) were recorded. The DYSKIMOT software also computed the angular accelerations (AccA X, Y, Z) in real-time by numerical differentiation (method) and the corrected angles (AngC X, Y, Z) by numerical integration and linear drift subtraction of the angular velocities. Typical traces are shown in Figure 2. The DYSKIMOT IMU casing was 3D printed using PLA (Polylactic Acid), the most widely used polymer in 3D printing. Other polymers may have been used, such as ABS (Acrylonitrile butadiene styrene) or TPU (Thermoplastic polyurethane). The latter choice made it possible to produce flexible parts that would presumably be more comfortable for the user.

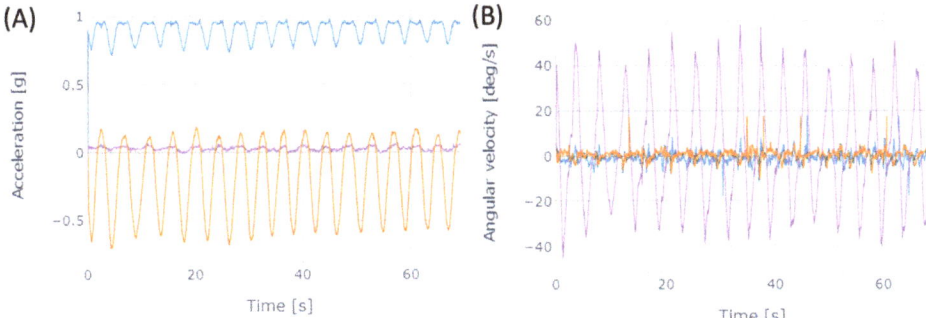

Figure 2. Typical traces of (**A**) Acc X (blue), Acc Y (purple), and Acc Z (orange) and (**B**) Gyr X (blue), Gyr Y (purple), and Gyr Z (orange) time series recorded with SENS1 during a b&r test in a healthy NLBP subject.

As in [2], we considered the first 10 s of the time series as the warm-up period, and any data collected after 70 s were omitted from analyses. Therefore, only data between 10 and 70 s were used for the analysis; all of the time series lasted 1 min.

2.3. SampEn and Complexity Factors

An R (v 4.1.0, R Core Team, Auckland, New Zealand) routine was developed to calculate SampEn for all recorded time series. In accordance with Yentes [19], we used the following parameters in the algorithm (R-Studio) for calculating the SampEn: vector length m = 2, tolerance r = 0.2 SD and the number of points in the data series N = 6000. The details can be found in [20]. The values obtained from Gyr and Acc, respectively, were referred to as SampEn Gyr X, Y, Z and SampEn Acc X, Y, Z.

In the case of the b&r test, the Gyr Y time series should have considerable practical implications since it follows the direction of the performed movement. Therefore, specific computations were performed for this time series. The Gyr Y of SENS2 was subtracted from the same time series of SENS1 (Gyr Y) and SENS3 (−Gyr Z; SENS3 has a different orientation, see Figure 1). SampEn was computed for the resulting time series. The calculation of SampEn using these data should provide a relevant estimation of the complexity of angular velocity variations in lumbar and hip -flexion during the b&r test. The SampEn values obtained in this way were termed the lumbar flexion complexity factor (LCF) and the hip flexion complexity factor (HCF), and together formed what we called complexity factors (CF).

Statistical comparisons between all SampEn and CF in CLBP patients and NLBP subjects were performed with a t-test or with a Mann–Whitney rank sum when the Shapiro–Wilk normality test failed. The mean, SD, standard error of measurement (**SEM** $= \frac{SD}{\sqrt{N}}$, where N is the sample size), 95% confidence interval (CI denotes half-width), and minimum detectable change (**MDC** $= 1.96\sqrt{2}$ **SEM**) were calculated for the differences in parameter values between the two groups. Statistical tests were performed with SigmaPlot software (v. 14.0, Systat Software, San Jose, CA, United States of America) with a significance level of 5%.

2.4. Machine Learning Analysis

2.4.1. Data Segmentation

The first way to apply ML is to use and analyze a given time series as a whole. A second way is to divide the time series into cycles and use them as independent data related to a particular participant. Since we have explored both options, further details on segmentation into cycles are provided below.

The different b&r cycles can be clearly seen in Figure 2. Each cycle corresponds to the repetition of b&r trunk movements carried out by a participant. The start and end of each cycle were determined by identifying the successive minima of the Acc Z time series for SENS1, i.e., the time series with the highest signal-to-noise ratio.

The segmentation algorithm, which divides the time series into distinct cycles, consists of five steps: (1) averaging the original Acc Z time series using a rolling centered window (width: 25 points or 0.25 s); (2) calculating the global amplitude and the exact value of the threshold (40% of the amplitude above the minimum); (3) extracting data below this threshold to avoid the processing of local minimum above this threshold; (4) detecting the minima and computing the cycle limits as the average position of two consecutive minima; (5) finally, all cycles were normalized by linear interpolation to 450 points, which is the maximum number of points for a cycle in our data set. The last 450 points were referred to as "itime".

In the Results section, ML analysis based on 1-min time series is referred to as "whole sequences", and ML analysis based on individual cycles is referred to as "cycle segmentation".

2.4.2. Discrimination of NLBP and CLBP Participants

The discriminating power of classification by the ML algorithm was assessed by computing accuracy and Area Under Curve (AUC) values for binary classification. Several classification algorithms were used, all belonging to the supervised ML, as each participant was labeled with either NLBP or CLBP condition. The ML algorithms studied were Linear Support Vector Machines (Linear SVM), Non-linear Support Vector Machine Radial Basis Function (SVM RBF), Random Forest (RF), Gaussian naive Bayes (GaussianNB), K-neighbors (KNN), Adaptive Boosting (AdaBoost), and Decision Tree (DT) [28]. The grid-search method [29] was used to optimize the hyperparameters for each ML algorithm. The hyperparameters are listed in Table 1. The ML algorithms and the grid search are implemented by the v1.1 Scikit-learn library.

Table 1. Classifier's hyperparameters.

ML Algorithm	Hyperparameters
BF KNN	number of neighbours (**3**, 5, 8, 10), weighting function (uniform, **distance**), algorithm (**Brute-Force** (BF KNN or BF KNN), kd_tree, auto, ball_tree)
Linear SVM	regularization parameter (**0.001**, 0.01, 0.1, 1, 10, 100, 1000)
SVM RBF	C-parameter (0.001, 0.01, 0.1, **1**, 10, 100), kernel coefficient Gamma (**0.001**, 0.01, 0.1, 1, 10, 100)
DT	maximum depth of the tree (1, 5, **10**, 100), function to measure the quality of the splits (**gini**, entropy), strategy to select the split nodes (**best**, random)
RF	maximum depth of the tree (1, 5, **10**, 100), number of trees in the forest (1, 5, 10, **100**), number of features considered in the search for the best split (**1**, 5, 10, 100)
AdaBoost	maximum number of estimators at which boosting stops (5, 10, **50**, 100, 500), weight applied to each classifier at each boosting iteration (0.000001, 0.001, 0.1, **1**, 5, 10, 100)
GaussianNB	ratio of the largest variance of all features added to the variances for computational stability (**0.0000001**, 0.01, 1, 10, 100)

BF KNN: Brute-Force K-Nearest Neighbors, SVM: Support Vector Machine, RBF: radial basis function, DT: Decision Tree, RF: Random Forest, AdaBoost: Adaptive boosting, GaussianNB: Gaussian naive Bayes; hyperparameters in bold are the selected ones by the grid-search function.

Statistical describers were maximum, minimum, mean, median, 1st quartile, 3rd quartile, and SD for each available time series (each component X, Y, and Z was treated as an independent time series). These parameters, referred to as raw data features, were used as discriminators for ML algorithms. The performance evaluation of each ML algorithm was measured after an n-fold cross-validation process, scaling of the time series, and 100 training repetitions with a random ordering of NLBP and CLBP.

The computed SampEn and CF were also included as features in the ML algorithms in a second step. The accuracy and AUC of the ML algorithms were computed using only raw data features and only SampEn or CF. The added value of SampEn and CF in identifying CLBP was assessed.

2.4.3. Most Discriminative Features

Two methods were used to identify the best discriminating feature: Sequential Feature Selector forward (SFS Forward) and Sequential Feature Selector backward (SFS Backward) [30]. The SFS Forward accumulates the best-performing features one by one and creates a hierarchy from the best-performing feature to the worst-performing feature. The SFS Backward starts with all features and removes the worst-performing features one by one. This results in a hierarchy from the longest-remaining feature to the least-remaining feature. Each SFS was run 700 times (7 algorithms × 100 training repetitions).

3. Results

3.1. SampEn & CF

Four of the 18 calculated SampEn values (six time series and 3 IMUs) showed significant differences between CLBP and NLBP groups. HCF showed significant differences between CLBP and NLBP groups, whereas LCF did not. These statistically significant results are shown in Table 2, while the others have been omitted for simplicity.

Table 2. Significative differences (T-test or Wilcoxon test depending on the normality or not of the distribution of the SampEn values) between CLBP and NLBP groups. All parameters are SampEn values defined in Section 2.3.

SampEn	Gyr Y SENS1		Gyr Z SENS2		HCF			Gyr Y SENS2		Acc X SENS2	
	CLBP	NLBP	CLBP	NLBP	CLBP	NLBP		CLBP	NLBP	CLBP	NLBP
Mean	0.161	0.208	0.625	0.516	0.272	0.326	Median	0.217	0.282	0.266	0.389
SD	0.05	0.072	0.168	0.144	0.053	0.100	Q1	0.187	0.220	0.227	0.312
SEM	0.011	0.016	0.038	0.032	0.012	0.022	Q3	0.261	0.343	0.407	0.523
p-value	0.021		0.035		0.044		p-value	0.021		0.047	
					Difference NLBP−CLBP						
Mean	0.035		−0.108		0.055		Mean	−0.034		0.097	
SD	0.168		0.254		0.111		SD	0.159		0.301	
CI	0.074		0.111		0.046		CI	0.070		0.132	
SEM	0.038		0.057		0.024		SEM	0.036		0.067	
MDC	0.104		0.157		0.070		MDC	0.099		0.187	

CI: 95% confidence interval; SEM: Standard Error of Measure; MDC: Minimal Detectable Change; SampEn value for: the Y-axis of the gyroscope from the sensor 1 (Gyr Y SENS1), the Z-axis of the gyroscope from the sensor 2 (Gyr Z SENS2), Hip Complexity Factor (HCF), the Y-axis of the gyroscope from the sensor 2 (Gyr Y SENS2), the X-axis of the accelerometer from the sensor 2 (Acc X SENS2).

3.2. Cycle Segmentation

The result of the segmentation process was a data set of 1678 cycles labeled with their respective index (CLBP patient or healthy NLBP subject). Figure 3 show the principle of segmentation. Figure 4 shows all the computed cycles for Gyr Y of SENS2 as a function of time in the form of a mean cycle and a shaded area indicating the cycle's SD.

3.3. Machine Learning

The optimal hyperparameter values for each ML algorithm are highlighted in bold in Table 1. The performance indicators of all the ML algorithms used are listed in Table 3.

Table 3. Comparison of prediction performance between the whole sequences and cycle segmentation procedures, for all considered ML algorithms.

	Whole Sequences		Cycle Segmentation	
Algorithms	Accuracy (%)	AUC	Accuracy (%)	AUC
BF KNN	0.63 ± 0.08	0.69 ± 0.09	0.65 ± 0.05	0.67 ± 0.06

Table 3. *Cont.*

Algorithms	Whole Sequences		Cycle Segmentation	
	Accuracy (%)	AUC	Accuracy (%)	AUC
Linear SVM	0.72 ± 0.07	0.79 ± 0.07	0.68 ± 0.06	0.71 ± 0.08
SVM RBF	0.52 ± 0.06	0.52 ± 0.09	0.64 ± 0.04	0.71 ± 0.06
DT	0.66 ± 0.08	0.65 ± 0.09	0.66 ± 0.06	0.65 ± 0.06
RF	0.78 ± 0.07	0.83 ± 0.08	0.72 ± 0.05	0.80 ± 0.06
AdaBoost	0.68 ± 0.07	0.74 ± 0.08	0.70 ± 0.06	0.74 ± 0.08
GaussianNB	**0.79 ± 0.08**	**0.85 ± 0.07**	0.69 ± 0.07	0.74 ± 0.07

BF KNN: Brute-Force K-Nearest Neighbors, SVM: Support Vector Machine, RBF: radial basis function, DT: Decision Tree, RF: Random Forest, AdaBoost: Adaptive boosting, GaussianNB: Gaussian Naive Bayes. Bold numbers indicate best prediction results.

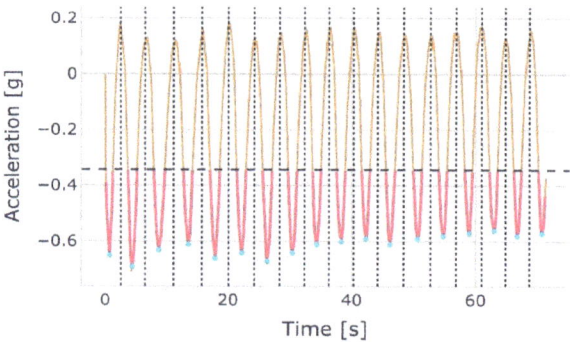

Figure 3. Principle of cycle segmentation based on minima of Acc Z. The dashed horizontal line represents the global threshold (40% above the global minima). The dotted vertical lines represent the cycle limits that lie in the middle of two consecutive local minima. The pink lines show the part of the time series that is below the threshold, the orange lines show the time series that is above the threshold, and the blue dots show the minima of the pink lines.

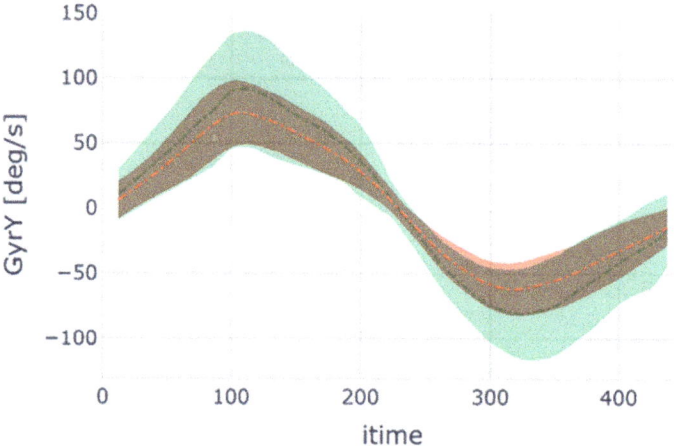

Figure 4. Mean Gyr Y of the SENS2 cycle as function of time is shown for NLBP subjects (green dashed dot line) and for CLBP patients (red dashed dot line). The colored areas correspond to the cycles SD for healthy NLBP subjects (green) and CLBP patients (red or brown when overlapped with green). Note that all cycles were normalized to the same number of points (n = 450) and that mean and SD refer to all cycle values at a given normalized time point (itime).

The best classification accuracy was obtained using the whole sequences with the GaussianNB algorithm. In this case, an accuracy of 79% and an AUC value of 0.85 were obtained. Gaussian naive Bayes process each feature, computing a normal distribution with their mean and standard deviation. To predict the class of a new subject, the algorithm computes the likelihood of the subject's raw data belonging to the gaussian distribution of NLBP and CLBP. The Gaussian naïve Bayes could compare the scores obtained for each class and decide the best-fitted class for the subject. As the raw data were on a times series, it seems reasonable that the data fit well with the GaussianNB algorithm.

Table 4 shows the effects of using SampEn or CF as features instead of raw IMU data for the whole sequences. The performance globally decreased with SampEn. The best algorithm (GaussianNB) achieved 64% Accuracy and an AUC value of 0.69. Using CF, the best algorithm (SVM RBF) achieved 74% Acc and an AUC value of 0.80. Overall, cycle segmentation produced the worst results, so for simplicity, we have omitted these data from the results table.

Table 4. Accuracy and AUC scores for CLBP-NLBP classification using the whole sequences with different features.

Whole Sequences	Raw Data		SampEn		CF	
Algorithms	Accuracy (%)	AUC	Accuracy (%)	AUC	Accuracy (%)	AUC
BF KNN	0.63 ± 0.08	0.69 ± 0.09	0.59 ± 0.10	0.62 ± 0.09	0.73 ± 0.06	0.78 ± 0.06
Linear SVM	0.72 ± 0.07	0.79 ± 0.07	0.53 ± 0.02	0.64 ± 0.10	0.68 ± 0.06	0.74 ± 0.07
SVM RBF	0.52 ± 0.06	0.52 ± 0.09	0.53 ± 0.02	0.64 ± 0.10	**0.74 ± 0.06**	**0.80 ± 0.08**
DT	0.66 ± 0.08	0.65 ± 0.09	0.58 ± 0.07	0.56 ± 0.07	0.60 ± 0.10	0.61 ± 0.10
RF	0.78 ± 0.07	0.83 ± 0.08	0.59 ± 0.08	0.64 ± 0.09	0.68 ± 0.07	0.71 ± 0.07
AdaBoost	0.68 ± 0.07	0.74 ± 0.08	0.55 ± 0.10	0.57 ± 0.10	0.62 ± 0.10	0.62 ± 0.11
GaussianNB	**0.79 ± 0.08**	**0.85 ± 0.07**	**0.64 ± 0.06**	**0.69 ± 0.07**	0.60 ± 0.08	0.60 ± 0.10

BF KNN: Brute-Force K-Nearest Neighbors, SVM: Support Vector Machine, RBF: radial basis function, DT: Decision Tree, RF: Random Forest, AdaBoost: Adaptive boosting, GaussianNB: Gaussian Naive Bayes. Bold numbers indicate best prediction results.

3.4. Most Discriminative Features

The minimum value of Gyr Y measured by SENS2 was the most discriminative feature (first 355 times in 700 runs), followed by the Q3 of Acc X measured by SENS3. The SD of Acc Y measured by SENS2 was the most discriminating feature of the second test (114 times in 700 runs). The complete results can be found in Table 5.

Table 5. Number of times the most discriminating characteristics are first and second out of 700 runs.

Feature	First	Feature	Second
Gyr Y SENS2 min	355	Acc Y SENS2 SD	114
Acc X SENS3 Q3	136	Gyr Y SENS2 min	112
Acc Y SENS2 SD	111	Acc X SENS3 Q3	103
Acc Y SENS2 SD	89	Acc Y SENS2 Q1	83
Acc X SENS3 Q1	64	Acc X SENS3 mean	71

Gyr: Gyroscope; Acc: Accelerometer; SENS: Sensor; min: minimum; SD: standard deviation; Q1: 1st quartile; Q3 3rd quartile.

4. Discussion

Our results showed that ML was able to discriminate CLBP patients from NLBP subjects with good accuracy, especially for the GaussianNB algorithm. The identification of the most discriminating features shows that Gyr Y SENS2 min is the best parameter: CLBP patients have a lower flexion angular velocity (in norm) in the return phase of the b&r test than NLBP subjects; the angular velocity was measured by a sensor placed in front of the second sacral vertebra. A wide variety of models for the kinematic analysis of the lumbar region are available in the literature [31]. Several authors have proposed positioning two sensors, one near T12 and the other near S2, to characterize the movements of the lumbar spine in the sagittal plane. Some used this model with an optoelectronic system [32], while others used IMUs with or without comparison to an optoelectronic system [9,11,32,33]. In the positioning of our IMUs, SENS2 (placed at S2) provided the maximum number of discriminative features. SENS1 (placed at T12) alone did not provide us with discriminative data, but the HCF, calculated from SENS2 (S2) and SENS3, did. The optimal number of sensors remains an open discussion, but SENS2 should be preferred for clinical applications. According to our results, the single SENS2 seems to be sufficient to clinically discriminate between CLBP and NLBP subjects; this result may seem attractive for clinical use by reason of its simplicity; however, due to the limited sample of our study, this finding should be treated with caution. Nonetheless, we advocate the use of multiple sensors to analyze lumbopelvic and hip movements in clinical research in order to expand our understanding of the disturbances of these movements in the clinical setting.

Due to the early onset of fatigue, the duration of the b&r test (70 s) could be a source of bias if a CLBP patient is severely physically deconditioned. However, the test can be interrupted after 20 s, and reliable SampEn values can be obtained despite a three-fold shorter time series [20]. Future clinical studies should be conducted to understand the effects of spinal erector muscle fatigue on the b&r test. The use of the b&r test in acute or sub-acute patients has also not been clinically studied.

Some values of SampEn and CF were significantly different between CLBP patients and NLBP subjects when the b&r test was performed. SampEn showed a significant difference for the Gyr Y of SENS1, located at the lower thoracic level, and Gyr Y SENS2, located at the upper sacral level. These differences suggest a lower complexity of variability in angular velocity measured about the transverse axis, which corresponds to the main b&r movement. In other words, CLBP patients show more stereotyped movements of the lumbo–pelvic complex, which is consistent with the optimal variability paradigm of [21,34]: the healthier an individual, the more variability they can show in performing a movement, which is an indication of their adaptability. HCF also showed a significant decrease in CLBP patients, as did SampEn for Acc X of SENS2. In contrast, SampEn for Gyr Z showed an increase. The former describes the complexity of the pelvic tilting movement about an antero–posterior axis, and the latter the complexity of the vertical pelvic displacement, which is an obvious part of the b&r test. As with lumbar muscle activity in a previous study [35], the observed behaviors suggest a tendency toward stereotyped movements in CLBP patients. The literature suggests that the increase or decrease in complexity may indicate two different pathological phenotypes: instability or hypercontrol [36]. It is quite possible that the observed phenomenon of either upward or downward changes in CF is responsible for the less and even non-discriminative results in distinguishing CLBP patients from NLBP participants. In future studies, it would be appropriate to pre-classify CLBP patients using existing relevant clinical tests [37–39] to investigate the ability of the b&r test to highlight these two phenotypes.

Despite these observed significant differences, the mean differences between SampEn and HCF in CLBP patients compared with NLBP subjects are so close to those of SEM and MDC that the clinical interest of SampEn can be questioned. Furthermore, although SampEn is easy to compute with any modern computer, a deviation of this parameter from a norm not yet established may be very difficult or impossible to detect by a clinician in practice. It is important to identify more standard kinematic parameters (position, velocity, acceleration) representative of the CLBP population. Visualization of all cycles performed during the b&r test in a single graphical representation has already shown that NLBP participants, for example, achieved overall higher values for angular velocity about the flexion axis than CLBP patients. This component of angular velocity proved to be the most discriminating feature in our study. Therefore, focusing on flexion movement velocity may be a good recommendation for clinicians when managing CLBP patients.

Regardless of the most discriminating features, the ML algorithms were able to accurately identify CLBP patients when performing a b&r test. The algorithm with the best performance is GaussianNB, which is supplied with the whole time series recorded by the IMUs. It achieves an accuracy of 79% and an AUC value of 0.85. It is worth noting that good accuracy can also be achieved when an SVM RBF algorithm is provided with CF from the whole time series. In this case, an accuracy of 74% and an AUC value of 0.80 are achieved. The better performance of the SVM algorithm might be related to a well-known property of this method, which tends to perform better than other ML algorithms when the number of features is small [40].

Abdollahi et al. were able to distinguish LBP patients from NLBP subjects during a kinematic test using ML analysis—specifically SVM—of time series collected via an IMU attached to the sternum [12]. They were also able to classify them according to the risk of chronicity [12]. Similar results with lower accuracy were obtained with the same test but using classical statistical analysis (linear discriminant analysis) [41]. In our study, we found that the SENS2 had higher discriminating power in both classical statistical analysis and ML analysis. However, we did not investigate whether our method is able to classify patients according to their risk of chronicity. The differences between [12] and our study are mainly due to the different experimental protocols. Although we use a sagittal plane test, our test is performed over a longer period of time (60 s of recording) with a sensor recording frequency (100 Hz) five times higher than [12]. The amount of data collected this way allowed us to analyze the complexity of the movement variation. In our study, we did not measure the center of mass motion, and our NLBP population consisted of only 20 subjects, which severely limits the learning ability of the ML process. However, both studies demonstrate the interest in using ML in spinal kinematic analysis to identify and assess CLBP patients. It remains to be shown that these tools are also useful for the therapeutic follow-up of these patients.

As a counterpoint to using biomechanics to better understand LBP conditions, a meta-model created with the help of a panel of 27 multidisciplinary experts is used to illustrate the number of factors that contribute to LBP, disability, quality of life, and other outcomes as well as the number and strength of their interactions [42]. With a problem as multifactorial and complex as LBP, the authors of this counterpoint emphasize the need to integrate the interactions of biopsychosocial factors into research to improve the management of patients with LBP. This suggests that in future works, it will be essential to integrate these biopsychosocial factors and the state of the internal environment into the raw IMU data and the variability indicators computed from them when performing a b&r test to better understand its discriminating power. This may be achieved via analysis from non-invasive portable electrochemical sensors [43] of fluids such as sweat and its relevant components. An ML algorithm can help achieve this goal, as both quantitative and qualitative data can be used.

5. Conclusions

The objective of this study was to evaluate the relevance of various machine ML algorithms and SampEn in the identification of LBP conditions. Using the raw data from three IMUs and the SampEn values obtained during a b&r test, the results showed better abilities to discriminate CLBP patients from NLBP subjects for the GaussianNB ML algorithm than the SampEn discriminant values alone. This study demonstrated that: supervised ML and a complexity assessment of trunk movement variability are useful in the identification of CLBP conditions, and that simple kinematic indicators are sensitive to the latter condition.

Regardless of the pathology studied, our study can shed light on the advantages and disadvantages of "standard" statistical analysis and ML-based approaches in clinical applications. In standard statistical analysis, the experimenter/clinician a priori identifies relevant indices and computes them. If the indices are well chosen, they will show statistically significant differences between groups, typically between healthy subjects and patients. By accepting arbitrariness in the choice of indices, such a methodology can show significant results for small populations, typically groups of 20 subjects, which can be easily recruited from a clinician's patients and acquaintances. One of the advantages of ML is that the algorithm itself finds the most discriminative indices in a non-arbitrary way, but the population has to be larger than in usual statistical analysis, which can make ML complicated to apply in daily clinical practice. What we have shown is that ML may already give good results in discriminating small but accurately selected groups and that it may also identify the main discriminative features of the performed measurements. The latter features might, in turn, be used in quick clinical tests based on the measurement of a single parameter and threshold value. Hence, ML may provide key parameters to be included in more standard approaches already used in daily clinical practice.

Author Contributions: Conceptualization, P.T., W.B., A.T., E.S.-B.; methodology, P.T., M.H., L.P., O.N.; software, P.T., M.H., L.P., O.N.; validation, P.T., F.B., F.D., R.S. and M.H.; data curation, P.T., M.H., L.P.; writing—original draft preparation, P.T., M.H., L.P., F.B.; writing—review and editing, P.T., F.B., F.D., R.S., M.H., A.T., E.S.-B., W.B., O.N. All authors have read and agreed to the published version of the manuscript.

Funding: The authors acknowledge financial support from the First Haute-Ecole program, project no 1610401, DYSKIMOT, in partnership with OMT-Skills (http://omtskills.be/—accessed on 8 october 2020), and from the European Regional Development Fund (Interreg FWVl 4.7.360 NOMADe).

Institutional Review Board Statement: The study was conducted according to the guidelines of the Declaration of Helsinki and approved by the Intercommunale de Santé Publique du Pays de Charleroi Ethics Committee (ISPPC/OM008) under the number B325-2020-43666.

Informed Consent Statement: Informed consent was obtained from all subjects involved in the study.

Data Availability Statement: Data are available at https://osf.io/t4dgr/ (accessed on 19 January 2022), folder "Low Back Pain vs Healthy". Source codes are available at https://github.com/martinhouryfors/IMU-and-IA-to-Assess-Chronic-Low-Back-Pain (accessed on 15 June 2022).

Conflicts of Interest: The authors declare no conflict of interest. The funders had no role in the design of the study; in the collection, analyses, or interpretation of data; in the writing of the manuscript, or in the decision to publish the results.

References

1. Vos, T.; Lim, S.S.; Abbafati, C.; Abbas, K.M.; Abbasi, M.; Abbasifard, M.; Abbasi-Kangevari, M.; Abbastabar, H.; Abd-Allah, F.; Abdelalim, A.; et al. Global Burden of 369 Diseases and Injuries in 204 Countries and Territories, 1990–2019: A Systematic Analysis for the Global Burden of Disease Study 2019. *Lancet* **2020**, *396*, 1204–1222. [CrossRef]
2. Ippersiel, P.; Teoli, A.; Wideman, T.H.; Preuss, R.A.; Robbins, S.M. The Relationship Between Pain-Related Threat and Motor Behavior in Nonspecific Low Back Pain: A Systematic Review and Meta-Analysis. *Phys. Ther.* **2022**, *102*, pzab274. [CrossRef] [PubMed]
3. André, M.; Lundberg, M. Thoughts on Pain, Physical Activity, and Body in Patients With Recurrent Low Back Pain and Fear: An Interview Study. *Phys. Ther.* **2022**, *102*, pzab275. [CrossRef] [PubMed]
4. Senba, E.; Kami, K. A New Aspect of Chronic Pain as a Lifestyle-Related Disease. *Neurobiol. Pain* **2017**, *1*, 6–15. [CrossRef]
5. Mahdavi, S.B.; Riahi, R.; Vahdatpour, B.; Kelishadi, R. Association between Sedentary Behavior and Low Back Pain; A Systematic Review and Meta-Analysis. *Health Promot. Perspect.* **2021**, *11*, 393–410. [CrossRef]
6. Cappelle, J.; Monteyne, L.; Van Mulders, J.; Goossens, S.; Vergauwen, M.; Van der Perre, L. Low-Complexity Design and Validation of Wireless Motion Sensor Node to Support Physiotherapy. *Sensors* **2020**, *20*, 6362. [CrossRef]
7. Poitras, I.; Dupuis, F.; Bielmann, M.; Campeau-Lecours, A.; Mercier, C.; Bouyer, L.; Roy, J.-S. Validity and Reliability of Wearable Sensors for Joint Angle Estimation: A Systematic Review. *Sensors* **2019**, *19*, 1555. [CrossRef]
8. Benson, L.C.; Clermont, C.A.; Bošnjak, E.; Ferber, R. The Use of Wearable Devices for Walking and Running Gait Analysis Outside of the Lab: A Systematic Review. *Gait Posture* **2018**, *63*, 124–138. [CrossRef]
9. Robert-Lachaine, X.; Mecheri, H.; Larue, C.; Plamondon, A. Validation of Inertial Measurement Units with an Optoelectronic System for Whole-Body Motion Analysis. *Med. Biol. Eng. Comput.* **2017**, *55*, 609–619. [CrossRef]
10. Cuesta-Vargas, A.I.; Galán-Mercant, A.; Williams, J.M. The Use of Inertial Sensors System for Human Motion Analysis. *Phys. Ther. Rev.* **2010**, *15*, 462–473. [CrossRef]
11. Bauer, C.M.; Heimgartner, M.; Rast, F.M.; Ernst, M.J.; Oetiker, S.; Kool, J. Reliability of Lumbar Movement Dysfunction Tests for Chronic Low Back Pain Patients. *Man. Ther.* **2016**, *24*, 81–84. [CrossRef] [PubMed]

12. Abdollahi, M.; Ashouri, S.; Abedi, M.; Azadeh-Fard, N.; Parnianpour, M.; Khalaf, K.; Rashedi, E. Using a Motion Sensor to Categorize Nonspecific Low Back Pain Patients: A Machine Learning Approach. *Sensors* **2020**, *20*, 3600. [CrossRef]
13. Mathew, B.; Norris, D.; Hendry, D.; Waddell, G. Artificial Intelligence in the Diagnosis of Low-Back Pain and Sciatica. *Spine* **1988**, *13*, 168–172. [CrossRef] [PubMed]
14. Tagliaferri, S.D.; Angelova, M.; Zhao, X.; Owen, P.J.; Miller, C.T.; Wilkin, T.; Belavy, D.L. Artificial Intelligence to Improve Back Pain Outcomes and Lessons Learnt from Clinical Classification Approaches: Three Systematic Reviews. *NPJ Digit. Med.* **2020**, *3*, 93. [CrossRef] [PubMed]
15. D'Antoni, F.; Russo, F.; Ambrosio, L.; Vollero, L.; Vadalà, G.; Merone, M.; Papalia, R.; Denaro, V. Artificial Intelligence and Computer Vision in Low Back Pain: A Systematic Review. *Int. J. Environ. Res. Public Health* **2021**, *18*, 10909. [CrossRef] [PubMed]
16. Galbusera, F.; Casaroli, G.; Bassani, T. Artificial Intelligence and Machine Learning in Spine Research. *JOR Spine* **2019**, *2*, e1044. [CrossRef]
17. Tack, C. Artificial Intelligence and Machine Learning | Applications in Musculoskeletal Physiotherapy. *Musculoskelet. Sci. Pract.* **2019**, *39*, 164–169. [CrossRef]
18. Girase, H.; Nyayapati, P.; Booker, J.; Lotz, J.C.; Bailey, J.F.; Matthew, R.P. Automated Assessment and Classification of Spine, Hip, and Knee Pathologies from Sit-to-Stand Movements Collected in Clinical Practice. *J. Biomech.* **2021**, *128*, 110786. [CrossRef]
19. Yentes, J.M.; Hunt, N.; Schmid, K.K.; Kaipust, J.P.; McGrath, D.; Stergiou, N. The Appropriate Use of Approximate Entropy and Sample Entropy with Short Data Sets. *Ann. Biomed. Eng.* **2013**, *41*, 349–365. [CrossRef]
20. Thiry, P.; Nocent, O.; Buisseret, F.; Bertucci, W.; Thevenon, A.; Simoneau-Buessinger, E. Sample Entropy as a Tool to Assess Lumbo-Pelvic Movements in a Clinical Test for Low-Back-Pain Patients. *Entropy* **2022**, *24*, 437. [CrossRef]
21. van Emmerik, R.E.A.; Ducharme, S.W.; Amado, A.C.; Hamill, J. Comparing Dynamical Systems Concepts and Techniques for Biomechanical Analysis. *J. Sport Health Sci.* **2016**, *5*, 3–13. [CrossRef]
22. Falk, J.; Aasa, U.; Berglund, L. How Accurate Are Visual Assessments by Physical Therapists of Lumbo-Pelvic Movements during the Squat and Deadlift? *Phys. Ther. Sport* **2021**, *50*, 195–200. [CrossRef] [PubMed]
23. Beange, K.H.E.; Chan, A.D.C.; Beaudette, S.M.; Graham, R.B. Concurrent Validity of a Wearable IMU for Objective Assessments of Functional Movement Quality and Control of the Lumbar Spine. *J. Biomech.* **2019**, *97*, 109356. [CrossRef] [PubMed]
24. Hage, R.; Buisseret, F.; Houry, M.; Dierick, F. Head Pitch Angular Velocity Discriminates (Sub-)Acute Neck Pain Patients and Controls Assessed with the DidRen Laser Test. *Sensors* **2022**, *22*, 2805. [CrossRef] [PubMed]
25. Bouhassira, D.; Attal, N.; Alchaar, H.; Boureau, F.; Brochet, B.; Bruxelle, J.; Cunin, G.; Fermanian, J.; Ginies, P.; Grun-Overdyking, A.; et al. Comparison of Pain Syndromes Associated with Nervous or Somatic Lesions and Development of a New Neuropathic Pain Diagnostic Questionnaire (DN4). *Pain* **2005**, *114*, 29–36. [CrossRef] [PubMed]
26. Cleland, C.L.; Hunter, R.F.; Kee, F.; Cupples, M.E.; Sallis, J.F.; Tully, M.A. Validity of the Global Physical Activity Questionnaire (GPAQ) in Assessing Levels and Change in Moderate-Vigorous Physical Activity and Sedentary Behaviour. *BMC Public Health* **2014**, *14*, 1255. [CrossRef]
27. Hage, R.; Detrembleur, C.; Dierick, F.; Pitance, L.; Jojczyk, L.; Estievenart, W.; Buisseret, F. DYSKIMOT: An Ultra-Low-Cost Inertial Sensor to Assess Head's Rotational Kinematics in Adults during the Didren-Laser Test. *Sensors* **2020**, *20*, 833. [CrossRef]
28. Géron, A. *Hands-on Machine Learning with Scikit-Learn, Keras, and TensorFlow: Concepts, Tools, and Techniques to Build Intelligent Systems*, 2nd ed.; O'Reilly Media: Sebastopol, CA, USA, 2019; ISBN 978-1-4920-3264-9.
29. Ndiaye, E.; Le, T.; Fercoq, O.; Salmon, J.; Takeuchi, I. Safe Grid Search with Optimal Complexity. In Proceedings of the 36th International Conference on Machine Learning, Long Beach, CA, USA, 9–15 June 2019; Volume 97, pp. 4771–4780.
30. Aha, D.W.; Bankert, R.L. A Comparative Evaluation of Sequential Feature Selection Algorithms. In *Learning from Data*; Fisher, D., Lenz, H.-J., Eds.; Lecture Notes in Statistics; Springer: New York, NY, USA, 1996; Volume 112, pp. 199–206. ISBN 978-0-387-94736-5.
31. Pourahmadi, M.R.; Ebrahimi Takamjani, I.; Jaberzadeh, S.; Sarrafzadeh, J.; Sanjari, M.A.; Bagheri, R.; Taghipour, M. Kinematics of the Spine During Sit-to-Stand Movement Using Motion Analysis Systems: A Systematic Review of Literature. *J. Sport Rehabil.* **2019**, *28*, 77–93. [CrossRef]
32. Pourahmadi, M.R.; Ebrahimi Takamjani, I.; Jaberzadeh, S.; Sarrafzadeh, J.; Sanjari, M.A.; Bagheri, R.; Jannati, E. Test-Retest Reliability of Sit-to-Stand and Stand-to-Sit Analysis in People with and without Chronic Non-Specific Low Back Pain. *Musculoskelet. Sci. Pract.* **2018**, *35*, 95–104. [CrossRef]
33. Shojaei, I.; Vazirian, M.; Salt, E.G.; Van Dillen, L.R.; Bazrgari, B. Timing and Magnitude of Lumbar Spine Contribution to Trunk Forward Bending and Backward Return in Patients with Acute Low Back Pain. *J. Biomech.* **2017**, *53*, 71–77. [CrossRef]
34. Goldberger, A.L.; Peng, C.-K.; Lipsitz, L.A. What Is Physiologic Complexity and How Does It Change with Aging and Disease? *Neurobiol. Aging* **2002**, *23*, 23–26. [CrossRef]
35. Falla, D.; Gizzi, L.; Tschapek, M.; Erlenwein, J.; Petzke, F. Reduced Task-Induced Variations in the Distribution of Activity across Back Muscle Regions in Individuals with Low Back Pain. *Pain* **2014**, *155*, 944–953. [CrossRef]
36. Stergiou, N.; Decker, L.M. Human Movement Variability, Nonlinear Dynamics, and Pathology: Is There a Connection? *Hum. Mov. Sci.* **2011**, *30*, 869–888. [CrossRef] [PubMed]
37. Laird, R.A.; Keating, J.L.; Kent, P. Subgroups of Lumbo-Pelvic Flexion Kinematics Are Present in People with and without Persistent Low Back Pain. *BMC Musculoskelet. Disord.* **2018**, *19*, 309. [CrossRef] [PubMed]

38. Tousignant-Laflamme, Y.; Cook, C.E.; Mathieu, A.; Naye, F.; Wellens, F.; Wideman, T.; Martel, M.; Lam, O.T. Operationalization of the New Pain and Disability Drivers Management Model: A Modified Delphi Survey of Multidisciplinary Pain Management Experts. *J. Eval. Clin. Pract.* **2020**, *26*, 316–325. [CrossRef] [PubMed]
39. Molgaard Nielsen, A.; Hestbaek, L.; Vach, W.; Kent, P.; Kongsted, A. Latent Class Analysis Derived Subgroups of Low Back Pain Patients—Do They Have Prognostic Capacity? *BMC Musculoskelet. Disord.* **2017**, *18*, 345. [CrossRef]
40. Li, X.; Cervantes, J.; Yu, W. A Novel SVM Classification Method for Large Data Sets. In Proceedings of the 2010 IEEE International Conference on Granular Computing, San Jose, CA, USA, 14–16 August 2010; pp. 297–302.
41. Davoudi, M.; Shokouhyan, S.M.; Abedi, M.; Meftahi, N.; Rahimi, A.; Rashedi, E.; Hoviattalab, M.; Narimani, R.; Parnianpour, M.; Khalaf, K. A Practical Sensor-Based Methodology for the Quantitative Assessment and Classification of Chronic Non Specific Low Back Patients (NSLBP) in Clinical Settings. *Sensors* **2020**, *20*, 2902. [CrossRef]
42. Cholewicki, J.; Breen, A.; Popovich, J.M.; Reeves, N.P.; Sahrmann, S.A.; van Dillen, L.R.; Vleeming, A.; Hodges, P.W. Can Biomechanics Research Lead to More Effective Treatment of Low Back Pain? A Point-Counterpoint Debate. *J. Orthop. Sports Phys. Ther.* **2019**, *49*, 425–436. [CrossRef]
43. Lu, H.; He, B.; Gao, B. Emerging Electrochemical Sensors for Life Healthcare. *Eng. Regen.* **2021**, *2*, 175–181. [CrossRef]

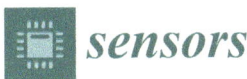

Article

Energy–Accuracy Aware Finger Gesture Recognition for Wearable IoT Devices

Woosoon Jung [1] and Hyung Gyu Lee [2,*]

[1] Department of Computer and Information Engineering, Daegu University, Gyeongsan-si 38453, Korea; quado.jung@gmail.com
[2] Department of Software, Duksung Women's University, Seoul 01369, Korea
* Correspondence: hglee@duksung.ac.kr

Abstract: Wearable Internet of Things (IoT) devices can be used efficiently for gesture recognition applications. The nature of these applications requires high recognition accuracy with low energy consumption, which is not easy to solve at the same time. In this paper, we design a finger gesture recognition system using a wearable IoT device. The proposed recognition system uses a lightweight multi-layer perceptron (MLP) classifier which can be implemented even on a low-end micro controller unit (MCU), with a 2-axes flex sensor. To achieve high recognition accuracy with low energy consumption, we first design a framework for the finger gesture recognition system including its components, followed by system-level performance and energy models. Then, we analyze system-level accuracy and energy optimization issues, and explore the numerous design choices to finally achieve energy–accuracy aware finger gesture recognition, targeting four commonly used low-end MCUs. Our extensive simulation and measurements using prototypes demonstrate that the proposed design achieves up to 95.5% recognition accuracy with energy consumption under 2.74 mJ per gesture on a low-end embedded wearable IoT device. We also provide the Pareto-optimal designs among a total of 159 design choices to achieve energy–accuracy aware design points under given energy or accuracy constraints.

Keywords: MLP; gesture recognition; flex sensor; model search; neural network

1. Introduction

Gesture recognition is among the popular issues for human–machine interface applications. In particular, hands are the parts that can move most accurately with relatively little energy, compared to other body parts. Thus, hand gesture recognition is used as an efficient interface for human–computer interaction (HCI) [1–8]. Traditionally, vision-based gesture recognition received much attention since it avoid the need to wear any tools or equipment on the body [1,2,6]. However, it is also known that the performance of vision-based gesture recognition is highly dependent on camera setup such as the angle to the object, the size of the image and the intensity of illumination [9]. In addition, high computation requirements and power consumption are needed to process and analyze multiple images in real time. Thus, it may not be feasible to implement vision-based gesture recognition applications on low-end embedded devices.

An alternative method of implementing gesture recognition is to use wearable sensors such as inertial measurement units (IMU), electromyography (EMG) sensors, flex sensors, and pressure sensors [3,8,10–13]. Unlike vision-based approaches, a wearable sensor-based approach is not only less sensitive to the perceived environments but also generates relatively small amounts of data with affordable (or even higher) recognition accuracy. In addition, this approach can recognize minimal body movements including small finger gestures. Most of all, its computation and power requirements may be less than vision-based approaches. In that sense, a wearable sensor-based approach is more suitable for

Citation: Jung, W.; Lee, H.G. Energy–Accuracy Aware Finger Gesture Recognition for Wearable IoT Devices. *Sensors* **2022**, *22*, 4801. https://doi.org/10.3390/s22134801

Academic Editors: Fabien Buisseret, Liesbet Van der Perre and Frédéric Dierick

Received: 12 May 2022
Accepted: 21 June 2022
Published: 25 June 2022

Publisher's Note: MDPI stays neutral with regard to jurisdictional claims in published maps and institutional affiliations.

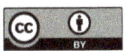

Copyright: © 2022 by the authors. Licensee MDPI, Basel, Switzerland. This article is an open access article distributed under the terms and conditions of the Creative Commons Attribution (CC BY) license (https://creativecommons.org/licenses/by/4.0/).

gesture recognition than a vision-based approach if we are targeting low-end wearable IoT devices.

Among various wearable sensors such as IMUs, EMG, and flex sensors, we focus on using a state-of-the-art flex sensor [14] which can measure bi-directionally in 2 axes of bending with a single sensor. This sensor is suitable for being implemented in low-end embedded devices because it provides low-power, drift-free, and path-independent sensing with high accuracy. In addition, the sensor is made from silicon, which is good for wearable implementations.

In this paper, we design a light-weight finger gesture recognition system that can be implemented in low-end embedded devices using a single flex sensor. To this end, we first design a framework for a finger gesture recognition system that recognizes 17 finger gestures. The framework consists of data collection, preprocessing filters, and a light-weight multi-layer perceptron (MLP)-based classifier. Then, we construct performance and energy models to find optimal design choices efficiently. We analyze and discuss the energy–accuracy aware system-level design issues, and explore the design choices of finger gesture recognition by considering computation requirements/memory resource targeting for four types of low-end micro controller units (MCUs). Finally, the functionality and feasibility of the proposed work are verified by implementing prototypes. The contributions of this paper are summarized as follows:

- Provide the full design for a finger gesture recognition system using a single flex sensor.
- Explore the design choices of a finger gesture recognition system in terms of performance, accuracy, and energy consumption using the conducted performance and energy consumption models.
- Demonstrate the functionality and feasibility of the proposed designs by implementing the prototypes using four commonly used low-end embedded MCUs.
- Show the energy–accuracy aware design which achieves up to 95.5% accuracy with an energy consumption of 2.74 mJ per gesture.
- Provide the energy–accuracy aware Pareto-optimal designs among a total of 159 design choices to find energy–accuracy aware design points under given energy or accuracy constraints.

The rest of this paper is organized as follows. The backgrounds are described in Section 2. In Section 3, the framework and component-level design for the finger gesture recognition system are described, while Section 4 discusses energy–accuracy aware design optimization. Finally, Section 5 demonstrates the experiment results, followed by the conclusion in Section 6.

2. Backgrounds

This section describes the backgrounds of this work which consists of the existing work related to gesture recognition and the basics of the flex sensor used in this work.

2.1. Related Work

An IMU sensor which embeds micro electro mechanical systems (MEMS) accelerometers, gyroscopes, and magnetometers was popularly used because it can capture the wide range of body movements. An IMU sensor can even be attached to a cane to detect falls in the elderly [10]. However, IMUs generally require high filtering resources because raw data contain a lot of noise and drifts [4]. In addition, a high sampling rate (higher than a few kilo samples per second) requirement for recognizing delicate movements and high recognition accuracy are major concerns for implementing on low-end embedded devices [15].

EMG sensors are used for body movement recognition as well. Instead of directly measuring the physical movements of the body, the sensor alternatively measures the biomedical signals using specially made probes attached to the skin surface. EMG sensors can detect the very fine movements of the body that cannot be detected by physical movement measuring sensors alone [3,16,17]. However, the acquired biomedical signals vary for different people even with the same movement and are noise sensitive depending on the condition of the skin surface even for the same person [18].

Conventional flex sensors based on conductive ink, fiber-optic, or conductive fabric technologies are used for various wearable IoT applications such as embedded device-based health care [19], sign language recognition [20,21], and posture correction [22]. Multiple sensors are attached to each joint of the body, and the measured bending information is used for recognizing the body movement. This method provides a low-cost and low-energy solution that can be easily implemented in low-end embedded devices. However, the recognized body activity is generally simple and must use multiple sensors to detect complex body movements. Recently, an advanced flex sensor that can measure two axes of bi-directional bending with a single sensor was developed [14]. The sensor embeds a low-power integrated analog front and generates digital angular data in degree. We use this advanced flex sensor for finger gesture recognition in this paper. Thus, the details on this flex sensor will be explained in Section 2.2.

In general, data collected from the wearable flex sensor for body movement recognition requires time-domain data analysis using machine learning (ML) techniques such as dynamic time warping (DTW) [20], hidden Markov models (HMMs) [21], recurrent neural networks (RNNs), and long short-term memory (LSTM). Although these techniques support relatively high recognition accuracy for time-series data, it is questionable whether these techniques can be efficiently implemented in a low-end wearable device [7,23] because of the not trivial size of memory requests. Since the data used in HCI applications generally have a small number of dimensions compared to the images, a simple MLP technique can be a sufficient solution if it satisfies the desired performance and accuracy. Therefore, this paper focuses on using an MLP technique where the computation requirements (processing time) are simply proportional to the size of MLP model. The optimal MLP structure was determined in terms of model size, accuracy, and energy consumption in this paper.

2.2. Basics of Flex Sensors

Flex sensors measure the amount of bending or deflection. There are three types of commonly used flex sensors, as shown in Figure 1. Depending on the material, the sensor is categorized as conductive ink, fiber-optic, or conductive fabric. The operating principle of the sensors utilizes a phenomenon where the electrical properties of a material used in the sensor change when the flex sensor is physically bending. Depending on the type of flex sensor, the maximum bending angle, durability, and stability of the measured value appear differently. For example, sensors made with conductive ink are widely used due to low cost, but accuracy is relatively low, and calibration or filtering is required because the measured values vary slightly depending on the measurement environment such as temperature and humidity. In addition, the physical length of the sensor is fixed without elasticity, which limits the wearability of the sensor.

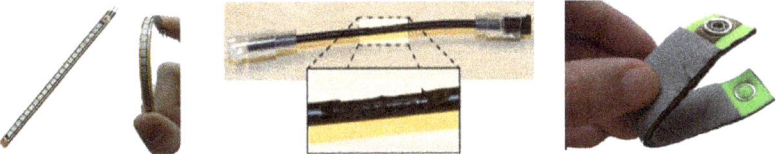

Figure 1. Types of flex sensors (from left, conductive ink, fiber-optic, and conductive fabric based).

Sensors made with an optical fiber support high accuracy and high durability. However, a pair of a light source and a detector is required, and only unidirectional sensing is possible [24]. Conductive fabric/polymers can be used for wearable applications due to the elasticity of the sensor compared to other technologies. The cost of these sensors is relatively high, compared with other types of sensors, and these sensors respond to pressure as well as bending, making it difficult to maintain high accuracy. Most of all, conventional flex sensors can measure one axis of bending. Thus, multiple sensors must be used to measure complex movements [13].

The advanced flex sensor introduced in the previous subsection is made with a silicone elastomer layered with a conductive and non-conductive material. This sensor not only measures the bending degree of two axes stably with a single sensor, but also has the advantage of being flexible and stretchable with silicon material. As mentioned, this sensor is not a simple variable resistor type but a sensor module that embeds a low-power integrated analog front, resulting much less noise over time compared with the other sensors. In addition, it generates digital data through an inter-integrated circuit (I^2C) standard communication interface. This means that power-hungry analog-to-digital converters (ADCs) are not necessary, which is good for wearable IoT devices.

Figure 2 shows the collected sample data from two users, repeating several gestures with their index fingers, where a single flex sensor is attached. The measured values indicate the angle changes according to the movement of the finger. Although there are slight deviations in the measured values of each repeated gesture, we observe specific patterns for each gesture regardless of the users. These patterns appear differently depending on the type of gesture. We also note that the duration of a single gesture—the number of sample data related to the gesture—varies depending on the type of the gesture and user. The duration of a single gesture also varies depending on the time even for the same gesture by the same person. Therefore, gesture recognition should be appropriately designed in consideration of these variations.

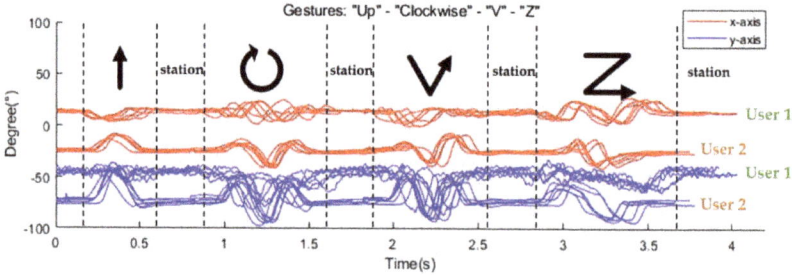

Figure 2. Example outputs of the flex sensor (four types of gestures from two users).

3. Designing the Finger Gesture Recognition System

This section mainly describes the design for a light-weight finger gesture recognition system using a wearable flex sensor, implemented in low-end wearable devices. To this end, the system-level design including its framework is proposed. Then, the component-level design consisting of designing preprocessing filters and an MLP-based classifier is described.

3.1. System Architecture

Figure 3 shows the framework for the proposed finger gesture recognition system. The system simply consists of three parts: raw data collection, preprocessing, and classification. The first step for finger gesture recognition is to collect motion data generated from a 2-axes flex sensor. The flex sensor attached to the index finger generates a series of 32-bit sample data. One set of sample data represents the X-axis (16 bits) and Y-axis (16 bits) bending degrees of the index finger at the moment of sampling. The flex sensor can operate at a sampling rate of up to 500 Hz. In this work, we set the maximum sampling frequency to 100 Hz, which is sufficient for finger gesture recognition applications.

Raw data collected from the flex sensor can be directly used as an input to the gesture classifier. However, in general, the raw data may include lots of measurement noise and there are non-negligible deviations in the raw data collected even for the same gestures depending on the time and user, as shown in Figure 2. Additionally, the group of data sent to the classifier for gesture recognition should not be mixed with other sample data related to past or future gestures. Without resolving these problems prior to classification, recognition accuracy can be degraded while the computation requirements and energy consumption during the classification process can be increased significantly. For this reason, we design preprocessing filters which will be described in detail in Section 3.2.

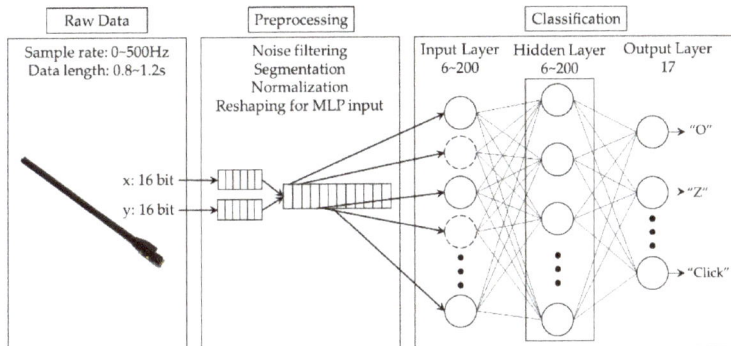

Figure 3. The framework for the proposed finger gesture recognition system.

Finally, the preprocessed group of data is sent to the classifier for recognizing the gesture among predefined ones. The main purpose of this study is to design and implement a gesture recognition system with high accuracy that can be implemented even on a low-end embedded device which operates with a limited energy resource such as a tiny battery or via energy harvesting. To this end, we design a light-weight MLP-based classifier to decrease computation requirements and energy consumption to as low as possible. The design and optimization of this MLP-based classifier will be explained in Section 3.3.

3.2. Designing Preprocessing Filters

In this section, we design preprocessing filters that convert the shape of data, as shown in Figure 4 by applying a noise filter, a segmentation filter, a normalization filter, and a reshape filter in order.

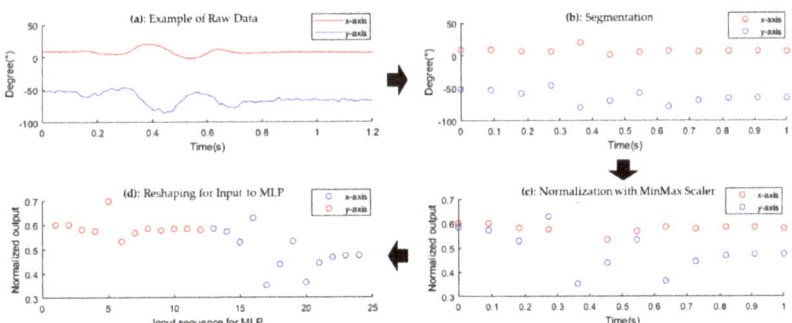

Figure 4. Preprocessing flow of the raw data collected.

Noise filter: No matter how well the sensor circuit is designed, it is unavoidable that the raw data contain a lot of noise during data collection from the sensor, as shown in Figure 4a. Noise is generated in a random and non-uniform pattern, which makes detecting the unique pattern of each gesture even more difficult, and finally requires more computation. To minimize the effect of noise, we use an infinite impulse response (IIR), where the input signal and output signal are applied recursively to perform filtering. This IIR filter is more suitable for our work than a finite impulse response (FIR) filter because of its low implementation cost and low latency.

Data segmentation filter: The segmentation filter first separates a group of data, only related to a single gesture among continuously collected data from the sensor. To design this segmentation function, we investigate an average rate of change in sampled data to indicate the start and end of collecting a group of data only related to a single gesture, assuming that the finger is not moving for a certain amount of the time before and after each gesture. The average rate of change can be simply calculated at the same time as executing the noise filter so that the overhead for calculating the average rate of change is minimized. Starting from a steady state, the collection is started if the average rate of change is over the predefined threshold, and the collection is stopped if the average rate of change is under the predefined threshold as well. We reasonably set this threshold empirically after intensive experiments.

The second role of the segmentation filter is to change the variable number of sampled data for a single gesture to the fixed number. As mentioned, the number of sample data grouped into a single gesture varies depending on gesture type, user, and time of trial. If this number varies, it is difficult to apply a simple MLP-based classifier. To resolve this issue, we interpolate the data if the number of data is smaller than the predefined number while we reduce the number of data by applying a smoothing function in the opposite case, so that the number of sampled data to the classifier is fixed with the predefined one, as shown in Figure 4b. Since the number of data to be sent to the classifier for a single gesture recognition is also tightly coupled with setting the sample rate of the flex sensor and designing a classifier as well, we discuss this issue in Section 4, separately.

Normalization and Reshaping: Normalization is an efficient method for an MLP-based classifier to increase recognition accuracy while reducing the computation requirements by adjusting the amplitude of data. We use a MinMax scaler, which normalizes the amplitude of data based on maximum and minimum values among the whole set of data, as shown in Figure 4c. Note that minimum and maximum values of the data are determined during the segmentation, the additional overhead of this process is almost negligible. The last process before sending the data to the classifier is reshaping the output of the sensor to fit the input of the MLP with a predefined size. Since the output of sensor data is 16 bits from the X-axis and 16 bits from the Y-axis, it is converted from 2D array to 1D array data, as shown in Figure 4d. This process is simple, with almost no computational overhead for this process if this process is performed with the normalization process.

3.3. Designing an MLP-Based Classifier

For recognizing hand gestures, we design a simple MLP-based classifier but support high recognition accuracy using minimal resources. This section only describes a classifier design and component-level optimization issue while system-level optimization issues will be discussed in Section 4.

Input Layer: In designing the input layer of an MLP-based classifier, the number of nodes is mainly determined by the size of the input data set. In our design, since the segmentation filter determines the size of the input data set with a predefined number, the number of nodes in the input layer is also designed to have the same number with the predefined one in the segmentation filter.

Hidden Layer: Determining the number of hidden layers and the number of nodes for each hidden layer is a main design issue because they are directly related to the amount of computing, memory space, and energy consumption, in addition to recognition accuracy. Huge design choices include selecting a proper structure for the hidden layer. In this work, the amount of data generated by the flex sensor is smaller compared with that of image processing. Thus, the number of hidden layers we consider is limited to a single or a double hidden layer. To find the best solution, we intensively explore the design choices of the MLP-based classifier by changing the number of nodes used for each layer in terms of recognition accuracy, energy consumption, and the feasibility of implementation considering the performance and memory size targeting low-end embedded devices. Each node in the hidden layer uses a rectified linear unit (ReLu) activation function. For each explored MLP model, we perform an independent training and testing process. The exploration in detail will be described with system-level optimization in Section 4, while the results will be described in Section 5.

Output Layer: The number of nodes in the output layer is generally determined by the number of recognized gestures. In this work, the number of gestures is set to 17. Thus, we design the output layer to have 17 nodes. Each node in the output layer uses a Softmax activation function to generate a probability value for each gesture so that the gesture with the highest probability is selected as the final result.

4. Energy–Accuracy Aware Design Optimization

Based on the design described in Section 3, this section analyzes the implementation issues of energy–accuracy aware system-level optimization targeting low-end embedded devices. We first analyze the practical issues of designing an entire system focusing on performance and power management. Then, we build performance and energy estimation models to find the energy–accuracy trade-offs. Finally, energy–accuracy aware system-level design optimization is described.

4.1. Performance (Timing) Estimation Models

In terms of the design components, the proposed system consists of data collection, preprocessing filters, and an MLP-based classifier. At the same time, in terms of hardware components, the system mainly consists of a flex sensor and an MCU board. Thus, management of these hardware components is a practical issue of the implementation. For example, activation/deactivation scheduling of the MCU and the sensor module is tightly coupled with the performance and energy consumption of the system. The MCU can be in a standby state synchronized with the operating frequency of the sensor. When the preprocessing and MLP classification tasks are executed in the MCU, the sensor can be entered into a standby state to minimize the power consumption of the sensor. To address these issues, we first build timing models of gesture recognition, as shown in Figure 5. Table 1 describes the parameters used in our timing models.

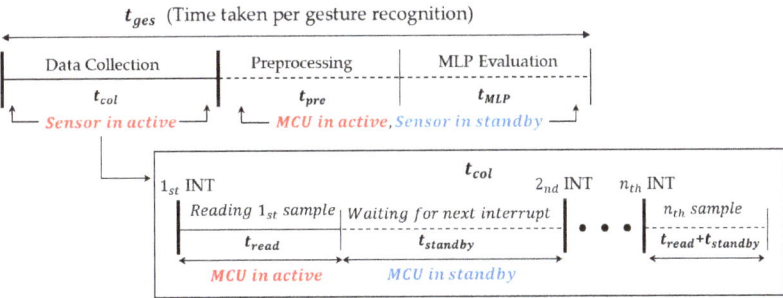

Figure 5. The routine (loop) that performs classification.

The time taken per single gesture recognition, t_{ges}, is defined as the sum of the time for executing data collection, t_{col}, which is equal to the duration of a gesture, the time for preprocessing, t_{pre}, and the time for MLP classification, t_{MLP}. Depending on the user and the type of gesture, t_{col} varies from 0.8 s to 1.2 s based on our experiences. t_{pre} and t_{MLP} vary from 33 µs to 1727 µs, and 284 µs to 3360 µs, respectively, depending on the number of sensor data, the size of MLP models, and the type of MCUs.

Looking at the data collection process which accounts for most of the time spent on gesture recognition, the MCU repeats the sensor data read with the sampling frequency f_s. At each period of read, the MCU reads a single data set, and then transits back to the standby state, waiting for the next interruption from the sensor. The time for reading a single set of data is defined as t_{read}, and the time spent in the standby state is defined as

$t_{standby}$. In our experiments, t_{read} is measured as 269 µs, which is determined by the I²C configuration when running at 400 KHz. Note that the sensor is always in the active state during t_{col}, while it is in the standby state during t_{pre} and t_{MLP}. Since t_{col} varies only with the type of gesture and user, and not with the design parameters, the number of sampled data per gesture to be recognized, N, is calculated as:

$$N = t_{col} * f_s \qquad (1)$$

When estimating t_{pre}, since we expect that it is proportional to N, we model it as a simple function of N. We also expect that t_{MLP} may be proportional to N because N determines the number of nodes in the input layer. However, since N varies depending on the gesture and user, we change N into N', which is a fixed number in the segmentation process. In addition to N', t_{MLP} is also tightly coupled with the size of MLP parameters, N_{MLP}. Thus, we model t_{MLP} as a function of N' and N_{MLP}. Based on the scenario described above, t_{ges} can be estimated as follows:

$$t_{ges} = N * \frac{1}{f_s} + t_{pre}(N) + t_{MLP}(N', N_{MLP}) \qquad (2)$$

Since our design considers N' as close to N as possible, t_{ges} is mainly affected by f_s and N_{MLP} because N is, in turn, determined by f_s, as shown in Equation (1). We find $t_{pre}(N)$ and $t_{MLP}(N', N_{MLP})$ from the extensive measurements using several low-end MCU prototypes which will be explained in Section 5.

Table 1. Description of the parameters used in the model.

Definition	Description
N	Number of sampled data per gesture to be recognized
N_{MLP}	Number of parameters used in the MLP classifier
f_s	Sensor frequency (sample rate)
t_{ges}	Time taken per gesture recognition $= t_{col} + t_{pre} + t_{MLP}$
t_{read}	Time taken to read one sample from the sensor 269 us (including time to wakeup, I²C transfer, time to sleep)
t_{pre}	Time taken to perform preprocessing Depends on f_s
t_{MLP}	Time taken to perform the MLP evaluation Depends on # of parameters in the f_s
t_{col}	Time taken to collect data $= \left(t_{read} + t_{standby}\right) \times N$

4.2. Energy Estimation Models

Figure 6 visualizes the power consumption of two main hardware components during t_{col}, t_{pre} and t_{MLP}. Considering the complexity of power management, our design only uses two power states—active and standby—for both the MCU and the sensor.

The energy consumption per single gesture recognition, E_{ges}, is defined as the sum of the energy consumption in the MCU, E_{mcu}, and the energy consumption in the sensor, E_{sensor}. The energy consumption of the MCU, in turn, consists of the energy consumption for executing three tasks—data collection, E_{mcu_col}, preprocessing, E_{mcu_pre}, and MLP classification, E_{MLP}—as follows:

$$E_{mcu} = E_{mcu\_col} + E_{mcu\_pre} + E_{mcu\_MLP}. \qquad (3)$$

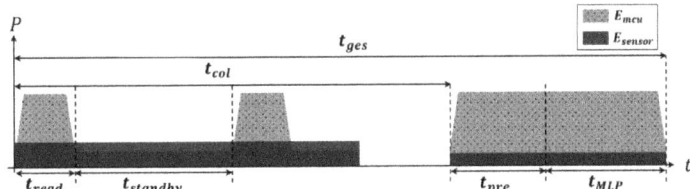

Figure 6. Visualized energy consumption over the time.

In the data collection task, the MCU operates periodically with the frequency of f_s to read data from the sensor, switching between the active and standby states. Thus, the energy consumed by the MCU for executing the data collection task is the sum of the energy consumption in the active and standby states as follows:

$$E_{mcu\_col} = t_{read} \cdot N \cdot P_{mcu\_active} + (t_{col} - t_{read} \cdot N) \cdot P_{mcu\_standby}, \quad (4)$$

where P_{mcu_active} and $P_{mcu\_statndby}$ indicate the power consumption of the MCU in the active and standby states, respectively.

The energy consumption for executing the preprocessing, E_{mcu_pre}, and the energy consumption for executing the MLP operation, E_{mcu_MLP}, are simply estimated by:

$$E_{mcu\_pre} = t_{pre} \cdot P_{mcu\_active}, \; E_{mcu\_MLP} = t_{MLP} \cdot P_{mcu\_active}. \quad (5)$$

As mentioned, the sensor is in the active state only during data collection for time t_{col}, and the E_{sensor} is defined as:

$$E_{sensor} = t_{col} \cdot P_{sensor\_active} + (t_{pre} + t_{MLP}) P_{sensor\_idle}, \quad (6)$$

where P_{sensor_active} and P_{sensor_idle} indicate the power consumption of the sensor in the active and standby states, respectively. Unlike the MCU, the power consumption of the sensor in the active state depends on the sampling frequency, f_s. To reflect the power consumption change by f_s, we build a power consumption model of the sensor by directly measuring the power consumption depending on f_s as follows:

$$P_{sensor\_active} = \alpha \cdot f_s, \quad (7)$$

where α is the coefficient, which is determined as 3.56, for the flex sensor we used in the design with a 3.3 V operating voltage.

Based on Equations (3)–(7), E_{ges} is finally estimated as below:

$$E_{ges} = (t_{read} \cdot N + t_{pre} + t_{MLP}) \cdot P_{mcu\_active} + (t_{col} - t_{read} \cdot N) \cdot P_{mcu\_standy} + \alpha \cdot t_{col} \cdot f_s + (t_{pre} + t_{MLP}) \cdot P_{sensor\_idle}. \quad (8)$$

Similar to Equation (2), only f_s and N_{MLP} are major optimizable design parameters among the parameters used in Equation (8), while the other parameters such as P_{mcu_active} and P_{mcu_standy} are determined by the type of MCU device. Note that we do not consider any dynamic frequency and voltage scaling in this work, thus P_{mcu_active} and P_{mcu_standy} are constant if the same MCU devices are used in the design.

4.3. Energy–Accuracy Aware System-Level Design

There are numerous design choices where the energy and accuracy are trade-off relations in general. This means that maximizing recognition accuracy while simultaneously minimizing energy consumption is not easy to solve. Thus, we first define accuracy- or energy-constrained objective functions as below:

$$\begin{array}{cc} \text{Minimize } E_{ges}(f_s, N_{MLP}) & \text{Maximize } Acc(f_s, N_{MLP}) \\ \text{Subject to } Acc(N_{MLP}) \geq T_A & \text{or} \quad \text{Subject to } E_{ges}(f_s) \leq T_E \end{array}$$

where T_A and T_E are the given thresholds for the minimum accuracy and for the maximum energy consumption, respectively. In addition to this, we also consider a resource constraint of the devices such as the memory size of the device.

As modeled in previous sections, the sampling frequency, f_s, is a primary design factor which affects all three tasks. In general, the lower the f_s, the lower the E_{ges}, while lowering f_s may negatively affect recognition accuracy. In addition to f_s, there are many other design choices as well as selecting a proper low-end device that can implement all the designs on it. For these reasons, we first discuss major system-level design choices, and then narrow down the design choices considering four types of commonly used low-end MCUs.

Using Equation (8), we can easily analyze and explore the design choices of f_s in terms of energy consumption. However, recognition accuracy cannot be simply explored with f_s and the other design parameters. For example, increasing f_s may enhance recognition accuracy because it provides more information to the MLP classifier. However, improvement in accuracy is not simply proportional to f_s, and there is a saturation point. Thus, we have to find an optimal setting of f_s through system-level design choice exploration.

In designing preprocessing filters, a simple design choice is whether each filter is adopted. We use a segmentation filter and a reshape filter for all design choices because they are indispensable while noise and normalization filters are optional. In designing a segmentation filter, determining N is tightly coupled with the setting of f_s, as shown in Equation (1), and the effects of this will be analyzed through design choice explorations as well. In terms of changing the number of sampled data from N to N' in the segmentation filter, if the difference between N and N' is larger, energy consumption in the sensor is relatively high, while the information provided to the MLP classifier is limited. Thus, we set the difference between the two numbers as close as possible by considering average t_{col}.

In designing a MLP classifier, finding the optimal number of parameters used in the MLP is important to find an energy–accuracy aware design. The higher the N_{MLP}, the higher the accuracy but the larger the energy consumption. Similar to f_s, the maximum achievable accuracy is also limited even when N_{MLP} is increasing continuously. Thus, we also explore the design choices of the MLP classifier by varying N_{MLP} and f_s, considering the constraint of memory space in the target device.

5. Evaluations

This section introduces experimental setups including the prototypes we implement to verify the energy–accuracy aware design points. Then, the results of design choice exploration and the Pareto-optimal energy–accuracy aware design points are presented with some findings and discussions.

5.1. Experimental Setup

To demonstrate the feasibility of the proposed designs, we implemented an in-house prototype tiny enough to wear on the body, as shown in Figure 7. The prototype consists of an MCU board and a flex sensor attached to the index finger. The MCU board embeds Bluetooth communication so that the recognized results can be transferred to PCs or smartphones. The flex sensor is connected through I^2C to the MCU board. We consider four commonly used low-end MCUs for targeting low-end embedded devices. Table 2 shows the operating clock frequency, on-chip memory size, type of architecture, and power consumption of four MCUs. CC2652R shows the highest computation speed and the largest memory, including a single-precision floating point unit (FPU), while the other three MCUs have lower computation requirements and memory resources without FPUs. Note that using a hardware FPU and a different bus width of each MCU may affect the precision of floating point operation slightly. However, this issue is beyond our work because the compiler provided from each MCU handles this issue separately. In terms of power consumption in the active state, Atmega2560 has the largest active power consumption per MHz even though it is an 8-bit reduced instruction set computer (RISC) processor. In the standby state, CC2652R consumes the largest amount of power, while Atmega2560 consumes the least amount of power among four MCUs. For the flex sensor, we use a 2-axes flex sensor [14].

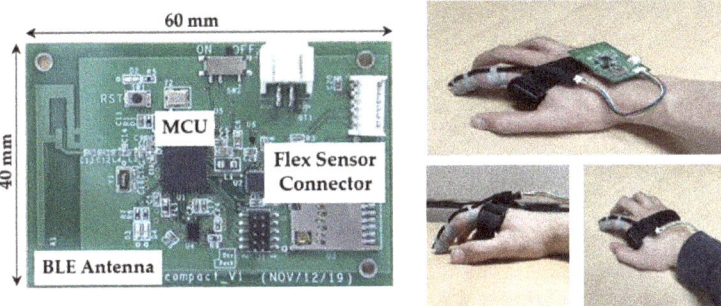

Figure 7. In-house prototype with CC2652R MCU.

Table 2. Characteristics of the low-end MCUs used in this work.

MCU	Clock Frequency (MHz)	On-Chip Memory (KB)	Max. N_{MLP}	Architecture	Active Current (mA/MHz)	Standby Current (uA)
CC2652R	48	80	18,100	CortexM4F 32 bit RISC	0.07	675
Atmega2560	16	8	1972	AVR 8 bit RISC	2.3	170
Atmega1284P	16	16	3960	AVR 8 bit RISC with picoPower	0.86	210
MSP430	16	4	900	16 bit RISC	0.13	420

The prototypes are used for two purposes—data collection and design verification—through real-time gesture recognition. In data collection, the raw data collected are directly sent to the PC so that the data are used for training and for testing the MLP classifier. The prototypes are also used to provide the timing information to the energy models defined in Section 4.3. While the timing information is directly measured from the prototype board, the power consumption of the MCU is acquired from the datasheet rather than the prototype to fairly estimate only energy consumption related to gesture recognition. This means that energy estimation is not affected by the type of board implementation.

In total, 17 types of gestures are defined as continuous motions, as shown in Figure 8. The gray circles in the figure indicate the finger positions at the start/end of each motion. We collected a total of 5100 gestures (300 sets) from 5 users. Each set consists of 17 different gestures, and each user repeated one set of gestures 60 times. The users consist of four males and one female, with ages from 20 s to 40 s and heights from 160 to 180 cm. In order to prevent the overfitting of the trained network model and to ensure generalization ability, the collected gestures were randomly mixed among the same gestures. Then, two-thirds of collected data were used for training with the cross-validation method, while the remaining one-third of collected data were used for evaluation.

MLP training is performed in the Pytorch environment. The hyper-parameters used for trainings are 0.0075 and 500 for the learning rate and epoch, respectively. No significant performance change is observed after the epoch of 500, so the maximum epoch is fixed at 500. For comparison purposes, we build one gated recurrent unit (GRU) and two tiny ML models generated using TensorFlow and Neuton's AutoML, which is commercially available from Google AI.

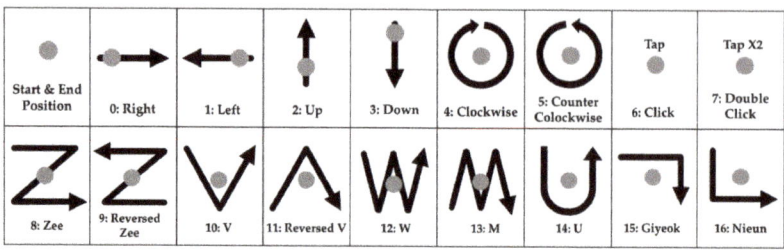

Figure 8. Definition of 17 finger gestures.

5.2. Results of Design Choice Exploration

Figure 9a shows the changes in t_{pre} for four types of MCUs by increasing f_s. As expected, t_{pre} is almost linearly proportional to f_s. Figure 9b shows the changes in t_{MLP} by increasing N_{MLP}. Note that we change N into N_{MLP} for simplification. Although it is not precisely linearly proportional to N_{MLP}, we can still use this approximate linear model based on our experiments. As shown in the graphs, the slopes are lower in the order of CC2652R, Atmega2560/1284P, and MSP430, which directly shows the computation power of each MCU.

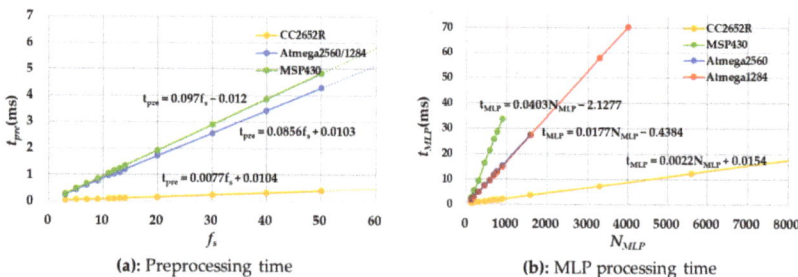

Figure 9. Comparison of preprocessing and MLP time.

Figure 10 presents the results of recognition accuracy by varying N_{MLP} for the single and double hidden layers of MLPs, and also with and without preprocessing filters. In this paper, N_{MLP} is calculated as:

$$N_{MLP} = i \cdot h_1 + \sum_{k=1}^{n-1}(h_k \cdot h_{k+1}) + h_n \cdot o + \sum_{k=1}^{n} h_k + o \qquad (9)$$

where i and o indicate the number of nodes in the input and output layers, respectively, while h_k is the number of nodes in the k-*th* hidden layer, and n is the number of hidden layers. Note that i is equal to N', which is affected by f_s. This means that N_{MLP} reflects the effect of f_s as well. For better understanding, we also mark the label of the X-axis with f_s.

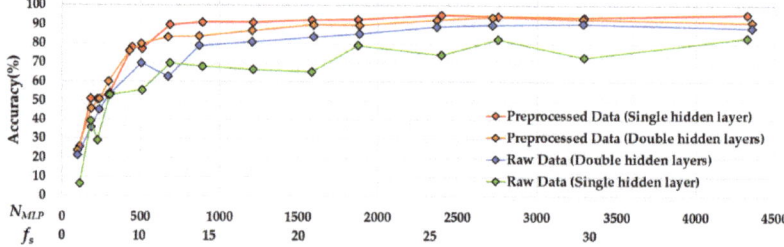

Figure 10. Recognition accuracy comparisons by increasing N_{MLP}.

As expected, recognition accuracy is highly correlated with N_{MLP} in all four configurations. Increasing N_{MLP} enhances recognition accuracy in all four configurations until N_{MLP} reaches 689. However, increased accuracy starts to saturate from N_{MLP} = 689 for the single hidden layer with preprocessing and from N_{MLP} = 1597 for the double hidden layer with preprocessing. Clearly, applying preprocessing filters enhances accuracy for both single- and double-hidden-layer configurations. The contributions of preprocessing filters are significant especially when N_{MLP} is in low regions—smaller than 900 in our experiments. In case of MSP430, which has a maximum 900 of N_{MLP}, the achievable maximum accuracy without a preprocessing filter is 78.7% in the single layer of MLP, while that of the one with a preprocessing filter is 91.0%.

The accuracy for the single hidden layer and double hidden layer of MLPs shows different behaviors depending on whether the preprocessing filter is applied. When preprocessing filters are not applied, the double-hidden-layer MLP shows better performance at most ranges of N_{MLP}. In general, it is known that using more hidden layers is useful to solve non-linear problems [25]. We observe that without preprocessing, the gesture data show more non-linearity. When processing filters are applied, the single-hidden-layer MLP shows better accuracy than the double hidden layer when N_{MLP} is not sufficient. As shown in the figure, the accuracy of the single-hidden-layer MLP increases rapidly as N_{MLP} increases, while that of the double-hidden-layer MLP increases relatively slowly. The accuracy of the single-hidden-layer MLP with preprocessing starts to saturate from 89.7% at N_{MLP} = 689, whereas the accuracy of the double-hidden-layer MLP starts to saturate from 92.3% at N_{MLP} = 1583, which uses 2.32-fold more resources. We found that applying preprocessing filters reduces the non-linearity of the data so that maximum accuracy is reached quickly to the saturation point in the single-hidden-layer MLP.

Based on comparisons of the four configurations, we conclude that the single-hidden-layer MLP with preprocessing is more suitable for devices that have limited resources.

5.3. Pareto-Optimal Energy–Accuracy Aware Design Points

We explored the design choices of the proposed finger gesture recognition system in terms of accuracy as well as the energy consumption by analyzing a total of 159 designs with varying design choices. Figure 11 shows the energy–accuracy results of each design choice as well as the Pareto-optimal designs. As shown in the figure, MSP430 and CC2652R quickly converge to peak accuracy by increasing the energy constraints. MSP430 consumes approximately half the energy compared to CC2652R while still reaching 91.0% accuracy. However, the maximum N_{MLP} of MSP430 is only 900, so it cannot reach the highest achievable accuracy of 95.5%, and only CC2652R can achieve maximum accuracy even though it consumes approximately twice the energy.

Atmega2560 has the worst energy–accuracy efficiency. We found that Atmega2560 is based on an 8-bit RISC architecture, and computation requirements during the preprocessing and forward propagation operations in the MLP needs more active time of the MCU, which increases energy consumption when f_s and N_{MLP} increase. We observe similar energy–accuracy behaviors in Atmega1284P but with lower energy consumption than that of Atmega2560 because the active power consumption of Atmega1284P is lower than Atmega2560. Nevertheless, neither can be a Pareto-optimal.

Figure 11 also includes the energy–accuracy information of three models (one GRU and two AutoML) which are generated by a commercial platform. Due to the memory limitation, all three models are only applicable to CC2652R. The accuracy of two AutoML models are comparable to our MLP model that has 891 to 3287 parameters. However, due to the energy consumption, those models cannot be selected as Pareto optimal. The GRU model shows slightly better accuracy than our design, with similar energy consumption. Thus, it can be selected as a Pareto-optimal solution if CC2562R or higher MCU is used for the target device. However, this GRU model cannot be a solution if the user wants to implement it on a low-end MCU such as MSP430 or lower.

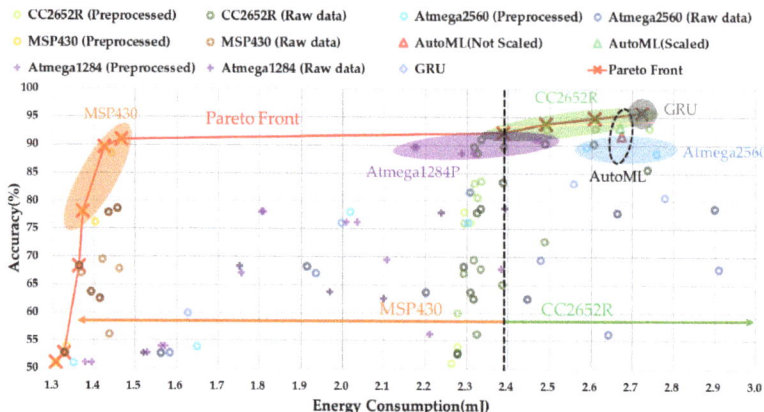

Figure 11. Pareto curve between energy consumption and accuracy for four types of MCUs.

Table 3 shows the design choices of each Pareto Front in detail. If the accuracy is given as a design constraint, MSP430 can be used if the given accuracy is under 91.0% while CC2652R MCU can be used over 91.0% of constraints. When energy consumption is a major constraint of the design, MSP430 is mostly used if the budget of the energy is under 2.39 mJ per gesture while CC2652R is used if the energy budget is over 2.39 mJ. ATmega2560/1284P can still be considered as a target MCU if the users want to reuse the hardware and software they have already developed. In this case, the results of our exploration could be useful as well.

Table 3. Details of the Pareto Front design choices.

MCU Type	Sample Rate	N_{MLP}	Memory Size (Byte)	MLP Layers	Accuracy (%)	E_{ges} (mJ)
MSP430	5	185	740	$10 \times 6 \times 17$	51.1	1.31
	7	297	1188	$14 \times 7 \times 7 \times 17$	60.1	1.33
	9	449	1796	$18 \times 12 \times 17$	78.1	1.36
	11	589	2356	$22 \times 11 \times 11 \times 17$	81.7	1.37
	12	689	2756	$24 \times 16 \times 17$	89.7	1.42
	14	891	3564	$28 \times 19 \times 17$	91.0	1.47
CC2652R	20	1583	6332	$40 \times 27 \times 17$	92.3	2.39
	30	3287	13,148	$60 \times 30 \times 30 \times 17$	92.9	2.49
	40	5603	22,412	$80 \times 57 \times 17$	94.8	2.61
	50	7787	31,148	GRU	95.8	2.72

A confusion matrix is useful for analyzing the patterns of mispredictions. Figure 12a shows the confusion matrix of a model using 891 parameters with an accuracy of 91.0% and an energy consumption of 1.47 mJ when using a MSP430. In this design, 21.0% of "Double Click" gestures (class 7) are mispredicted as "Click" gestures (class 6). As defined in Figure 8, "Click" moves the finger up and down once, while "Double Click" moves the finger up and down in the same way but twice. Figure 13 shows the raw data collected on two gestures directly from the sensors. As shown in the figures, the patterns of the two gestures are similar, thus the model with 891 parameters is not enough to distinguish them clearly.

Figure 12b shows the confusion matrix of the classifier using 8513 parameters, which is 9.55-fold greater than using 891 parameters. This design achieves 95.5% accuracy with an energy consumption of 2.74 mJ when using CC2652R. Nevertheless, 14.0% of "Double Click" gestures (class 7) are mispredicted as "Click" gestures (class 6). This may indicate that simple MLP may not be a perfect solution to completely distinguish these two gestures. Although this design shows a lower number of mispredictions than the design with 891 parameters, energy consumption is increased by 1.86 fold, while improvement in accuracy is only 4.4%. In addition, this design cannot be implemented in MSP430 because of memory shortage. Table 4 summarizes and compares this work with existing hand/finger gesture recognition designs, in terms of the sensors, classification models with size information, the number of recognized classes, accuracy, and implementation. We do not directly compare recognition accuracy because the target applications, type of sensor, the number of recognized classes, and the dataset used for training and testing are different in each work. As shown in the table, most studies only provide the design and performance analysis without details on implementation issues. The work in [3,7] tried to reduce model size and can be implemented in MCU devices, but not on low-end MCUs with only a few tens of KB memory and low computing resources. The work in [8] was implemented on an Arduino Due board. However, the Arduino board only collects and preprocesses the collected data while classifications are performed on Field Programmable Gate Arrays (FPGAs). Most of all, none of the existing studies considers energy–accuracy design choices, which is very important for designing wearable IoT devices.

Table 4. Comparisons of existing hand gesture recognition studies.

	[1]	[3]	[5]	[6]	[7]	[8]	[13]	[23]	[26]	This Work
Used sensors	Camera	EMG (Myo)	Depth camera	Optical and IMU	Flex Sensor	IMU	Pressure, flex, gyro, IMU, etc.	Accelerometer	Flex sensor	2-axes flex sensor
Models (num. of parmas or mem. size)	CNN + RNN (N/A)	CNN (34 K)	Custom (600 MB)	HMM (N/A)	GRU + MAP (50 K~)	RCE (274.3 Kb)	LSTM (N/A)	RNN (69 K)	AL[1] (N/A)	MLP (185~8513)
Classes	4	7	124	26	4	10	31	8	4	17
Accuracy (%)	96.4	98.8	91.9	98.1	97.3	98.6	90.0	88.6	88.3	95.5
Implementation	N/A	N/A	Inter i5, GPU (GTX750)	N/A	Raspberry Pi 3	Arduino + FPGA	N/A	N/A	N/A	CC2652R, Atmega, MSP430

[1] AL: adversarial learning.

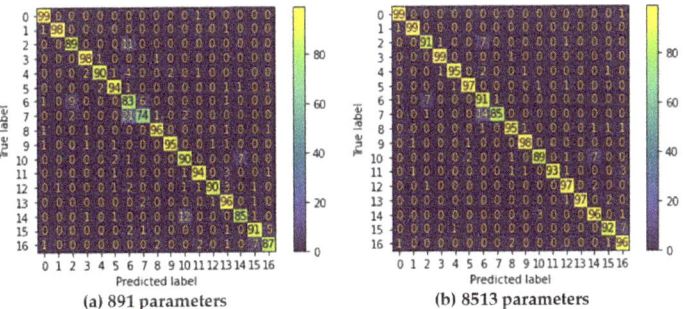

(a) 891 parameters (b) 8513 parameters

Figure 12. Confusion matrices of two Pareto Fronts.

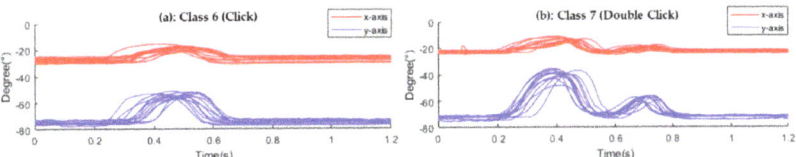

Figure 13. Raw data collected on gestures 6 and 7 from the flex sensor.

6. Conclusions

In this paper, we implemented a finger gesture recognition system based on a lightweight MLP-based classifier using a low-end MCU and a 2-axes flex sensor. In order to find energy–accuracy aware design points, we first designed a full process of finger gesture recognition and its system-level performance and energy models. Then, we analyzed system-level design issues including sensor operating frequency and the size of the MLP classifier. Finally, we explored the numerous design choices based on accuracy and energy constraints. Considering four commonly used MCUs, a total of 159 design points were determined according to the configuration of the sensor operating frequency, the presence of preprocessing filters, and the size of the MLP classifier. As a result of Pareto Fronts, the proposed design achieved up to 95.5% accuracy with an energy consumption of 2.74 mJ, which shows up to 10% higher accuracy than previous studies [26] with similar low-end MCUs. Collectively, this study details how to achieve energy–accuracy aware design points under given energy or accuracy constraints.

In this work, we do not address the effect of using AI accelerators such as digital signal processors (DSPs), FPGAs or application-specific integrated chips (ASICs). Since these accelerators will greatly affect performance as well as energy efficiency, considering these components will be our future work to find energy–accuracy aware design choices for wearable IoT devices.

Author Contributions: Conceptualization, W.J.; methodology, W.J.; software, W.J.; validation, W.J.; formal analysis, W.J. and H.G.L.; investigation, W.J.; resources, W.J.; data curation, W.J.; writing—original draft preparation, W.J.; writing—review and editing, W.J. and H.G.L.; visualization, W.J.; supervision, H.G.L.; project administration, H.G.L.; funding acquisition, H.G.L. All authors have read and agreed to the published version of the manuscript.

Funding: This research was funded by the National Research Foundation of Korea (NRF) grant number NRF-2020R1F1A1076533.

Conflicts of Interest: The authors declare no conflict of interest.

References

1. Gunawan, M.R.; Djamal, E.C. Spatio-Temporal Approach using CNN-RNN in Hand Gesture Recognition. In Proceedings of the 2021 4th International Conference of Computer and Informatics Engineering (IC2IE), Depok, Indonesia, 14–15 September 2021; pp. 385–389. [CrossRef]
2. Chen, X.; Guo, H.; Wang, G.; Zhang, L. Motion feature augmented recurrent neural network for skeleton-based dynamic hand gesture recognition. In Proceedings of the 2017 IEEE International Conference on Image Processing (ICIP), Beijing, China, 17–20 September 2017; pp. 2881–2885. [CrossRef]
3. Chen, L.; Fu, J.; Wu, Y.; Li, H.; Zheng, B. Hand Gesture Recognition Using Compact CNN via Surface Electromyography Signals. *Sensors* **2020**, *20*, 672. [CrossRef] [PubMed]
4. Mendes, N.; Ferrer, J.; Vitorino, J.; Safeea, M.; Neto, P. Human Behavior and Hand Gesture Classification for Smart Human-robot Interaction. *Procedia Manuf.* **2017**, *11*, 91–98. [CrossRef]
5. Alam, S.; Kwon, K.-C.; Kim, N. Implementation of a Character Recognition System Based on Finger-Joint Tracking Using a Depth Camera. *IEEE Trans. Hum.-Mach. Syst.* **2021**, *51*, 229–241. [CrossRef]
6. Chen, M.; AlRegib, G.; Juang, B.-H. Air-Writing Recognition—Part I: Modeling and Recognition of Characters, Words, and Connecting Motions. *IEEE Trans. Hum.-Mach. Syst.* **2015**, *46*, 403–413. [CrossRef]
7. Chuang, W.-C.; Hwang, W.-J.; Tai, T.-M.; Huang, D.-R.; Jhang, Y.-J. Continuous Finger Gesture Recognition Based on Flex Sensors. *Sensors* **2019**, *19*, 3986. [CrossRef] [PubMed]
8. Kim, M.; Cho, J.; Lee, S.; Jung, Y. IMU Sensor-Based Hand Gesture Recognition for Human-Machine Interfaces. *Sensors* **2019**, *19*, 3827. [CrossRef] [PubMed]
9. Dang, L.M.; Min, K.; Wang, H.; Piran, J.; Lee, C.H.; Moon, H. Sensor-based and vision-based human activity recognition: A comprehensive survey. *Pattern Recognit.* **2020**, *108*, 107561. [CrossRef]
10. Fernandez, I.G.; Ahmad, S.A.; Wada, C. Inertial Sensor-Based Instrumented Cane for Real-Time Walking Cane Kinematics Estimation. *Sensors* **2020**, *20*, 4675. [CrossRef] [PubMed]
11. Côté-Allard, U.; Fall, C.L.; Drouin, A.; Campeau-Lecours, A.; Gosselin, C.; Glette, K.; Laviolette, F.; Gosselin, B. Deep Learning for Electromyographic Hand Gesture Signal Classification Using Transfer Learning. *IEEE Trans. Neural Syst. Rehabil. Eng.* **2019**, *27*, 760–771. [CrossRef] [PubMed]

12. Lin, B.-S.; Hsiao, P.-C.; Yang, S.-Y.; Su, C.-S.; Lee, I.-J. Data Glove System Embedded With Inertial Measurement Units for Hand Function Evaluation in Stroke Patients. *IEEE Trans. Neural Syst. Rehabil. Eng.* **2017**, *25*, 2204–2213. [CrossRef] [PubMed]
13. Chan, J.; Veas, E.; Simon, J. Designing a Sensor Glove Using Deep Learning. In Proceedings of the 26th International Conference on Intelligent User Interfaces, College Station, TX, USA, 14–17 April 2021; pp. 150–160. [CrossRef]
14. Bendlabs. 2-Axis Soft Flex Sensor. Available online: https://www.bendlabs.com/products/2-axis-soft-flex-sensor/ (accessed on 30 August 2018).
15. Laput, G.; Harrison, C. Sensing Fine-Grained Hand Activity with Smartwatches. In Proceedings of the ACM Conference on Human Factors in Computing Systems (CHI'19), Glasgow, UK, 4–9 May 2019. [CrossRef]
16. Ketykó, I.; Kovács, F.; Varga, K.Z. Domain Adaptation for sEMG-based Gesture Recognition with Recurrent Neural Networks. In Proceedings of the 2019 International Joint Conference on Neural Networks (IJCNN), Budapest, Hungary, 14–19 July 2019; pp. 1–7. [CrossRef]
17. Hao, J.; Yang, P.; Chen, L.; Geng, Y. A gait recognition approach based on surface electromyography and triaxial acceleration signals. *Chin. J. Tissue Eng. Res.* **2019**, *23*, 5164. [CrossRef]
18. Roland, T.; Amsuess, S.; Russold, M.F.; Baumgartner, W. Ultra-Low-Power Digital Filtering for Insulated EMG Sensing. *Sensors* **2019**, *19*, 959. [CrossRef] [PubMed]
19. Ponraj, G.; Ren, H. Sensor Fusion of Leap Motion Controller and Flex Sensors Using Kalman Filter for Human Finger Tracking. *IEEE Sens. J.* **2018**, *18*, 2042–2049. [CrossRef]
20. Lichtenauer, J.F.; Hendriks, E.A.; Reinders, M.J. Sign Language Recognition by Combining Statistical DTW and Independent Classification. *IEEE Trans. Pattern Anal. Mach. Intell.* **2008**, *30*, 2040–2046. [CrossRef] [PubMed]
21. Vijayalakshmi, P.; Aarthi, M. Sign language to speech conversion. In Proceedings of the 2016 International Conference on Recent Trends in Information Technology (ICRTIT), Chennai, India, 8–9 April 2016; pp. 1–6. [CrossRef]
22. Hu, Q.; Tang, X.; Tang, W. A Smart Chair Sitting Posture Recognition System Using Flex Sensors and FPGA Implemented Artificial Neural Network. *IEEE Sens. J.* **2020**, *20*, 8007–8016. [CrossRef]
23. Shin, S.; Sung, W. Dynamic hand gesture recognition for wearable devices with low complexity recurrent neural networks. In Proceedings of the 2016 IEEE International Symposium on Circuits and Systems (ISCAS), Montréal, QC, Canada, 22–25 May 2016; pp. 2274–2277. [CrossRef]
24. Wang, L.; Meydan, T.; Williams, P.; Wolfson, K.T. A proposed optical-based sensor for assessment of hand movement. In Proceedings of the 2015 IEEE Sensors, Busan, Korea, 1–4 November 2015; pp. 1–4. [CrossRef]
25. Shafi, I.; Ahmad, J.; Shah, S.I.; Kashif, F.M. Impact of Varying Neurons and Hidden Layers in Neural Network Architecture for a Time Frequency Application. In Proceedings of the 2006 IEEE International Multitopic Conference, Islamabad, Pakistan, 23–24 December 2006; pp. 188–193. [CrossRef]
26. Panda, A.K.; Chakravarty, R.; Moulik, S. Hand Gesture Recognition using Flex Sensor and Machine Learning Algorithms. In Proceedings of the 2020 IEEE-EMBS Conference on Biomedical Engineering and Sciences, Langkawi Island, Malaysia, 1–3 March 2021; pp. 449–453. [CrossRef]

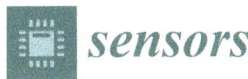

Article

Home-Based Measurements of Dystonia in Cerebral Palsy Using Smartphone-Coupled Inertial Sensor Technology and Machine Learning: A Proof-of-Concept Study

Dylan den Hartog [1], Marjolein M. van der Krogt [1,2], Sven van der Burg [3], Ignazio Aleo [4], Johannes Gijsbers [4], Laura A. Bonouvrié [1,2], Jaap Harlaar [5], Annemieke I. Buizer [1,2,6] and Helga Haberfehlner [1,2,7,*]

1. Rehabilitation Medicine, Amsterdam UMC Location Vrije Universiteit Amsterdam, 1081 HZ Amsterdam, The Netherlands; dylan.den.hartog@hotmail.com (D.d.H.); m.vanderkrogt@amsterdamumc.nl (M.M.v.d.K.); l.bonouvrie@amsterdamumc.nl (L.A.B.); ai.buizer@amsterdamumc.nl (A.I.B.)
2. Amsterdam Movement Sciences, Rehabilitation and Development, 1081 BT Amsterdam, The Netherlands
3. Netherlands eScience Center, 1098 XH Amsterdam, The Netherlands; s.vanderburg@esciencecenter.nl
4. Moveshelf Labs B.V., 3521 AL Utrecht, The Netherlands; ignazio.aleo@moveshelf.com (I.A.); johannes.gijsbers@moveshelf.com (J.G.)
5. Department Biomechanical Engineering, TU Delft, 2628 CD Delft, The Netherlands; j.harlaar@tudelft.nl
6. Emma Children's Hospital, Amsterdam UMC Location University of Amsterdam, 1105 AZ Amsterdam, The Netherlands
7. Department of Rehabilitation Sciences, KU Leuven, Campus Bruges, 8200 Bruges, Belgium
* Correspondence: h.haberfehlner@amsterdamumc.nl

Abstract: Accurate and reliable measurement of the severity of dystonia is essential for the indication, evaluation, monitoring and fine-tuning of treatments. Assessment of dystonia in children and adolescents with dyskinetic cerebral palsy (CP) is now commonly performed by visual evaluation either directly in the doctor's office or from video recordings using standardized scales. Both methods lack objectivity and require much time and effort of clinical experts. Only a snapshot of the severity of dyskinetic movements (i.e., choreoathetosis and dystonia) is captured, and they are known to fluctuate over time and can increase with fatigue, pain, stress or emotions, which likely happens in a clinical environment. The goal of this study was to investigate whether it is feasible to use home-based measurements to assess and evaluate the severity of dystonia using smartphone-coupled inertial sensors and machine learning. Video and sensor data during both active and rest situations from 12 patients were collected outside a clinical setting. Three clinicians analyzed the videos and clinically scored the dystonia of the extremities on a 0–4 scale, following the definition of amplitude of the Dyskinesia Impairment Scale. The clinical scores and the sensor data were coupled to train different machine learning models using cross-validation. The average F1 scores (0.67 ± 0.19 for lower extremities and 0.68 ± 0.14 for upper extremities) in independent test datasets indicate that it is possible to detected dystonia automatically using individually trained models. The predictions could complement standard dyskinetic CP measures by providing frequent, objective, real-world assessments that could enhance clinical care. A generalized model, trained with data from other subjects, shows lower F1 scores (0.45 for lower extremities and 0.34 for upper extremities), likely due to a lack of training data and dissimilarities between subjects. However, the generalized model is reasonably able to distinguish between high and lower scores. Future research should focus on gathering more high-quality data and study how the models perform over the whole day.

Keywords: cerebral palsy; dystonia; choreoathetosis; machine learning; home-based; inertial measurement unit; wearable device

1. Introduction

Cerebral palsy (CP) is the most common physically disabling condition in childhood, associated with a lifelong movement disability [1]. CP is caused by brain malformation or brain injury acquired pre- or perinatally, or early in the postnatal period [1]. Three different subtypes of motor disorder are distinguished within CP: spastic, dyskinetic and ataxic CP [1]. Dyskinetic CP accounts for 6–15%, with a prevalence of about 0.12–0.3 in every 1000 live births in Europe [2]. On average, dyskinetic CP is the most disabling form of CP [3].

Dyskinetic movements and postures are characterized by two features, which often co-exist in the same patient: dystonia, which is described by abnormal patterns of posture and/or slow movements; and choreoathetosis, which is characterized by faster involuntary, uncontrolled, jerky, and contorting movements [3]. Dystonia and choreoathetosis can seriously hamper everyday activities of patients.

Several new invasive treatments have been developed in recent decades to reduce dyskinesia and thereby improve daily live function [3]. These neuromodulation treatments include intrathecal baclofen treatment provided via an implanted microinfusion pump, and deep brain stimulation [4]. Intrathecal baclofen treatment has been shown to effective in achieving personal treatment goals in children with dyskinetic CP, however only a small effect on dystonia and choreoathetosis could be shown [5,6]. Deep brain stimulation can be effective in a selected group of individuals with dyskinetic CP. For patient selection, an in-depth understanding of dyskinetic movements is required [7].

Accurate and reliable measurements of the severity of the movement disorder are essential for indication, evaluation, monitoring and fine-tuning of these treatments (i.e., indication, dosage of medication and location and dosage of stimulation). However, it remains a huge challenge to capture the severity of the dyskinetic movements and postures in an objective way.

Assessment of dystonia and choreoathetosis in children and adolescents is now commonly performed by visual evaluation either directly in the doctor's office or from video recordings using standardized scales [8]. These assessments are both lacking objectivity and require much time and effort of clinical experts. Furthermore, only a snapshot of the severity of dyskinetic movements is captured, and they are known to fluctuate over time and can increase with fatigue, pain or emotions (e.g., stress), which likely happens in a clinical environment [9].

The gold standard for the analysis of upper and lower extremity movements in individuals with CP is a collection of 3D kinematics (rotations of multiple joints and segments during reaching, grasping and walking) [10,11]. However, the collection of data for 3D kinematics requires advanced motion capture systems, which do not allow outside-lab measurements. To enable measurements at home and in daily life environments, for CP, there is an increasing interest in using simpler systems for data collection, such as video-based markerless motion tracking (e.g., OpenPose) [12] and Inertial Measurements Units (IMUs) [13,14]. These easily applicable measurement systems, combined with machine learning models trained by algorithms (e.g., traditional such as logistic regression, random forest, support vector machine, or deep learning algorithms) may significantly contribute to the early detection of CP [15] and the monitoring of daily life functions [12,13]. Within other neurological diseases such as Parkinson's disease [16–18] and Huntington's disease [19], wearable sensors in combination with machine learning techniques are also increasingly used in monitoring of movement disorders. Specifically, in the last decade, IMUs became an attractive and accurate solution, with an increased battery life of several hours, or days, small form-factors, and low cost, making them a very suitable option for home-based measurements for the assessment of movement disorders in childhood. Inertial motion quantities, such as accelerations and angular velocities, combined with an algorithm that automatically assess the presence and amplitude of dystonia and choreoathetosis, would yield meaningful information without manual and time investment. However, no algorithm specific for automatic evaluation of dystonia and choreoathetosis from sensor data is available for dyskinetic CP. As dystonia and choreoathetosis can be significantly variable in dyskinetic CP between as well as within subjects concerning involved body parts, and dependent on environmental factors and the activity performed [20–22], the automatic evaluation is a challenging machine learning task.

Monitoring of movement disorders of children and young adults with dyskinetic CP for a longer period of time within a well-known environment would provide a realistic and reliable evaluation of dystonia and choreoathetosis and can serve treatment decision and monitoring for this complex group. Within this proof-of-concept study, we used four IMUs coupled to a smartphone, allowing the collection of IMUs data and time-synchronized video recordings at home. We aim (1) to show the feasibility of data collection in a natural environment in children and young adults with dyskinetic CP and (2) to train a machine learning model that can detect and score dystonia using IMU data.

2. Materials and Methods

The flowchart in Figure 1 summarizes the dataflow from home measurements (IMUs and videos) towards the final evaluation of the picked classification models. Below, a detailed description of the methods is provided.

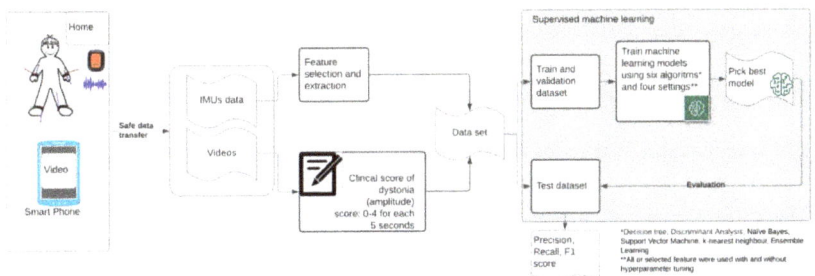

Figure 1. Flowchart of used methodology—measurements of dyskinesia at home (MODYS@home).

2.1. Participants

Participants were recruited from the pediatric outpatient rehabilitation department during regular appointments from 1 March till 31 October 2021. Patients were included if they had: (1) a clinical diagnosis of dyskinetic CP [23,24], (2) were 4–24 years old, and (3) if parents/caregivers were able to follow the instructions for the home-based measurements.

In total, 12 participants were included; Participants had following characteristics (mean ± Standard deviation (range)):

- Age 14.9 ± 4.4 (10.2–21.4) years;
- Weight: 37.3 ± 17.2 (21.7–76.9) kg;
- Height: 145.41 ± 23.5 (116–190) cm;
- 4 females/8 males;
- Gross Motor Function Classification System (GMFCS): II ($n=2$), IV ($n=5$) or V ($n=5$);
- Manual Ability Classification System (MACS): II ($n=1$), III ($n=3$), IV ($n=2$), V ($n=6$).

The study was approved by the Medical Ethics Committee of the VU University Medical Center Amsterdam (The Netherlands). Written informed consent was obtained from participants and, if applicable, their parents for participation in this study.

2.2. Measurements

2.2.1. Materials

The following materials were used for the experiments:

(1) Mobile phone: Samsung A71 (Samsung Electronics, Daegu, South-Korea), with;
(2) MODYS@home app (developed by Rutgers Engineering, Norg, The Netherlands): a custom mobile application for Android, using the Xsens DOT Software Development

Kit (SDK). The app automatically links recorded videos with corresponding time stamps in the sensor data;

(3) Four IMUs (Xsens DOT, Xsens Technologies B.V., Enschede, The Netherlands). Xsens DOT is a wearable sensor incorporating 3D accelerometers, gyroscopes and magnetometers to provide acceleration, angular velocity, and the Earth's magnetic field. Combined with Xsens, sensor fusion algorithms, 3D orientation and free acceleration are provided [10]. Inertial and orientation data outputs of the Xsens DOT sensor are presented in Table 1. The Xsens DOT sensors were set to measure with a sampling frequency of 60 Hz with an accelerometer range of ±16 g and a gyroscope range of ±2000 dps;

(4) Fixation material (Xsens DOT Adhesive patches (Xsens DOT, Xsens Technologies B.V., Enschede, The Netherlands), FabriFoam NuStim Wrap (Fabrifoam, Exton, PA, USA), 3m Coban self-adherent wrap (3M, St. Paul, MN, USA).

Table 1. Inertial and orientation data outputs of Xsens DOT sensors.

Output	Unit
Free acceleration	m/s^2
Angular velocity	degree/s
Euler angles	degree. Roll, pitch, yaw (ZYX Euler Sequence. Earth fixed type, also known as Cardan or aerospace sequence)

2.2.2. Procedure

For the measurements within this proof-of-concept study, participants could choose between measurements at home or in the hospital. For home measurements, participants received a measurement set containing a mobile phone with the MODYS@home app installed, four IMUs, chargers for the phone and sensors, fixation material and a manual. The four Xsens DOT sensors were attached towards the forearm (palmar on the forearm, proximal of processus styloideus ulnae) and lower leg (proximal of the lateral malleolus) (Figure 2). The method of fixation on the attachment site was individually determined. Participants and parents/caregivers were instructed on how to place the IMUs on the participant and how to use the MODYS@home app to record videos and collect sensor data. They were asked to record 10 videos of about 1 minute each day, for both active and resting situations for 7 days within a period of 2 weeks. After the period of 2 weeks, the measurements set was picked up by the researcher and data was transferred by USB-connection for further analysis. For the individuals measured in the hospital, activities and rest data were collected, mimicking a home-based environment. Examples of activities performed at home as well as in the hospital are wheelchair driving, walking, stair climbing, cycling, eating/drinking, sport activities, gaming, computer use, playing music, playing a board game, reading, watching a video/television, using a communication device and resting in a chair or lying down. Activities were chosen by parents/caregivers and participants dependent on the functional level of the individual. Videos during passive movements, e.g., caregiving, transfers were excluded in the current analysis.

2.3. Software

Clinical scoring was done using an open-source tool for video annotation, ELAN version 6.2, Max Planck Institute for Psycholinguistics, Nijmegen, The Netherlands, sourced from: https://archive.mpi.nl/tla/elan/download (accessed on 3 May 2022); MATLAB (Mathworks Inc., Natick, MA, USA) release R2018b was used for processing the data and developing the machine learning models. The code used in the current study is made available (Supplementary S1).

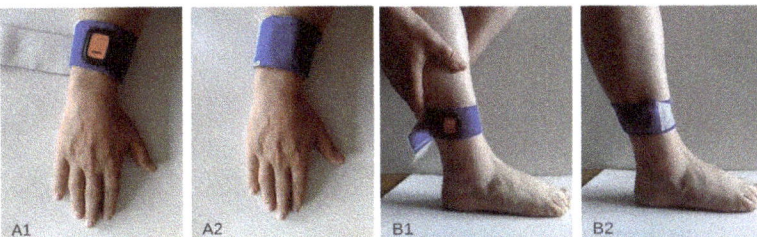

Figure 2. Attachment sites of the inertial sensor units on the upper extremity (**A1**,**A2**) and the lower extremity (**B1**,**B2**).

2.4. Clinical Scoring

Three clinicians assessed the videos. For each time window of 5 seconds, a score between 0–4 was assigned for dystonia for the left and right arm and the left and right leg, separately, following the definition of amplitude of the Dyskinesia Impairment Scale (DIS) [25] for scoring dystonia. Within Parkinson's disease, a 5 s time windows was found to be optimal to achieve the minimum estimation error when estimating the severity of tremor, bradykinesia and dyskinesia using accelerometers and machine learning [26]. The DIS distinguishes between proximal and distal segments of the extremities when scoring amplitude. This score was summarized within the current scoring. Thus, each clinician provided four scores for dystonia for each time window of each video. The median of the three scores was calculated as the final score for the machine learning.

2.5. Data Pre-Processing

Data from the IMUs required pre-processing to serve as input for machine learning. As some time stamps were missing with different sensors, the sensor data from the four sensors was synchronized using linear interpolation with the values from adjacent timestamps.

For each sensor, the resultant free acceleration (a) and resultant angular velocity (ω) at each time stamp was calculated using Equations (1) and (2) respectively:

$$a_r = \sqrt{a_x^2 + a_y^2 + a_z^2} \tag{1}$$

$$\omega_r = \sqrt{\omega_x^2 + \omega_y^2 + \omega_z^2} \tag{2}$$

Each sensor therefore provided 11 signals: 4 accelerations, 4 angular velocities and 3 Euler angles. A single timestamp containing data from all four sensors consisted of 4 × 11 = 44 signals. Each 5 s time window contained 300 timestamps.

In MATLAB, the videos were automatically linked to the sensor data, cutting out parts of the sensor data where a video was recorded. These cut-out parts of sensor data were segmented into time windows of 5 s, equal to the clinical windows. Finally, the clinical scores were automatically linked to the corresponding time windows. Figure 3 shows an example of the sensor signals togethers with the clinical scoring.

Per subject, two tables containing input data and output were created for machine learning. Tables were created for both upper and lower extremities, by adding the data from the left and right extremities.

2.6. Feature Selection and Extraction

Research has shown that feature selection is an effective way to improve the learning process and recognition accuracy, and decreases the complexity and computational cost [27]. We used a method recently described by Den Hartog et al. [28]. In brief, time domain and frequency domain features were tested on the data from all subjects. A Fast Fourier Transform was used to extract frequency-domain features. Initially, 32 different feature classes were tested for usability. For each time window, a single feature class was extracted per IMU signal, creating 11-dimensional feature vectors (1 feature class × 11 signals). These feature vectors were then fed to six different machine learning algorithms (Decision Tree, Discriminant Analysis, Naïve Bayes, Support Vector Machine, k-nearest neighbors, and Ensemble Learning), to test the feature classes' predictive power. Feature classes were only selected if they were capable of achieving an F1 score of at least 0.7 with a machine learning algorithm, indicating a strong correlation with the output. A total of 10 feature classes passed the selection round (Table 2).

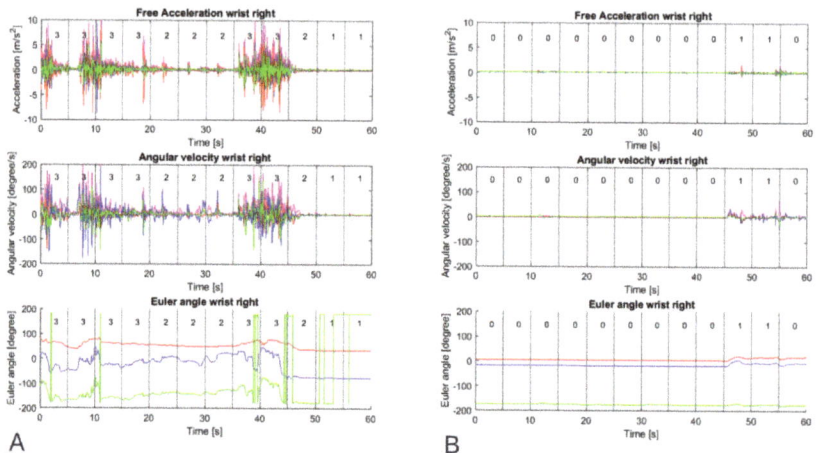

Figure 3. Example of data of one participant's right wrist during a resting activity showing inertial sensor output: free acceleration, angular velocity and Euler angle, (**A**) with a high level of dystonia and (**B**) with a low level of dystonia. The number within the time windows of 5 s is the median clinical score of three raters for upper extremity dystonia of the right wrist.

Table 2. Overview of the 10 feature classes passed the feature selection round.

Nr	Feature Class
1	Absolute harmonic mean
2	Absolute maximum
3	Bandpower
4	Geometric mean
5	Maximum
6	Median
7	Minimum
8	Root-mean-square
9	Root-sum-of-squares
10	Shannon entropy

Next, for each time window, all 10 feature classes were extracted for each of the 11 IMU signals, creating 10-dimensional feature vectors (10 classes × 11 signals). This means that for each time window there are 110 features that could describe the characteristics of that window.

Next, sequential feature selection (SFS) as described by MATLAB (Sequential Feature Selection—MATLAB & Simulink—MathWorks Benelux) was used, as this is an effective way to identify redundant and irrelevant features. Sequential feature selection is a wrapper-type feature selection algorithm that starts training using a subset of features and then adds or removes a feature using a selection criterion. The selection criterion directly measures the change in model performance that results from adding or removing a feature. The algorithm repeats training and improving a model until its stopping criteria are satisfied.

In this study, sequential feature selection (SFS), with a maximum number of objective evaluation of 20, was used. SFS sequentially adds features to an empty candidate set until the addition of further features does not decrease the objective function. In this study, misclassification rate was set as the objective function.

Finally, the extracted features were normalized to rescale the data to a common scale. Supervised machine learning algorithms learn the relationship between input and output and the unit, scale, and distribution of the input data may vary from feature to feature. This will impact the classification accuracy of the models. In this work, the data was normalized by scaling each input variable to a range of 0 to 1.

2.7. Machine Learning and Algorithms

After processing the data and extracting features, the next step is to feed the feature vectors to machine learning algorithms. In this study, six types of supervised machine learning algorithms were tested: Decision Tree, Discriminant Analysis, Naïve Bayes, Support Vector Machine, k-nearest neighbors, and Ensemble Learning.

2.8. Training, Validating and Testing

For an objective evaluation of the machine learning algorithms, the datasets were divided into a training dataset, validation dataset and testing dataset.

Since the datasets were small, a 5-fold cross-validation was used to evaluate the performance of the models. For each iteration, 80% of the data was used for training and validation, and 20% was used for testing. For training the machine learning models, another 5-fold cross-validation was also used within the training and validation data.

The validation dataset provides an evaluation of a model fit on the training dataset while tuning the model's hyperparameters [29]. After training and validating, the trained models were evaluated with the testing data containing 20% of the data. The testing dataset was used to provide an unbiased evaluation of a final model fit on the training dataset [29]. This testing dataset was not used for training. Since a 5-fold cross-validation was used, all samples were tested in the testing dataset. The models' predicted clinical scores of the testing data were compared with the true clinical scores, to calculate the precision, recall and F1 score of the model when used on unseen data [29].

Most datasets contain a severe skew in the class distribution, which could lead to the machine learning algorithms performing poorly on the minority classes. To address this problem, the training data was oversampled to equalize the number of samples per score.

Different models were trained, validated, and tested using four different settings for each type of the six machine learning algorithms. This was done for both the upper extremities dataset and the lower extremities dataset. Models were trained (1) using all features (ALL), (2) using all features and hyperparameter tuning to find the optimal set of hyperparameters (ALL + HYP), (3) with selected features (SFS) and (4) using selected features and hyperparameter tuning (SFS + HYP) (Table 3).

Table 3. Types of models used for training, validating, and testing.

Model	Features	Hyperparameter Tuning
ML model (ALL)	All features	no
ML model (ALL + HYP)	All features	yes
ML model (SFS)	Selected features with SFS	no
ML model (SFS + HYP)	Selected features with SFS	yes

ML = machine learning; ALL = all features; SFS = Sequential feature selection; HYP = hyperparameter tuning.

For the ALL + HYP and SFS + HYP, the hyperparameters were determined using a Bayesian optimization algorithm with 15 iterations during the first fold (Table 3). The found hyperparameters were then used during the remaining folds to test for the model's precision, recall and F1 score.

Individual models (i.e., using the data of one participant only) as well as generalized models (i.e., using all data) were trained. The performance for each model was calculated. The trained individual models were tested on holdout testing data using 5-fold cross-validation. Generalized models were evaluated using leave-two-subjects-out cross-validation (6-fold). For each of the 6 folds, data from 10 subjects was used for training and validating (5-fold cross-validation), and tested on the data from the two left-out subjects.

As main performance metric the F1 score was computed, which used the precision and recall (Equations (3)–(5)), calculated from 'True positive' (TP), 'False positive' (FP), and 'False negative' (FN) scores. F1 scores were calculated after training and validating, and after testing the models on the holdout test data. Per patient, the models with the highest F1 scores were selected as the final models for that patient. In addition, for the generalized models the root mean square errors (RMSE) was calculated and confusion matrix plotted for better interpretation of the model performance.

$$\text{precision} = \frac{\text{TP}}{\text{TP} + \text{FP}} \tag{3}$$

$$\text{recall} = \frac{\text{TP}}{\text{TP} + \text{FN}} \tag{4}$$

$$\text{F1 score} = 2 \cdot \frac{\text{precision} \cdot \text{recall}}{\text{precision} + \text{recall}} \tag{5}$$

3. Results

3.1. Datasets

Two patients were measured within the movement laboratory mimicking a home environment and activities, the other ten patients were measured at home by parents/caregivers. Even though parents/caregivers were instructed to record 10 one-minute videos each day, there were large differences in the number of samples (5-s time windows) in the final datasets for each subject. Not all parents/caregivers filmed as many videos as they were instructed. One participant stopped after one measurement due to uncomfortableness while attaching and wearing the sensors. The data of this subject were excluded for the individual trained models. Furthermore, errors in the sensors occurred for some measurements, resulting in loss of data. The most common errors were failure of one or more sensors and an error in the synchronization between the sensors. Moreover, not all windows could be scored because certain body parts were not visible on the videos. These factors led to different sizes of datasets for each subject. Table 4 lists the number of samples in each dataset of each subject. See Supplementary S2 for an overview of the distribution of the scores for each patient. The full dataset is available (Supplementary S3).

Table 4. Overview of best individual model per dataset for each patient.

Subject	Dataset	Samples	Best Algorithm	Model	F1 Score Validation	F1 Score Test	Precision Test	Recall Test
Subject 1	dys lower	720	KNN	ALL + HYP	1	0.50	0.98	0.33
	dys upper	726	KNN	SFS	0.92	0.74	0.74	0.75
Subject 2	dys lower	189	KNN	ALL	0.94	0.93	0.93	0.93
	dys upper	186	KNN	SFS + HYP	0.88	0.75	0.73	0.77
Subject 4	dys lower	120	KNN	ALL	1	0.74	0.87	0.64
	dys upper	125	KNN	SFS	0.97	0.70	0.85	0.60
Subject 5	dys lower	338	KNN	ALL	1	0.66	0.96	0.50
	dys upper	441	KNN	SFS	0.98	0.96	0.95	0.98
Subject 6	dys lower	66	n/a	n/a	n/a	n/a	n/a	n/a
	dys upper	66	KNN	ALL + HYP	0.96	0.60	0.65	0.73

Table 4. Cont.

Subject	Dataset	Samples	Best Algorithm	Model	F1 Score Validation	F1 Score Test	Precision Test	Recall Test
Subject 7	dys lower	334	KNN	ALL	0.95	0.82	0.81	0.83
	dys upper	336	NB	ALL + HYP	0.97	0.59	0.73	0.50
Subject 8	dys lower	336	NB	ALL + HYP	1	0.62	0.81	0.50
	dys upper	298	KNN	SFS	0.93	0.64	0.73	0.58
Subject 9	dys lower	588	KNN	ALL + HYP	0.93	0.85	0.84	0.85
	dys upper	583	KNN	ALL	0.97	0.75	0.86	0.66
Subject 10	dys lower	514	n/a	n/a	n/a	n/a	1	1
	dys upper	510	KNN	SFS	0.97	0.53	0.53	0.54
Subject 11	dys lower	478	KNN	ALL + HYP	0.97	0.37	0.43	0.33
	dys upper	444	ENS	ALL	0.84	0.76	0.75	0.77
Subject 12	dys lower	775	KNN	SFS	0.93	0.51	0.61	0.44
	dys upper	1237	ENS	ALL	0.85	0.46	0.54	0.41

Dys lower = dystonia of lower extremity; Dys upper = Dystonia of upper extremity; NB = Naïve Bayes; KNN = k-nearest neighbors; ENS = Ensemble Learning; ALL = all features; SFS = Sequential feature selection; HYP = hyperparameter tuning.

3.2. Individual Clinical Scores Classification

Table 4 gives an overview of the best models (algorithm and model type) of each patient, together with the corresponding F1 scores, precision and recall. k-nearest neighbors algorithms led to the highest F1 validation score in most datasets and were therefore most often chosen as final model. Table 5 gives and overview of the mean F1 scores, precision and recall of all best models combined. High F1 scores (0.97 ± 0.03 for lower extremity dystonia and 0.93 ± 0.06 for upper extremity dystonia) were observed during validation of the individual models. In the independent test datasets, the F1 scores (0.67 ± 0.19 for lower extremity dystonia and 0.68 ± 0.14 for upper extremity dystonia) were lower (Table 5).

Table 5. Overview of mean F1 score, precision and recall.

Dataset	Mean F1 Score Validation	Mean F1 Score Test	Mean Precision Test	Mean Recall Test
dys lower	0.97 ± 0.03	0.67 ± 0.19	0.82 ± 0.18	0.66 ± 0.26
dys upper	0.93 ± 0.06	0.68 ± 0.14	0.73 ± 0.13	0.66 ± 0.16

Dys lower = dystonia of lower extremity; Dys upper = Dystonia of upper extremity.

3.3. Generalized Clinical Scores Classification

See Table 6 for an overview of the best models per dataset. Figures 4 and 5 show the confusion matrices of the datasets. The generalized model showed lower F1 scores (0.45 for the lower extremities and 0.34 for the upper extremities) in the test datasets than the individual models. F1 scores were high in the validation data sets, but significantly lower in the test data sets, indicating the model does not work equally as well on unseen data. The majority of misclassifications occurred in neighbouring clinical scores, since they present similar behaviours. The RMSE were 1.07 for dystonia lower extremties and 0.98 for dystonia upper extremites, respectively. A clinical score of 4 in the dystonia upper extremities data set was never correcly classified, likely due to a lack of training samples during training of the models.

Table 6. Overview of best generalized model per dataset.

Dataset	Samples	Best Algorithm	Model	F1 Score Validation	F1 Score Test	Precision Test	Recall Test
dys lower	4533	ENS	SFS	0.93	0.45	0.43	0.48
dys upper	4976	KNN	SFS	0.91	0.34	0.32	0.36

Dys lower = dystonia of lower extremity; Dys upper = Dystonia of upper extremity; KNN = k-nearest neighbors; ENS = Ensemble Learning; SFS = Sequential feature selection.

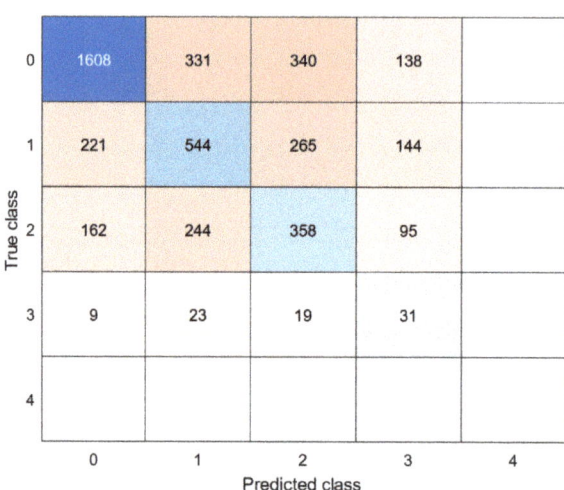

Figure 4. Confusion matrix: generalized model of lower extremities dystonia.

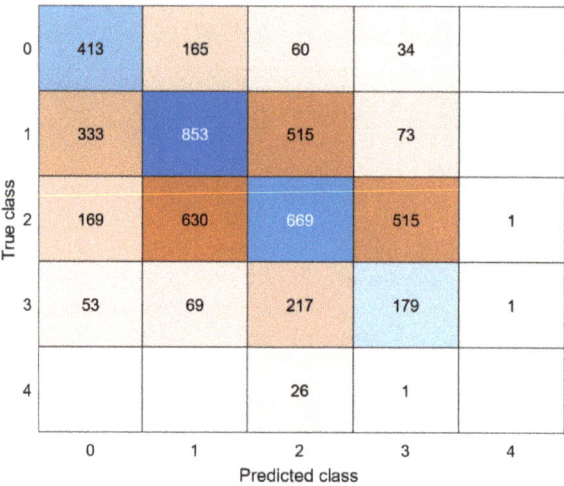

Figure 5. Confusion matrix: generalized model of upper extremities dystonia.

4. Discussion

Within this study, the feasibility was assessed to train machine learning models with a sufficient performance within dyskinetic CP by using home-based measured IMU and video data, collected by parents/caregivers.

In summary, most of the parents/caregivers were able to collect enough data to clinically score the videos and use IMUs data for feature calculation. For 1 patient out of 12, discomfort due to the fixation of sensors was reported. We consider the performance (i.e., F1 score) of the individual trained model as moderate and the overall performance of the generalized models as low. However, when looking at the confusion matrices, the misclassifications were most often observed in neighboring classes, indicating that these models are reasonably able to correlate between the severity of the disorder and the clinical score. This observation is confirmed by the RMSEs of about 1 on a 4-point scale.

The current results are in line with previous studies using wearable IMUs or accelerometers within other patient populations (e.g., Parkinson's disease [30–32] and Huntington's disease [19], showing that it is feasible to automatically predict the severity of movement disorders such as tremor, bradykinesia and dyskinesia. Most studies using wearables to monitor movement disorders have been performed within Parkinson's disease including steps towards clinical implementation (i.e., assessment of measurement properties of methods). However, widespread clinical use is still lacking [16,18]. When relating the current results to studies in Parkinson's disease, reported performance are comparable: e.g., Tsipouras et al. [31] used IMUs to automatically classify lepodova-induced dyskinesia within standardized tasks on a 0–4 scale, using machine learning algorithms and multiple combinations of sensors and features. A generalized model within this study achieved an average accuracy (79% $\pm$ 11%) [31]. However, the results need to be interpreted with care as no independent test set was used and no F1 scores were computed. Another study used sensors placed on the upper and lower extremities. A high correlation between the estimated dyskinesia severity scores was found between the model prediction and the expert-rated scores on (r = 0.77 ($p < 0.001$)) [33]. Although the population of Parkinson's disease and dyskinetic CP are not directly comparable, it indicates the potential of the proposed methodology for individuals with dyskinetic CP. A current study suggested that IMUs can be used as a mobile alternative for marker-based motion capture (omitting the need for an advanced movement laboratory) within upper extremity movements analysis of standardize movements in dyskinetic CP [14]. The proposed methodology goes one step further by using home-based collected IMUs data within unstandardized situations. This methodology is especially interesting for individuals who cannot perform standardized movements (such as gait and reaching/grasping), where instrumented methods are lacking [34]. In addition, the methodology gives the opportunity to capture the variability within dystonia for a longer period of time. The results show that within an individual, dystonia is 'consistent' enough to be detected within unseen data. However, this is not true for all individuals (i.e., subject 11 and subject 12 showed lower F1 scores within the test set). The same applies to the generalized models. A possible inconsistency within data of individuals as well as between individuals could be explained by, on the one hand, the challenge for clinicians to score home-based videos consistently and, on the other hand, the variation of dystonia concerning velocity and position that can occur within and between individuals [20]. As the performance of machine learning models greatly depends on the amount, the coverage and quality of the data, the performance of individual model would most likely increase with the collection of more data from each individual, as well as measures from more patients.

A limitation of this study is the low number of subjects included, which limits the amount of data used to train and test the generalized models. Another limitation of this study is that data was collected only at certain fixed moments, which were mainly standing, sitting, and lying down. The developed models are therefore not properly trained with data from other everyday activities. This is likely to lead to inaccuracies in the predictions if the models are used to predict data over an entire day. Future research should focus on gathering more types of movements and activities, to train even more accurate predictive models. The model might also improve by adding IMUs data from children and young adults without a movement disorder, especially as it has been hypothesized that overflow movements seen in dystonia may contain a small repertoire of involuntary movements within a more variable repertoire of intended voluntary movements [35]. As collection of more and variable data might be difficult to perform on large scale, possible data augmentation techniques for time series should be considered in future studies [36]. In addition, it could be an option to perform a 'calibration measurement' for each individual before using sensors in a home environment [16], add some extra clinical scores on time windows and use transfer learning (i.e., adding the individual scored data to the pre-trained generalized model) to improve the performance of the generalized models for each patient individually.

Since the results of this study demonstrated the feasibility of monitoring dystonia at home, it would be interesting to study the use of the models for treatment assessment (e.g., how the clinical scores vary before and after intrathecal baclofen treatment), with the hypothesis that the clinical scores will decline after the treatment. Moreover, the methods described in this paper could also be used to classify choreoathetosis, which also occurs in dyskinetic CP. However, there was too little variation in the scores in the current data to train models to classify choreoathetosis.

5. Conclusions

The results of this study indicate that it is feasible to assess dystonia in dyskinetic CP outside a clinical setting, using home measurements and individually trained machine learning models and thereby provide clinical useful information about the progression of dystonia during a longer period of time. The findings are in line with previous research on automatic assessment of dyskinesia in Parkinson's disease. To enhance clinical care, future studies should evaluate how standard dyskinetic CP measures can be complemented by providing frequent, objective, real-world assessments. Even though the generalized models achieved low F1 scores, they are reasonably able to link high clinical scores to high severity of the disorder and vice versa, even though they were trained with a limited amount of data. Future research should focus on gathering more high-quality data and study how the models perform over longer periods of time.

Supplementary Materials: The following supporting information can be downloaded at: https://www.mdpi.com/article/10.3390/s22124386/s1, Supplementary S1: Matlabcode to train machine learning models from data: https://doi.org/10.5281/zenodo.6379348 (accessed on 3 May 2022); Supplementary S2: Samples per clinical score for each subject. Supplementary S3: Dataset: Inertial sensor data and appertaining clinical scores: https://doi.org/10.5281/zenodo.6379451 (accessed on 3 May 2022).

Author Contributions: Methodology, validation, design, writing—original draft preparation, D.d.H. and H.H.; supervision, A.I.B., M.M.v.d.K. and L.A.B.; writing—critical review, interpretation and editing, M.M.v.d.K., S.v.d.B., I.A., J.G., L.A.B., J.H. and A.I.B. All authors have read and agreed to the published version of the manuscript.

Funding: The project was funded by the Netherlands Organization for Health Research and Development (ZonMW, Innovative medical device initiative (IMDI) project number 104022005). Moveshelf Labs B.V. (Utrecht, NL) provided support and in-kind contribution to the project. Support is provided by the Small-Scale Initiatives in Machine Learning (OpenSSI 2021) of the Netherlands eScience Center. Helga Haberfehlner is funded by the Postdoctoral Fellow Marie Skłodowska-Curie Actions—Seal of Excellence of the Research Foundation—Flanders (SoE fellowship_12ZZW22N).

Institutional Review Board Statement: Ethical review and approval were waived for this study by the Medical Ethics Committee of the VU University Medical Center (registered with the US Office for Human Research Projections (OHRP) as IRB00002991), as the Medical Research Involving Human Subjects Act (Wet Medisch-wetenschappelijk Onderzoek met mensen, WMO) does not apply to the current study.

Informed Consent Statement: Informed consent was obtained from all subjects involved in the study.

Data Availability Statement: The dataset analyzed during the current study and code is available on zenodo. Dataset: https://doi.org/10.5281/zenodo.6379451 (accessed on 3 May 2022); Code: https://doi.org/10.5281/zenodo.6379348 (accessed on 3 May 2022).

Acknowledgments: The authors wish to express their gratitude to the people involved in the user committee for their insightful comments and feedback, as well as to the enrolled subjects who voluntarily participated in this study. The authors acknowledge the contribution to the presented work of Constance Pieters and Nienke Heida, who clinically scored the videos, Karen Lagendijk and Benaja Feijter for their help in including patients, Simone Berkelmans and Karen Stolk, who helped in the preparation of the protocols and performed pilot measurements for the study.

Conflicts of Interest: Ignazio Aleo is the CEO of Moveshelf Labs B.V. (Utrecht, NL). Johannes Gijsbers is the VP of Product of the same company. Moveshelf Labs B.V. develops and commercializes Moveshelf for Movement Science, an Information system for Clinical Movement Analysis. They contributed to the conception and design of the study, revised the article for intellectual content, and provided approval of the submitted version. They were not involved with the data collection, analysis and with the interpretation of the results, or in the decision to publish the results.

References

1. Graham, H.K.; Rosenbaum, P.; Paneth, N.; Dan, B.; Lin, J.P.; Damiano, D.L.; Becher, J.G.; Gaebler-Spira, D.; Colver, A.; Reddihough, D.S.; et al. Cerebral Palsy. *Nat. Rev. Dis. Primers* **2016**, *2*, 15082. [CrossRef] [PubMed]
2. Himmelmann, K.; McManus, V.; Hagberg, G.; Uvebrant, P.; Krägeloh-Mann, I.; Cans, C.; on behalf of the SCPE Collaboration. Dyskinetic Cerebral Palsy in Europe: Trends in Prevalence and Severity. *Arch. Dis. Child.* **2009**, *94*, 921–926. [CrossRef] [PubMed]
3. Monbaliu, E.; Himmelmann, K.; Lin, J.P.; Ortibus, E.; Bonouvrié, L.; Feys, H.; Vermeulen, R.J.; Dan, B. Clinical Presentation and Management of Dyskinetic Cerebral Palsy. *Lancet. Neurol.* **2017**, *16*, 741–749. [CrossRef]
4. Bohn, E.; Goren, K.; Switzer, L.; Falck-Ytter, Y.; Fehlings, D. Pharmacological and Neurosurgical Interventions for Individuals with Cerebral Palsy and Dystonia: A Systematic Review Update and Meta-Analysis. *Dev. Med. Child. Neurol.* **2021**, *63*, 1038–1050. [CrossRef] [PubMed]
5. Bonouvrié, L.A.; Becher, J.G.; Vles, J.S.; Vermeulen, R.J.; Buizer, A.I.; Idys Study Group. The Effect of Intrathecal Baclofen in Dyskinetic Cerebral Palsy: The Idys Trial. *Ann. Neurol.* **2019**, *86*, 79–90. [CrossRef] [PubMed]
6. Bonouvrié, L.A.; Haberfehlner, H.; Becher, J.G.; Vles, J.S.; Vermeulen, R.J.; Buizer, A.I.; Idys Study Group. Attainment of Personal Goals in the First Year of Intrathecal Baclofen Treatment in Dyskinetic Cerebral Palsy: A Prospective Cohort Study. *Disabil. Rehabil.* **2022**, 1–8. [CrossRef]
7. Sanger, T.D. Deep Brain Stimulation for Cerebral Palsy: Where Are We Now? *Dev. Med. Child. Neurol.* **2020**, *62*, 28–33.
8. Stewart, K.; Harvey, A.; Johnston, L.M. A Systematic Review of Scales to Measure Dystonia and Choreoathetosis in Children with Dyskinetic Cerebral Palsy. *Dev. Med. Child. Neurol.* **2017**, *59*, 786–795. [CrossRef]
9. Sanger, T.D.; Delgado, M.R.; Gaebler-Spira, D.; Hallett, M.; Mink, J.W.; Task Force on Childhood Motor Disorders. Classification and Definition of Disorders Causing Hypertonia in Childhood. *Pediatrics* **2003**, *111*, e89–e97. [CrossRef]
10. States, R.A.; Krzak, J.J.; Salem, E.M.; Bodkin, A.W.; McMulkin, M.L. Instrumented Gait Analysis for Management of Gait Disorders in Children with Cerebral Palsy: A Scoping Review. *Gait Posture* **2021**, *90*, 1–8. [CrossRef]
11. Francisco-Martínez, C.; Prado-Olivarez, J.; Padilla-Medina, J.A.; Díaz-Carmona, J.; Pérez-Pinal, F.J.; Barranco-Gutiérrez, A.I.; Martínez-Nolasco, J.J. Upper Limb Movement Measurement Systems for Cerebral Palsy: A Systematic Literature Review. *Sensors* **2021**, *21*, 7884. [CrossRef] [PubMed]
12. Kidzinski, L.; Yang, B.; Hicks, J.L.; Rajagopal, A.; Delp, S.L.; Schwartz, M.H. Deep neural networks enable quantitative movement analysis using single-camera videos. *Nat. Commun.* **2020**, *11*, 4054. [CrossRef] [PubMed]
13. Khaksar, S.; Pan, H.; Borazjani, B.; Murray, I.; Agrawal, H.; Liu, W.; Elliott, C.; Imms, C.; Campbell, A.; Walmsley, C. Application of Inertial Measurement Units and Machine Learning Classification in Cerebral Palsy: Randomized Controlled Trial. *JMIR Rehabil. Assist. Technol.* **2021**, *8*, e29769. [CrossRef] [PubMed]
14. Vanmechelen, I.; Bekteshi, S.; Konings, M.; Feys, H.; Desloovere, K.; Aerts, J.M.; Monbaliu, E. Upper limb movement characteristics of children and youth with dyskinetic cerebral palsy—A sensor approach. *Gait Posture* **2020**, *81*, 377–378. [CrossRef]
15. Silva, N.; Zhang, D.; Kulvicius, T.; Gail, A.; Barreiros, C.; Lindstaedt, S.; Kraft, M.; Bolte, S.; Poustka, L.; Nielsen-Saines, K.; et al. The future of General Movement Assessment: The role of computer vision and machine learning—A scoping review. *Res. Dev. Disabil.* **2021**, *110*, 103854. [CrossRef] [PubMed]
16. Ancona, S.; Faraci, F.D.; Khatab, E.; Fiorillo, L.; Gnarra, O.; Nef, T.; Bassetti, C.L.A.; Bargiotas, P. Wearables in the home-based assessment of abnormal movements in Parkinson's disease: a systematic review of the literature. *J. Neurol.* **2022**, *269*, 100–110. [CrossRef]
17. Pulliam, C.L.; Heldman, D.A.; Brokaw, E.B.; Mera, T.O.; Mari, Z.K.; Burack, M.A. Continuous Assessment of Levodopa Response in Parkinson's Disease Using Wearable Motion Sensors. *IEEE Trans. Biomed. Eng.* **2018**, *65*, 159–164. [CrossRef]
18. Del Din, S.; Kirk, C.; Yarnall, A.J.; Rochester, L.; Hausdorff, J.M. Body-Worn Sensors for Remote Monitoring of Parkinson's Disease Motor Symptoms: Vision, State of the Art, and Challenges Ahead. *J. Parkinsons Dis.* **2021**, *11*, S35–S47. [CrossRef]
19. Bennasar, M.; Hicks, Y.A.; Clinch, S.P.; Jones, P.; Holt, C.; Rosser, A.; Busse, M. Automated Assessment of Movement Impairment in Huntington's Disease. *IEEE Trans. Neural. Syst. Rehabil. Eng.* **2018**, *26*, 2062–2069. [CrossRef]

20. Sanger, T.D. Arm trajectories in dyskinetic cerebral palsy have increased random variability. *J. Child. Neurol.* **2006**, *21*, 551–557. [CrossRef]
21. Monbaliu, E.; de Cock, P.; Ortibus, E.; Heyrman, L.; Klingels, K.; Feys, H. Clinical patterns of dystonia and choreoathetosis in participants with dyskinetic cerebral palsy. *Dev. Med. Child. Neurol.* **2016**, *58*, 138–144. [CrossRef] [PubMed]
22. Vanmechelen, I.; Bekteshi, S.; Konings, M.; Feys, H.; Desloovere, K.; Aerts, J.-M.; Monbaliu, E. Psychometric properties of upper limb kinematics during functional tasks in children and adolescents with dyskinetic cerebral palsy. *medRxiv* **2022**. [CrossRef]
23. Rosenbaum, P.; Paneth, N.; Leviton, A.; Goldstein, M.; Bax, M.; Damiano, D.; Dan, B.; Jacobsson, B. A report: The definition and classification of cerebral palsy April 2006. *Dev. Med. Child. Neurol.* **2007**, *109*, 8–14.
24. SCPE. Prevalence and characteristics of children with cerebral palsy in Europe. *Dev. Med. Child. Neurol.* **2002**, *44*, 633–640.
25. Monbaliu, E.; Ortibus, E.; de Cat, J.; Dan, B.; Heyrman, L.; Prinzie, P.; De Cock, P.; Feys, H. The dyskinesia Impairment Scale: A new instrument to measure dystonia and choreoathetosis in dyskinetic cerebral palsy. *Dev. Med. Child. Neurol.* **2012**, *54*, 278–283. [CrossRef]
26. Patel, S.; Lorincz, K.; Hughes, R.; Huggins, N.; Growdon, J.; Standaert, D.; Akay, M.; Dy, J.; Welsh, M.; Bonato, P. Monitoring motor fluctuations in patients with Parkinson's disease using wearable sensors. *IEEE Trans. Inf. Technol. Biomed.* **2009**, *13*, 864–873. [CrossRef]
27. Kuhn, M.; Johnson, K. An Introduction to Feature Selection. In *Applied Predictive Modeling*; Kuhn, M., Johnson, K., Eds.; Springer: New York, NY, USA, 2013; pp. 487–519.
28. Hartog, D.D.; Harlaar, J.; Smit, G. The Stumblemeter: Design and Validation of a System That Detects and Classifies Stumbles during Gait. *Sensors* **2021**, *21*, 6636. [CrossRef]
29. Halilaj, E.; Rajagopal, A.; Fiterau, M.; Hicks, J.L.; Hastie, T.J.; Delp, S.L. Machine learning in human movement biomechanics: Best practices, common pitfalls, and new opportunities. *J. Biomech.* **2018**, *81*, 1–11. [CrossRef]
30. Keijsers, N.L.; Horstink, M.W.; Gielen, S.C. Automatic assessment of levodopa-induced dyskinesias in daily life by neural networks. *Mov. Disord.* **2003**, *18*, 70–80. [CrossRef]
31. Tsipouras, M.G.; Tzallas, A.T.; Rigas, G.; Tsouli, S.; Fotiadis, D.I.; Konitsiotis, S. An automated methodology for levodopa-induced dyskinesia: Assessment based on gyroscope and accelerometer signals. *Artif. Intell. Med.* **2012**, *55*, 127–135. [CrossRef]
32. Rodriguez-Molinero, A.; Perez-Lopez, C.; Sama, A.; Rodriguez-Martin, D.; Alcaine, S.; Mestre, B.; Quispe, P.; Giuliani, B.; Vainstein, G.; Browne, P.; et al. Estimating dyskinesia severity in Parkinson's disease by using a waist-worn sensor: Concurrent validity study. *Sci. Rep.* **2019**, *9*, 13434. [PubMed]
33. Hssayeni, M.D.; Jimenez-Shahed, J.; Burack, M.A.; Ghoraani, B. Dyskinesia estimation during activities of daily living using wearable motion sensors and deep recurrent networks. *Sci. Rep.* **2021**, *11*, 7865. [CrossRef] [PubMed]
34. Haberfehlner, H.; Goudriaan, M.; Bonouvrie, L.A.; Jansma, E.P.; Harlaar, J.; Vermeulen, R.J.; Van der Krogt, M.M.; Buizer, A.I. Instrumented assessment of motor function in dyskinetic cerebral palsy: A systematic review. *J. Neuroeng. Rehabil.* **2020**, *17*, 39. [CrossRef] [PubMed]
35. Sanger, T.D.; Ferman, D. Similarity of Involuntary Postures between Different Children with Dystonia. *Mov. Disord. Clin. Pract.* **2017**, *4*, 870–874. [CrossRef] [PubMed]
36. Yeomans, J.; Thwaites, S.; Robertson, W.S.P.; Booth, D.; Ng, B.; Thewlis, D. Simulating Time-Series Data for Improved Deep Neural Network Performance. *IEEE Access* **2019**, *7*, 131248–131255.

Acknowledgments: The authors wish to express their gratitude to the people involved in the user committee for their insightful comments and feedback, as well as to the enrolled subjects who voluntarily participated in this study. The authors acknowledge the contribution to the presented work of Constance Pieters and Nienke Heida, who clinically scored the videos, Karen Lagendijk and Benaja Feijter for their help in including patients, Simone Berkelmans and Karen Stolk, who helped in the preparation of the protocols and performed pilot measurements for the study.

Conflicts of Interest: Ignazio Aleo is the CEO of Moveshelf Labs B.V. (Utrecht, NL). Johannes Gijsbers is the VP of Product of the same company. Moveshelf Labs B.V. develops and commercializes Moveshelf for Movement Science, an Information system for Clinical Movement Analysis. They contributed to the conception and design of the study, revised the article for intellectual content, and provided approval of the submitted version. They were not involved with the data collection, analysis and with the interpretation of the results, or in the decision to publish the results.

References

1. Graham, H.K.; Rosenbaum, P.; Paneth, N.; Dan, B.; Lin, J.P.; Damiano, D.L.; Becher, J.G.; Gaebler-Spira, D.; Colver, A.; Reddihough, D.S.; et al. Cerebral Palsy. *Nat. Rev. Dis. Primers* **2016**, *2*, 15082. [CrossRef] [PubMed]
2. Himmelmann, K.; McManus, V.; Hagberg, G.; Uvebrant, P.; Krägeloh-Mann, I.; Cans, C.; on behalf of the SCPE Collaboration. Dyskinetic Cerebral Palsy in Europe: Trends in Prevalence and Severity. *Arch. Dis. Child.* **2009**, *94*, 921–926. [CrossRef] [PubMed]
3. Monbaliu, E.; Himmelmann, K.; Lin, J.P.; Ortibus, E.; Bonouvrié, L.; Feys, H.; Vermeulen, R.J.; Dan, B. Clinical Presentation and Management of Dyskinetic Cerebral Palsy. *Lancet. Neurol.* **2017**, *16*, 741–749. [CrossRef]
4. Bohn, E.; Goren, K.; Switzer, L.; Falck-Ytter, Y.; Fehlings, D. Pharmacological and Neurosurgical Interventions for Individuals with Cerebral Palsy and Dystonia: A Systematic Review Update and Meta-Analysis. *Dev. Med. Child. Neurol.* **2021**, *63*, 1038–1050. [CrossRef] [PubMed]
5. Bonouvrié, L.A.; Becher, J.G.; Vles, J.S.; Vermeulen, R.J.; Buizer, A.I.; Idys Study Group. The Effect of Intrathecal Baclofen in Dyskinetic Cerebral Palsy: The Idys Trial. *Ann. Neurol.* **2019**, *86*, 79–90. [CrossRef] [PubMed]
6. Bonouvrié, L.A.; Haberfehlner, H.; Becher, J.G.; Vles, J.S.; Vermeulen, R.J.; Buizer, A.I.; Idys Study Group. Attainment of Personal Goals in the First Year of Intrathecal Baclofen Treatment in Dyskinetic Cerebral Palsy: A Prospective Cohort Study. *Disabil. Rehabil.* **2022**, 1–8. [CrossRef]
7. Sanger, T.D. Deep Brain Stimulation for Cerebral Palsy: Where Are We Now? *Dev. Med. Child. Neurol.* **2020**, *62*, 28–33.
8. Stewart, K.; Harvey, A.; Johnston, L.M. A Systematic Review of Scales to Measure Dystonia and Choreoathetosis in Children with Dyskinetic Cerebral Palsy. *Dev. Med. Child. Neurol.* **2017**, *59*, 786–795. [CrossRef]
9. Sanger, T.D.; Delgado, M.R.; Gaebler-Spira, D.; Hallett, M.; Mink, J.W.; Task Force on Childhood Motor Disorders. Classification and Definition of Disorders Causing Hypertonia in Childhood. *Pediatrics* **2003**, *111*, e89–e97. [CrossRef]
10. States, R.A.; Krzak, J.J.; Salem, Y.; Godwin, E.M.; Bodkin, A.W.; McMulkin, M.L. Instrumented Gait Analysis for Management of Gait Disorders in Children with Cerebral Palsy: A Scoping Review. *Gait Posture* **2021**, *90*, 1–8. [CrossRef]
11. Francisco-Martínez, C.; Prado-Olivarez, J.; Padilla-Medina, J.A.; Díaz-Carmona, J.; Pérez-Pinal, F.J.; Barranco-Gutiérrez, A.I.; Martínez-Nolasco, J.J. Upper Limb Movement Measurement Systems for Cerebral Palsy: A Systematic Literature Review. *Sensors* **2021**, *21*, 7884. [CrossRef] [PubMed]
12. Kidzinski, L.; Yang, B.; Hicks, J.L.; Rajagopal, A.; Delp, S.L.; Schwartz, M.H. Deep neural networks enable quantitative movement analysis using single-camera videos. *Nat. Commun.* **2020**, *11*, 4054. [CrossRef] [PubMed]
13. Khaksar, S.; Pan, H.; Borazjani, B.; Murray, I.; Agrawal, H.; Liu, W.; Elliott, C.; Imms, C.; Campbell, A.; Walmsley, C. Application of Inertial Measurement Units and Machine Learning Classification in Cerebral Palsy: Randomized Controlled Trial. *JMIR Rehabil. Assist. Technol.* **2021**, *8*, e29769. [CrossRef] [PubMed]
14. Vanmechelen, I.; Bekteshi, S.; Konings, M.; Feys, H.; Desloovere, K.; Aerts, J.M.; Monbaliu, E. Upper limb movement characteristics of children and youth with dyskinetic cerebral palsy—A sensor approach. *Gait Posture* **2020**, *81*, 377–378. [CrossRef]
15. Silva, N.; Zhang, D.; Kulvicius, T.; Gail, A.; Barreiros, C.; Lindstaedt, S.; Kraft, M.; Bolte, S.; Poustka, L.; Nielsen-Saines, K.; et al. The future of General Movement Assessment: The role of computer vision and machine learning—A scoping review. *Res. Dev. Disabil.* **2021**, *110*, 103854. [CrossRef] [PubMed]
16. Ancona, S.; Faraci, F.D.; Khatab, E.; Fiorillo, L.; Gnarra, O.; Nef, T.; Bassetti, C.L.A.; Bargiotas, P. Wearables in the home-based assessment of abnormal movements in Parkinson's disease: A systematic review of the literature. *J. Neurol.* **2022**, *269*, 100–110. [CrossRef]
17. Pulliam, C.L.; Heldman, D.A.; Brokaw, E.B.; Mera, T.O.; Mari, Z.K.; Burack, M.A. Continuous Assessment of Levodopa Response in Parkinson's Disease Using Wearable Motion Sensors. *IEEE Trans. Biomed. Eng.* **2018**, *65*, 159–164. [CrossRef]
18. Del Din, S.; Kirk, C.; Yarnall, A.J.; Rochester, L.; Hausdorff, J.M. Body-Worn Sensors for Remote Monitoring of Parkinson's Disease Motor Symptoms: Vision, State of the Art, and Challenges Ahead. *J. Parkinsons Dis.* **2021**, *11*, S35–S47. [CrossRef]
19. Bennasar, M.; Hicks, Y.A.; Clinch, S.P.; Jones, P.; Holt, C.; Rosser, A.; Busse, M. Automated Assessment of Movement Impairment in Huntington's Disease. *IEEE Trans. Neural. Syst. Rehabil. Eng.* **2018**, *26*, 2062–2069. [CrossRef]

20. Sanger, T.D. Arm trajectories in dyskinetic cerebral palsy have increased random variability. *J. Child. Neurol.* **2006**, *21*, 551–557. [CrossRef]
21. Monbaliu, E.; de Cock, P.; Ortibus, E.; Heyrman, L.; Klingels, K.; Feys, H. Clinical patterns of dystonia and choreoathetosis in participants with dyskinetic cerebral palsy. *Dev. Med. Child. Neurol.* **2016**, *58*, 138–144. [CrossRef] [PubMed]
22. Vanmechelen, I.; Bekteshi, S.; Konings, M.; Feys, H.; Desloovere, K.; Aerts, J.-M.; Monbaliu, E. Psychometric properties of upper limb kinematics during functional tasks in children and adolescents with dyskinetic cerebral palsy. *medRxiv* **2022**. [CrossRef]
23. Rosenbaum, P.; Paneth, N.; Leviton, A.; Goldstein, M.; Bax, M.; Damiano, D.; Dan, B.; Jacobsson, B. A report: The definition and classification of cerebral palsy April 2006. *Dev. Med. Child. Neurol.* **2007**, *109*, 8–14.
24. SCPE. Prevalence and characteristics of children with cerebral palsy in Europe. *Dev. Med. Child. Neurol.* **2002**, *44*, 633–640.
25. Monbaliu, E.; Ortibus, E.; de Cat, J.; Dan, B.; Heyrman, L.; Prinzie, P.; De Cock, P.; Feys, H. The dyskinesia Impairment Scale: A new instrument to measure dystonia and choreoathetosis in dyskinetic cerebral palsy. *Dev. Med. Child. Neurol.* **2012**, *54*, 278–283. [CrossRef]
26. Patel, S.; Lorincz, K.; Hughes, R.; Huggins, N.; Growdon, J.; Standaert, D.; Akay, M.; Dy, J.; Welsh, M.; Bonato, P. Monitoring motor fluctuations in patients with Parkinson's disease using wearable sensors. *IEEE Trans. Inf. Technol. Biomed.* **2009**, *13*, 864–873. [CrossRef]
27. Kuhn, M.; Johnson, K. An Introduction to Feature Selection. In *Applied Predictive Modeling*; Kuhn, M., Johnson, K., Eds.; Springer: New York, NY, USA, 2013; pp. 487–519.
28. Hartog, D.D.; Harlaar, J.; Smit, G. The Stumblemeter: Design and Validation of a System That Detects and Classifies Stumbles during Gait. *Sensors* **2021**, *21*, 6636. [CrossRef]
29. Halilaj, E.; Rajagopal, A.; Fiterau, M.; Hicks, J.L.; Hastie, T.J.; Delp, S.L. Machine learning in human movement biomechanics: Best practices, common pitfalls, and new opportunities. *J. Biomech.* **2018**, *81*, 1–11. [CrossRef]
30. Keijsers, N.L.; Horstink, M.W.; Gielen, S.C. Automatic assessment of levodopa-induced dyskinesias in daily life by neural networks. *Mov. Disord.* **2003**, *18*, 70–80. [CrossRef]
31. Tsipouras, M.G.; Tzallas, A.T.; Rigas, G.; Tsouli, S.; Fotiadis, D.I.; Konitsiotis, S. An automated methodology for levodopa-induced dyskinesia: Assessment based on gyroscope and accelerometer signals. *Artif. Intell. Med.* **2012**, *55*, 127–135. [CrossRef]
32. Rodriguez-Molinero, A.; Perez-Lopez, C.; Sama, A.; Rodriguez-Martin, D.; Alcaine, S.; Mestre, B.; Quispe, P.; Giuliani, B.; Vainstein, G.; Browne, P.; et al. Estimating dyskinesia severity in Parkinson's disease by using a waist-worn sensor: Concurrent validity study. *Sci. Rep.* **2019**, *9*, 13434. [PubMed]
33. Hssayeni, M.D.; Jimenez-Shahed, J.; Burack, M.A.; Ghoraani, B. Dyskinesia estimation during activities of daily living using wearable motion sensors and deep recurrent networks. *Sci. Rep.* **2021**, *11*, 7865. [CrossRef] [PubMed]
34. Haberfehlner, H.; Goudriaan, M.; Bonouvrie, L.A.; Jansma, E.P.; Harlaar, J.; Vermeulen, R.J.; Van der Krogt, M.M.; Buizer, A.I. Instrumented assessment of motor function in dyskinetic cerebral palsy: A systematic review. *J. Neuroeng. Rehabil.* **2020**, *17*, 39. [CrossRef] [PubMed]
35. Sanger, T.D.; Ferman, D. Similarity of Involuntary Postures between Different Children with Dystonia. *Mov. Disord. Clin. Pract.* **2017**, *4*, 870–874. [CrossRef] [PubMed]
36. Yeomans, J.; Thwaites, S.; Robertson, W.S.P.; Booth, D.; Ng, B.; Thewlis, D. Simulating Time-Series Data for Improved Deep Neural Network Performance. *IEEE Access* **2019**, *7*, 131248–131255.

Article
Head Pitch Angular Velocity Discriminates (Sub-)Acute Neck Pain Patients and Controls Assessed with the DidRen Laser Test

Renaud Hage [1,2,3,*], Fabien Buisseret [1,4], Martin Houry [5] and Frédéric Dierick [1,3,6]

1. CeREF Technique, Chaussée de Binche 159, 7000 Mons, Belgium; buisseretf@helha.be (F.B.); frederic.dierick@gmail.com (F.D.)
2. Traitement Formation Thérapie Manuelle (TFTM), Private Physiotherapy/Manual Therapy Center, Avenue des Cerisiers 211A, 1200 Brussels, Belgium
3. Faculté des Sciences de la Motricité, UCLouvain, Place Pierre de Coubertin 1, 1348 Ottignies-Louvain-la-Neuve, Belgium
4. Service de Physique Nucléaire et Subnucléaire, UMONS, Research Institute for Complex Systems, Place du Parc 20, 7000 Mons, Belgium
5. Centre de Recherche FoRS, Haute-Ecole de Namur-Liège-Luxembourg (Henallux), Rue Victor Libert 36H, 6900 Marche-en-Famenne, Belgium; martin.houry@henallux.be
6. Laboratoire d'Analyse du Mouvement et de la Posture (LAMP), Centre National de Rééducation Fonctionnelle et de Réadaptation–Rehazenter, Rue André Vésale 1, 2674 Luxembourg, Luxembourg
* Correspondence: renaudhage@gmail.com

Abstract: Understanding neck pain is an important societal issue. Kinematic data from sensors may help to gain insight into the pathophysiological mechanisms associated with neck pain through a quantitative sensorimotor assessment of one patient. The objective of this study was to evaluate the potential usefulness of artificial intelligence with several machine learning (ML) algorithms in assessing neck sensorimotor performance. Angular velocity and acceleration measured by an inertial sensor placed on the forehead during the DidRen laser test in thirty-eight acute and subacute non-specific neck pain (ANSP) patients were compared to forty-two healthy control participants (HCP). Seven supervised ML algorithms were chosen for the predictions. The most informative kinematic features were computed using Sequential Feature Selection methods. The best performing algorithm is the Linear Support Vector Machine with an accuracy of 82% and Area Under Curve of 84%. The best discriminative kinematic feature between ANSP patients and HCP is the first quartile of head pitch angular velocity. This study has shown that supervised ML algorithms could be used to classify ANSP patients and identify discriminatory kinematic features potentially useful for clinicians in the assessment and monitoring of the neck sensorimotor performance in ANSP patients.

Keywords: artificial intelligence; supervised machine learning; kinematics; head rotation test; neck pain

1. Introduction

Understanding neck pain is an important societal issue [1,2]. The overall prevalence of neck pain in the general population ranges from 0.4% to 86.8% and is higher in women than in men [3]. It ranks fourth in terms of years lived with a disability [1,2]. The majority of patients with neck pain are now classified as experiencing a "non-specific" neck disorder [4–6], meaning neck pain that occurs without trauma, signs or symptoms of major structural pathology, neurologic signs or specific pathology [4]. Acute or subacute non-specific neck pain (ANSP) means that the pain has been present for less than three months [4,7]. The assessment of sensorimotor function, a generic term for tests that encompass all afferent and efferent information flows and central integration mechanisms that contribute to joint stability [8], has demonstrated its importance for a better understanding of the pathophysiological mechanisms associated with chronic neck pain [9]. Indeed, the assessment of sensorimotor function, especially through kinematics of the head rotations, seems promising for the identification of chronic neck pain [10] but also of acute-subacute neck pain as shown by our previous results, which suggested that sensorimotor changes may also occur rapidly after pain resolution [11]. Nevertheless, identification based on sensorimotor evaluation requires the ability to know what would characterize neck pain in terms of the kinematic features of movement. Sensorimotor assessment of neck motion based not only on position degrees of freedom but also on velocity and acceleration features (e.g., peak and average velocity) appears promising because it has high sensitivity and specificity [10,12].

Identifying kinematic features from time series and comparing them between groups, e.g., to evaluate treatments or classify neck pain motion across ageing, is a widely used method [11–15]. Here, we focus on a peculiar test called DidRen laser test, designed to assess sensorimotor control of the neck and about which the interested reader will find detailed information in [11,15,16]. The DidRen laser test consists of a standardized task in which yaw rotations of the head are performed from "target to target" in the same sequence. These are fast, accurate, and small-amplitude rotations ($\pm 30°$) of the head in response to real visual targets to be hit by a laser beam placed on the subject's head [17]. However, such a methodology removes a substantial amount of information from the raw time series. The DidRen laser test did not cause pain in the patients (probably because of the too low amplitude of the rotation $< 30°$). Since the relationship between pain and sensorimotor control is well-established [18–21], if the test had caused pain when performed, it could have increased the kinematic difference between ANSP patients and healthy subjects.

Resorting to artificial intelligence (AI) techniques may lead to another type of analysis, i.e., "the machine" should find the relevant specifications of time series. The present study is devoted to the latter case. AI is defined as a field of science and engineering concerned with the computational understanding of what is commonly referred to as intelligent behavior and the creation of artefacts that exhibit such behavior [22]. Machine learning (ML) is defined as a subfield of AI as follows: "Machine learning is a branch of artificial intelligence that systematically applies algorithms to synthesize the underlying relationships among data and information" [23]. ML provides an experiential "learning" that can be related to human intelligence as ML can improve its analyses by using computer algorithms. There are two main forms of ML: supervised and unsupervised [24]. In supervised ML (SML), the algorithms are provided with training data that are analyzed for the features that are important for classification and labelled. The model is then "trained" on these data before being tested on unlabeled data. In our case, the data will be measured in head rotations. In SML, data must first be labelled by a clinician (painful or not, for example) so that the model can learn to interpret them through pattern recognition. Then, the model is tested with unlabeled data to obtain an interpretation result [25,26]. Several algorithms can be trained for pattern recognition, such as logistic regression, support vector machine, decision tree, random forest, naïve Bayes or K-nearest neighbor [24]. Patterns may be representative of various features, among which pathology and pain, see e.g., [27].

The first aim of this work was to evaluate the discriminative ability of AI and SML methods in sensorimotor assessment of yaw angular displacement of the head in patients with ANSP compared with healthy control participants (HCP) with data from a previous study [11] obtained during the DidRen laser test [15–17]. A second aim of this work was to illustrate the potential of SML for clinicians in musculoskeletal physiotherapy [28]. In ecological situations, neck kinematics should be quickly assessed by a therapist using thresholds designed to identify relevant impairments in the history of patients with neck pain. We test whether SML can provide such kinematic values and therefore has predictive value for ANSP.

2. Materials and Methods

2.1. Patients and Participants

This study included 80 subjects (38 ANSP patients and 42 HCP) from a previous study [11]. Data were collected from February to December 2019. ANSP patients diagnosed by general practitioners were recruited from a consecutive sample in a private manual therapy center in Brussels, Belgium. Inclusion criteria for ANSP patients were acute-subacute (<3 months) non-specific neck pain with a Neck Disability Index (NDI) $\geq$ 8% [29] and a Numeric Pain Rating Scale (NPRS) > 3 [30–34]. HCP were recruited by one of the authors (RH) from a sample of convenience from colleagues at the university hospital and from acquaintances. They were included if they reported no neck symptoms: NDI < 8% [29], NPRS = 0 [30], and no pain on active head rotation and/or manual spinal assessment [35]. Characteristics of the ANSP patients and HCP are listed in Table 1. All subjects signed an informed consent form. The study was approved by the Academic Bioethics Committee (https://www.a-e-c.eu, (accessed on 30 January 2019) Brussels, B200-2018-103) and conducted in accordance with the Declaration of Helsinki. The authors confirm that all ongoing and related trials for this drug/intervention are registered (ClinicalTrials.gov: 04407637).

Table 1. Characteristics of the acute and subacute non-specific neck pain (ANSP) patients and healthy control participants (HCP). *p*-values resulted from *t*-test for age and BMI, Mann–Whitney U-test for NDI and NPRS, and Chi-2 for gender.

	ANSP Patients (*n* = 38)	HCP (*n* = 42)	*p*-Values
Age (years), mean ± SD	46.2 ± 16.3	24.3 ± 6.8	<0.001
Gender *n* (men/women), (%)	21 (55%)/17 (45%)	27 (64%)/15 (36%)	0.55
BMI (kg m^{-2}), mean ± SD	23.5 ± 3.2	21.5 ± 4.2	0.014
NDI (100), median [Q1–Q3]	22 [16–31.5]	0 [0–0]	<0.001
NPRS, median [Q1–Q3]	6 [4–7]	0 [0–0]	<0.001

BMI: body mass index, NDI: neck disability index, NPRS: numeric pain rating scale.

2.2. Protocol

The protocol was described in a previous study [11]. It essentially involved assessment of fast neck yaw rotations with the DidRen laser test [15,16] for ANSP patients and HCP, completed by manual examination of the painful spinal region for segmental tenderness. For ANSP patients, the manual examination served to confirm familiar pain and guide the treatment. For HCP, thanks to its high sensitivity (92%), the manual examination was used to exclude HCP if they had pain at one or more levels of the cervical spine and confirm that they are not healthy in the neck [35]. The DidRen laser test was used to standardize the rotational yaw movements of the participant's head. Briefly, participants wore a helmet to which a laser was attached. They pointed the laser as fast as possible at three targets equipped with photosensitive sensors (Figure 1A,B). The angular separation of targets is 30°, and the sequence was fixed: center-left-center-right-center. Participants were asked to perform the sequence as fast as possible.

During the DidRen laser test, head angular displacement kinematics were recorded in 3D (yaw, pitch, and roll) using the DYSKIMOT inertial sensor [36]. The detailed description of the sensor can be found in the study by Hage et al. [36]. The sensor consists of a 3-axis accelerometer, a gyroscope and magnetometer, and a temperature sensor. These internal components respectively measure acceleration (in g, ±16 g), angular velocity (in °/s, ±2000°/s), and magnetic field (in gauss, ±16 gauss). The sensor recorded the motion at a sampling frequency of 100 Hz. The DYSKIMOT sensor was placed in front of the helmet (Figure 1C), with the yaw-axis (or X) in the vertical direction. The pitch-axis (or Y) was aligned with subject's medio-lateral axis at the start of the test and the roll-axis (or Z) was aligned with the antero-posterior axis. The head rotation demanded in the DidRen laser test is oriented along the yaw-axis. Note that the subjects were not instructed to realize pitch or roll rotations of the head during the test.

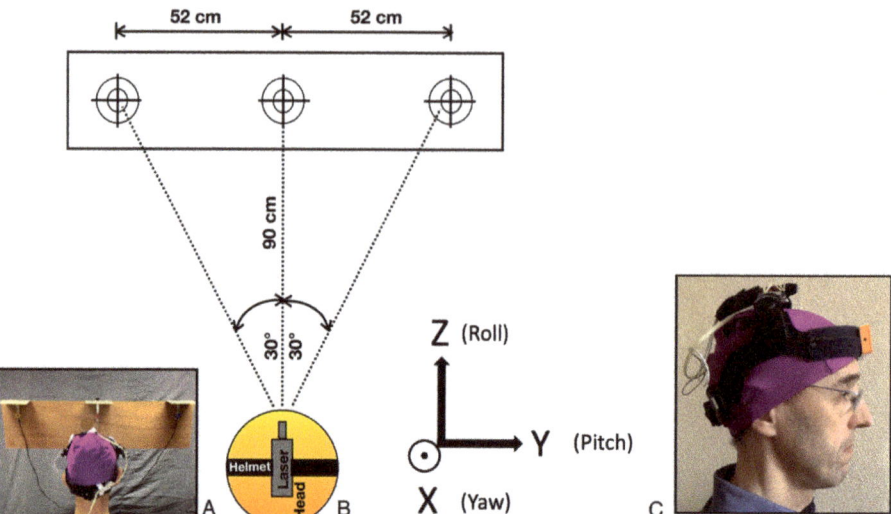

Figure 1. Description of the DidRen laser test. (**A**) Rear view of head position in front of the targets. (**B**) Schematic top view of the experimental setup with the three photosensitive sensors. The reference frame of the sensor is displayed when the head is in rest position. Coordinate system used in the study is also shown with the yaw (X-axis), pitch (Y-axis), and roll (Z-axis) rotations of the head during the test. (**C**) Helmet worn by an HCP (here RH) with laser on the top of the head and DYSKIMOT inertial sensor on the forehead.

2.3. Data Analysis

2.3.1. Dataset and Pre-Processing

In our previous papers [11,15], we analyzed the same dataset by resorting to "standard" statistical tests: we calculated several kinematical features of the angular position, speed, and acceleration time series (e.g., peak speed, time to reach peak, etc.). Then we showed that some parameters were significantly different between ANSP and HCP [11], and that age also had a significant impact on the parameters [15]. In the present study, we re-analyse the same dataset by using the raw sensor data to train various ML algorithms with the goal of finding an algorithm able to separate ANSP and HCP. To our knowledge, it is the first time that such ML techniques are used in the field of neck pain. The dataset consists of 7 time series for each participant: time, angular velocity (three components labelled GyrX, GyrY, GyrZ), and acceleration (AccX, AccY, AccZ). Then, a pre-processing procedure was applied to convert each time series into a summary format for all participants. Each time series is summarized with 7 statistical descriptors: 1st, 2nd, and 3rd quartiles, mean, minimum, maximum, and standard deviation. The result is a dataset with 186 inputs and 42 features (6 time series × 7 descriptors). Each set of statistical descriptors is labeled as ANSP (value 1) or HCP (value 0).

2.3.2. ML Algorithms and Determination of the Best Performer

It is generally difficult to determine a priori which ML algorithm performs best on a given dataset [37]. Therefore, several algorithms were tested to determine the most appropriate for classifying ANSP patients and HCP: K-Nearest Neighbor (KNN), Linear Support Vector Machine (Linear SVM), Non-linear Support Vector Machine Radial Basis Function (SVM RBF), Decision Tree (DT), Random Forest (RF), Adaptive Boosting (AdaBoost), and Gaussian Naive Bayes (GaussianNB).

The comparison between selected algorithms was based on metrics such as accuracy and the Area Under Curve (AUC) score, computed from the Receiver Operating Characteristic (ROC) curve. These metrics are only meaningful if the predictions are based on data that the ML algorithms have never learned. Therefore, the dataset was randomly split into two parts. The first part is the "training set", which consists of 80% of the dataset used to train the ML algorithms. The second part (remaining 20%) is the "test set" used to make the predictions with the trained ML algorithms. The validation of the ML algorithms is performed by n-fold cross-validation [38]. To minimize the biases associated with the training dataset, 100 different cross-validations were performed on mixed data for each selected ML algorithm. The hyperparameters of the ML algorithms were optimized using the Grid Search method [39] that finds the best combination of fixed hyperparameters based on n-fold cross-validation.

For KNN, the optimized parameters were the following: the number of neighbors (n_neighbors: 3, 5, 8, 10), the weighting function (weights: uniform, distance) and the algorithms used to compute the nearest neighbors (algorithms: Brute-Force (BF KNN or BF KNN), kd_tree, auto, ball_tree). For Linear SVM, different values for the regularization parameter or C-parameter (0.1, 1, 10, 100, 1000) were used in the evaluation to test the dependence of the approach on the C-parameter. For SVM RBF, the C-parameter (0.001, 0.01, 0.1, 1, 10, 100) and the kernel coefficient Gamma (0.001, 0.01, 0.1, 1, 10, 100) parameter were optimized. For DT, the optimized parameters were the maximum depth of the tree (max_depth: 1, 5, 10, 100), the function to measure the quality of the splits (criterion: gini, entropy), and the strategy to select the split nodes (splitter: best, random). For RF, the optimized parameters were the maximum depth of the tree (max_depth: 1, 5, 10, 100), the number of trees in the forest (n_estimators: 1, 5, 10, 100), and the number of features considered in the search for the best split (max_features: 1, 5, 10, 100). For Adaboost, the optimized parameters were the maximum number of estimators at which boosting stops (n_estimators: 1, 5, 10, 50, 100, 500) and the weight applied to each classifier at each boosting iteration (learning_rate: 0.000001, 0.001, 0.1, 1, 5, 10, 100). For GaussianNB, the optimized parameter was the ratio of the largest variance of all features added to the variances for computational stability (var_smoothing: 0.0000001, 0.01, 1, 10, 100).

All the computations related to the determination of the best performer were made in Python 3.8 and SciKit-Learn 1.0.2 software.

2.3.3. Determination of Most Informative Kinematic Features and Logistic Regressions

The most informative kinematic features, i.e., the features that trigger the most predictions, were computed by using the Sequential Feature Selector (SFS) forward and backward [40]. The backward SFS removes the poorest features one by one, while the forward SFS identifies the best combination of features. In both cases, the result is a list of kinematic features that performed best according to the AUC score. Each SFS was run 700 times (7 ML algorithms $\times$ 100 random data repartitions). Once the most informative kinematic feature was identified, a logistic regression was performed by using it, and the accuracy of this logistic regression was computed. Another logistic regression on total DidRen laser test duration was also performed to compare the present results to the unique outcome of the original DidRen laser test [17].

All the computations related to the determination of the most informative features and ML algorithms were made in Python 3.8 and SciKit Learn 1.0.2 software.

3. Results

3.1. Optimal Hyperparameters and Performance Metrics of ML Algorithms

Optimal hyperparameters are presented in Table 2. Performance metrics of the selected ML algorithms are given in Table 3. The least performing ML algorithm is the KNN, and the best performing one is the linear SVM with an accuracy of 82% and AUC of 84%. We show in Figure 2 the ROC curve of the Linear SVM, which is the best ML algorithm we found to classify ANSP patients and HCP.

Table 2. Optimal hyperparameter values: Number of neighbors (n_neighbors), Regularization parameter (C-parameter), Kernel coefficient (gamma), maximum depth of the tree (max_depth), number of trees in the forest (n_estimators), and number of features to consider when looking for the best split (max_features).

ML Algorithm	Hyperparameters
BF KNN	n_neighbors = 5, weights = "distance"
Linear SVM	kernel = "linear", C = 10
SVM RBF	gamma = 0.001, C = 100
DT	max_depth = 1, criterion = "entropy", splitter = "best"
RF	max_depth = 10, n_estimators = 100, max_features = 10

BF KNN: Brute-Force K-Nearest Neighbors, SVM: Support Vector Machine, RBF: radial basis function, DT: Decision Tree, RF: Random Forest.

Table 3. Performance metrics of the selected ML algorithms.

ML Algorithm	Accuracy	AUC Score
BF KNN	0.66 ± 0.03	0.51 ± 0.07
Linear SVM	0.82 ± 0.03	0.84 ± 0.04
SVM RBF	0.65 ± 0.05	0.57 ± 0.09
DT	0.74 ± 0.03	0.70 ± 0.04
RF	0.76 ± 0.03	0.76 ± 0.04
AdaBoost	0.75 ± 0.04	0.76 ± 0.05
GaussianNB	0.77 ± 0.03	0.82 ± 0.03

BF KNN: Brute-Force K-Nearest Neighbors, SVM: Support Vector Machine, RBF: radial basis function, DT: Decision Tree, RF: Random Forest, AdaBoost: Adaptive Boosting, GaussianNB: Gaussian Naive Bayes, AUC: area under curve.

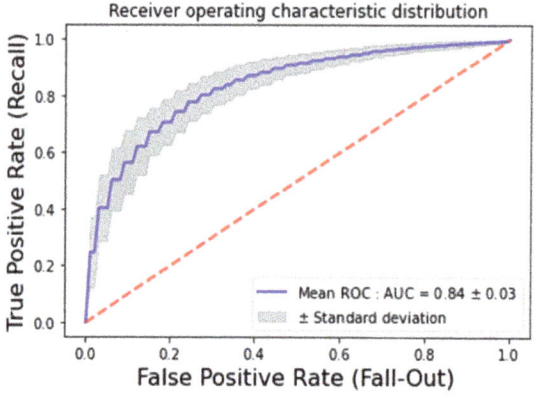

Figure 2. Receiver Operating Characteristic (ROC) curve of Linear SVM (in blue). The dotted red line represents the worst possible scenario, a random classifier.

The ROC curve plots the False Positive Rate ($\frac{FP}{FP+TN}$) and the True Positive Rate ($\frac{TP}{TP+FN}$) at all thresholds of Linear SVM classification.

3.2. Most Discriminative Features and Logistic Regressions

The most discriminative feature, regardless of the ML algorithm and SFS, was the first quartile of head pitch angular velocity (or GyrY), which ranked first 813 times in 1400. The second most discriminative feature was the median of head pitch angular velocity (ranked first 444 times in 1400). Thus, the pitch angular velocity appears to be the best discriminating feature to differentiate ANSP patients and HCP assessed with the DidRen laser test.

A logistic regression based on the median of head pitch angular velocity led to an accuracy of 77%. A logistic regression based on total duration of the DidRen test led to an accuracy of 63%.

4. Discussion

Our findings showed the effectiveness of the kernel linear SVM classifier in distinguishing ANSP patients from HCP. The accuracy of the linear SVM was 82% and the AUC score was 84%. The interpretation of the AUC score should be evaluated in terms of the importance given to its accuracy. We can assume that the medical community in the field of oncology prefers an AUC score close to 100%. Considering, on the one hand, the musculoskeletal field and, on the other hand, in relation to the non-specific pathology, the comparison between ANSP patients and HCP, which shows a great variability of the results [41], an AUC score higher than 80% can be considered satisfactory. As mentioned in the Introduction, the DidRen laser test did not cause pain in ANSP patients. This feature may help ANSP patients to show kinematic features such as HCP, which may increase the number of false negatives. Therefore, a larger rotation amplitude than 30° may decrease the false-negative rate.

Seven time series (time and kinematic data) related to yaw, pitch, and roll angular displacement and velocity of the head, which can be easily acquired with a single inertial sensor, were used to train the selected ML algorithms. However, regardless of the ML algorithm and SFS, not all axes of head motion have good discriminative information, as the two best discriminating kinematic features were related to head pitch. The accuracy was best with the linear SVM and lowest with all other selected ML algorithms, such as the non-linear SVM (RBF). The same finding regarding the superiority of linear SVM over RBF has already been observed in a study with limited sample size (17 young and 17 old subjects) aimed at detecting age-related changes in running kinematics [42]. For use in future clinical trials with kinematic variables with limited sample size, linear SVM may thus be a suitable option.

Like other studies using ML algorithms to detect kinematic changes in healthy or pathological subjects [42–45], our study is based on a rather small dataset in terms of typical AI calculations, but the results are consistent with the conclusions of [46]. While conducting observational sensorimotor assessment studies with large datasets holds promise for improving the understanding and management of various pathologies, here, the pathophysiological mechanisms associated with neck pain, the use of small datasets may also allow for a reduction in selection bias [46]. In addition, it is worth noting that an SVM has already been used in the musculoskeletal field to compare temporomandibular patients with control subjects [47]. With a smaller sample (10 patients and 10 control subjects), they achieved an average predictive accuracy of 60% ($p = 0.10$) [47]. The linear SVM algorithm is affordable with today's standard devices: a tablet computer could efficiently post-process the data from any wearable inertial sensor. Note also that a logistic regression based on head pitch angular velocity could be easily implemented on any smartphone, but with a lower accuracy of 77%.

The main discriminatory information used by the linear SVM algorithm to distinguish ANSP patients from HCP are the first quartile and the median of head pitch angular velocity. The two best kinematic discriminating features differed from those obtained by inferential statistical analysis, suggesting that ML approaches are complementary and clinically useful to detect kinematic changes in patients with ANSP.

HCP have larger medians and quartiles for head pitch angular velocity (computed from GyrY time series) than ANSP patients, making the Y-axis a highly discriminatory direction that should be prioritized for future clinical trials with the DidRen laser test. Our results may seem counterintuitive at first, because the DidRen laser test consists of a sensorimotor assessment organized around the Z-axis, i.e., during the execution of yaw rotations of the head. Thus, it would stand to reason that the GyrX time series should contain most of the discriminative information. Nevertheless, it is interesting to note that the sensorimotor disturbances in ANSP patients may be highlighted by the stronger secondary coupled motion during yaw rotations. There seems to be a reason for this, because biomechanically, coupled bending rotations in the cervical spine lead to a compensatory roll rotation, which compensates for the yaw rotation of the head, and the associated coupled movements observed during pitch head movements [48]. Indeed, in HCP, we can observe that yaw head rotation ($55.5 \pm 10.8°$) is coupled with a larger pitch motion ($16.3 \pm 11.4°$) than roll motion ($4.6 \pm 6.2°$) [48]. If we apply these considerations to patient assessment, this information may be of clinical interest because 3D motion analysis may be a useful tool for assessing postural changes in the cervical spine during sitting, but also because altered kinematics are associated with decreased performance, e.g., neck velocity and neck motion fluidity in functional movement tasks, in people with neck pain [49].

The present discussion suggests that the ML algorithms can provide relevant functional variables and thus optimize the prediction of ANSP status during the DidRen laser test. To further illustrate this point, we mention that total test duration was the only parameter measured in the original version of the DidRen laser test [17]. Logistic regression performed with duration yields lower accuracy than that obtained with the median of pitch head rotation alone, the latter parameter being favored by linear SVM.

In experimental studies, control and experimental groups are usually formed in such a way that no significant difference is observed in parameters such as age, ethnicity, gender, and degeneration/maturation stage, except for the variable of interest. In our case, this means that ANSP patients and HCP groups should differ only in terms of NDI and NPRS. Age is also significantly different in our groups, but we do not believe this is problematic for our purpose. Indeed, ML algorithms are designed to distinguish between HCP and ANSP patients. To find out the characteristics of ANSP patients, it is logical to compare them with the "healthiest" subjects, i.e., our HCP group. On the other hand, a control group with too young subjects would also have led to bias, since we have shown in a previous study that the kinematic behaviors recorded with the DidRen laser test have a U-shaped or inverted U-shaped age profile, making the differences between young and old particularly clear [16]. Because the prevalence of degenerative joint changes increases with age [4,50], possibly leading to movement limitations (yaw rotation steadily decreases between the ages of 30 and 60) [51], we selected HCP using a very sensitive manual examination [35]. After this examination, positive control subjects (with potential neck disorders) were excluded, and because their average age was higher (see [11]: the mean age of the excluded control subjects was 43.3 years), the average age of our HCP group decreased compared with the ANSP group. It is worth noting that a significant age difference between control and disease subjects was already found in a study aimed at developing and determining the predictive performance of ML models to distinguish between different subtypes of low-back pain and healthy control subjects [52]. For this purpose, as we did, they did not include age as a predictor when constructing the model [52].

It has already been shown by authors of the present study that several kinematic features of head rotation movements were significantly different in HCP and ANSP patients in terms of statistical tests comparing means [11]. The novelty of our results can also be outlined by comparing them with similar studies. The next logical step in the kinematical analysis of head rotation movements is to investigate whether some kinematic parameters can be used as predictors of neck pain or not. Bahat et al. performed simple logistic regressions on all selected kinematic parameters and found that it was the case [10]. For example, they found a sensitivity of 91% (right) and 94% (left) and a specificity of 95% (right and left) for head peak yaw angular velocity, and the maximum AUC was obtained with head peak pitch angular velocity [10]. Note that the discriminative power of head peak yaw angular velocity was shown in [11,13], where a test in a virtual (VR) environment was performed. The extent to which our current results hold in a VR environment is an open problem that we leave for future work.

We reach the same conclusion as [10] regarding pitch angular velocity by using a more model-independent approach, i.e., by allowing machine learning algorithms to sort out the most discriminant features from the raw data. We also go beyond simple logistic regressions by including all relevant features in a single ML algorithm. Indeed, converting time series into scalar variables may remove a substantial amount of information contained in the original time series that could lead to extra false negative results or inaccurate predictions [53]. Roijezon et al. used linear discriminant analysis to identify neck-pain patients, i.e., the same kind of methodology as ours, but obtained lower sensitivity and specificity than in the present study: they found a sensitivity of 74.6% and a specificity of 73.5% for classification based on head peak yaw angular velocity [12]. Thus, to our knowledge, this is the first time that ML algorithms have been applied to the raw sensor data recorded during head rotation to find a multi-feature classification algorithm for identifying ANSP patients. A clear advantage of this type of algorithm, in addition to the high accuracy currently achieved, is that it can be systematically improved by increasing the size of the data set and allowing the algorithm to "learn" from the new data.

In summary, we have shown that AI can help identify patients suffering from neck pain using the DidRen laser test augmented by an inertial sensor. In our approach, the accuracy and AUC scores are computed from inertial sensor's kinematic data. The obtained ML algorithm can be implemented in any tablet or smartphone and lead to an "augmented DidRen laser test"; hence, our results may be transferred to daily clinical practice. In our opinion, the best way to merge the DidRen laser test and an inertial sensor is to develop a VR version of the test: it will improve the standardization of the test through the standardization of the environment, and any VR device has at least one inertial sensor able to collect the needed data. Such a work is in progress, see e.g., [54]. Using AI to interpret sensor data can in principle be used in other movements than the rotation demanded in the DidRen laser test, but then the AI training must be made for each different motion, which outlines the necessity of defining standardized movements in clinical tests. Today, there is still no clinical gold standard for diagnosing acute neck pain, but the use of the DidRen laser test and AI appears to be a promising candidate to provide clinically useful information that can improve patient management. The diagnostic ability of our framework has been proven in the present study, but it is worth mentioning the possibility of data storage offered by sensor technology. The more data that will be stored, the more the ML accuracy will be refined, i.e., our diagnostic algorithm is systematically improvable over time. Moreover, the same test can be performed at various points of one patient's treatment to assess his/her evolution. One last feature of our approach is that it identifies key kinematic parameters (such as peak angular speed) on which therapists can focus to follow one patient's evolution.

Author Contributions: Conceptualization, R.H., F.D.; methodology, R.H., M.H.; software, R.H., M.H.; validation, R.H., F.B., F.D. and M.H.; data curation, R.H., M.H.; writing—original draft preparation, R.H., M.H.; writing—review and editing, R.H., F.B., F.D. and M.H. All authors have read and agreed to the published version of the manuscript.

Funding: CeREF acknowledges the financial support from the First Haute-Ecole program, project no 1610401, DYSKIMOT, in partnership with OMT-Skills (http://omtskills.be/, accessed on 12 March 2022), and from the European Regional Development Fund (Interreg FWVl NOMADe): 4.7.360.

Institutional Review Board Statement: The study was conducted according to the guidelines of the Declaration of Helsinki and approved by the Academic Bioethics Committee (https://www.a-e-c.eu/, accessed on 30 January 2019) under the number B200-2018-103. The authors confirm that all ongoing and related trials for this drug/intervention are registered (ClinicalTrials.gov: 04407637).

Informed Consent Statement: Informed consent was obtained from all participants involved in the study.

Data Availability Statement: Data are available at https://osf.io/rsuh2/ (accessed on 12 March 2022).

Conflicts of Interest: The authors declare no conflict of interest. The funders had no role in the design of the study; in the collection, analyses, or interpretation of data; in the writing of the manuscript, or in the decision to publish the results.

References

1. GBD 2015 Disease and Injury Incidence and Prevalence Collaborators. Global, regional, and national incidence, prevalence, and years lived with disability for 301 acute and chronic diseases and injuries in 188 countries, 1990–2013: A systematic analysis for the Global Burden of Disease Study 2013. *Lancet* **2015**, *386*, 743–800. [CrossRef]
2. Hoy, D.G.; Protani, M.; De, R.; Buchbinder, R. The epidemiology of neck pain. *Best Pract. Res. Clin. Rheumatol.* **2010**, *24*, 783–792. [CrossRef] [PubMed]
3. Kazeminasab, S.; Nejadghaderi, S.A.; Amiri, P.; Pourfathi, H.; Araj-Khodaei, M.; Sullman, M.J.M.; Kolahi, A.A.; Safiri, S. Neck pain: Global epidemiology, trends and risk factors. *BMC Musculoskelet. Disord.* **2022**, *23*, 26. [CrossRef] [PubMed]
4. Blanpied, P.R.; Gross, A.R.; Elliott, J.M.; Devaney, L.L.; Clewley, D.; Walton, D.M.; Sparks, C.; Robertson, E.K. Neck Pain: Revision 2017. *J. Orthop. Sports Phys. Ther.* **2017**, *47*, A1–A83. [CrossRef]
5. Childs, J.D.; Cleland, J.A.; Elliott, J.M.; Teyhen, D.S.; Wainner, R.S.; Whitman, J.M.; Sopky, B.J.; Godges, J.J.; Flynn, T.W.; American Physical Therapy Association. Neck pain: Clinical practice guidelines linked to the International Classification of Functioning, Disability, and Health from the Orthopedic Section of the American Physical Therapy Association. *J. Orthop. Sports Phys. Ther.* **2008**, *38*, A1–A34. [CrossRef]
6. Coulter, I.D.; Crawford, C.; Vernon, H.; Hurwitz, E.L.; Khorsan, R.; Booth, M.S.; Herman, P.M. Manipulation and Mobilization for Treating Chronic Nonspecific Neck Pain: A Systematic Review and Meta-Analysis for an Appropriateness Panel. *Pain Physician* **2019**, *22*, e55–e70. [CrossRef]
7. Pool, J.J.; Ostelo, R.W.; Knol, D.; Bouter, L.M.; de Vet, H.C. Are psychological factors prognostic indicators of outcome in patients with sub-acute neck pain? *Man Ther.* **2010**, *15*, 111–116. [CrossRef]
8. de Zoete, R.M.J.; Osmotherly, P.G.; Rivett, D.A.; Farrell, S.F.; Snodgrass, S.J. Sensorimotor Control in Individuals With Idiopathic Neck Pain and Healthy Individuals: A Systematic Review and Meta-Analysis. *Arch. Phys. Med. Rehabil.* **2017**, *98*, 1257–12571. [CrossRef]
9. Sjolander, P.; Michaelson, P.; Jaric, S.; Djupsjobacka, M. Sensorimotor disturbances in chronic neck pain—Range of motion, peak velocity, smoothness of movement, and repositioning acuity. *Man Ther.* **2008**, *13*, 122–131. [CrossRef]
10. Sarig Bahat, H.; Chen, X.; Reznik, D.; Kodesh, E.; Treleaven, J. Interactive cervical motion kinematics: Sensitivity, specificity and clinically significant values for identifying kinematic impairments in patients with chronic neck pain. *Man Ther.* **2015**, *20*, 295–302. [CrossRef]
11. Hage, R.; Detrembleur, C.; Dierick, F.; Brismée, J.M.; Roussel, N.; Pitance, L. Sensorimotor performance in acute-subacute non-specific neck pain: A non-randomized prospective clinical trial with intervention. *BMC Musculoskelet. Disord.* **2021**, *22*, 1017. [CrossRef] [PubMed]
12. Roijezon, U.; Djupsjobacka, M.; Bjorklund, M.; Hager-Ross, C.; Grip, H.; Liebermann, D.G. Kinematics of fast cervical rotations in persons with chronic neck pain: A cross-sectional and reliability study. *BMC Musculoskelet. Disord.* **2010**, *11*, 222. [CrossRef] [PubMed]
13. Sarig Bahat, H.; Weiss, P.L.; Laufer, Y. The effect of neck pain on cervical kinematics, as assessed in a virtual environment. *Arch. Phys. Med. Rehabil.* **2010**, *91*, 1884–1890. [CrossRef]
14. Bahat, H.S.; Igbariya, M.; Quek, J.; Treleaven, J. Cervical Kinematics of Fast Neck Motion across Age. *J. Nov. Physiother.* **2016**, *6*, 306. [CrossRef]
15. Hage, R.; Dierick, F.; Roussel, N.; Pitance, L.; Detrembleur, C. Age-related kinematic performance should be considered during fast head-neck rotation target task in individuals aged from 8 to 85 years old. *PeerJ* **2019**, *7*, e7095. [CrossRef] [PubMed]
16. Hage, R.; Buisseret, F.; Pitance, L.; Brismée, J.M.; Detrembleur, C.; Dierick, F. Head-neck rotational movements using DidRen laser test indicate children and seniors' lower performance. *PLoS ONE* **2019**, *14*, e0219515. [CrossRef]
17. Hage, R.; Ancenay, E. Identification of a relationship between cervical spine function and rotational movement control. *Ann. Phys. Rehabil. Med.* **2009**, *52*, 653–667. [CrossRef]
18. Falla, D.; Farina, D. Neural and muscular factors associated with motor impairment in neck pain. *Curr. Rheumatol. Rep.* **2007**, *9*, 497–502. [CrossRef]
19. Falla, D.; Farina, D. Neuromuscular adaptation in experimental and clinical neck pain. *J. Electromyogr. Kinesiol.* **2008**, *18*, 255–261. [CrossRef]
20. Treleaven, J. Sensorimotor disturbances in neck disorders affecting postural stability, head and eye movement control. *Man Ther.* **2008**, *13*, 2–11. [CrossRef]
21. Kristjansson, E.; Treleaven, J. Sensorimotor function and dizziness in neck pain: Implications for assessment and management. *J. Orthop. Sports Phys. Ther.* **2009**, *39*, 364–377. [CrossRef] [PubMed]
22. Ramesh, A.N.; Kambhampati, C.; Monson, J.R.; Drew, P.J. Artificial intelligence in medicine. *Ann. R. Coll. Surg. Engl.* **2004**, *86*, 334–338. [CrossRef] [PubMed]
23. Awad, M.; Khanna, R. *Machine Learning. Efficient Learning Machines: Theories, Concepts, and Applications for Engineers and System Designers*; Apress: Berkeley, CA, USA, 2015; pp. 1–18.

24. Uddin, S.; Khan, A.; Hossain, M.E.; Moni, M.A. Comparing different supervised machine learning algorithms for disease prediction. *BMC Med. Inform. Decis. Mak.* **2019**, *19*, 281. [CrossRef] [PubMed]
25. Biswas, M.; Kuppili, V.; Saba, L.; Edla, D.R.; Suri, H.S.; Cuadrado-Godia, E.; Laird, J.R.; Marinhoe, R.T.; Sanches, J.M.; Nicolaides, A.; et al. State-of-the-art review on deep learning in medical imaging. *Front. Biosci.* **2019**, *24*, 392–426.
26. Kohli, M.; Prevedello, L.M.; Filice, R.W.; Geis, J.R. Implementing Machine Learning in Radiology Practice and Research. *AJR Am. J. Roentgenol.* **2017**, *208*, 754–760. [CrossRef] [PubMed]
27. Jin, R.; Luk, K.D.; Cheung, J.P.Y.; Hu, Y. Prognosis of cervical myelopathy based on diffusion tensor imaging with artificial intelligence methods. *NMR Biomed.* **2019**, *32*, e4114. [CrossRef]
28. Tack, C. Artificial intelligence and machine learning | applications in musculoskeletal physiotherapy. *Musculoskelet. Sci. Pract.* **2019**, *39*, 164–169. [CrossRef]
29. Vernon, H. The Neck Disability Index: State-of-the-art, 1991–2008. *J. Manip. Physiol. Ther.* **2008**, *31*, 491–502. [CrossRef]
30. Cleland, J.A.; Childs, J.D.; Whitman, J.M. Psychometric properties of the Neck Disability Index and Numeric Pain Rating Scale in patients with mechanical neck pain. *Arch. Phys. Med. Rehabil.* **2008**, *89*, 69–74. [CrossRef]
31. Meisingset, I.; Stensdotter, A.K.; Woodhouse, A.; Vasseljen, O. Neck motion, motor control, pain and disability: A longitudinal study of associations in neck pain patients in physiotherapy treatment. *Man Ther.* **2016**, *22*, 94–100. [CrossRef]
32. Meisingset, I.; Woodhouse, A.; Stensdotter, A.K.; Stavdahl, Ø.; Lorås, H.; Gismervik, S.; Andresen, H.; Austreim, K.; Vasseljen, O. Evidence for a general stiffening motor control pattern in neck pain: A cross sectional study. *BMC Musculoskelet. Disord.* **2015**, *16*, 56. [CrossRef] [PubMed]
33. Salaffi, F.; Stancati, A.; Silvestri, C.A.; Ciapetti, A.; Grassi, W. Minimal clinically important changes in chronic musculoskeletal pain intensity measured on a numerical rating scale. *Eur. J. Pain* **2004**, *8*, 283–291. [CrossRef] [PubMed]
34. Boonstra, A.M.; Stewart, R.E.; Köke, A.J.; Oosterwijk, R.F.; Swaan, J.L.; Schreurs, K.M.; Schiphorst Preuper, H.R. Cut-Off Points for Mild, Moderate, and Severe Pain on the Numeric Rating Scale for Pain in Patients with Chronic Musculoskeletal Pain: Variability and Influence of Sex and Catastrophizing. *Front. Psychol.* **2016**, *7*, 1466. [CrossRef] [PubMed]
35. Schneider, G.M.; Jull, G.; Thomas, K.; Smith, A.; Emery, C.; Faris, P.; Cook, C.; Frizzell, B.; Salo, P. Derivation of a clinical decision guide in the diagnosis of cervical facet joint pain. *Arch. Phys. Med. Rehabil.* **2014**, *95*, 1695–1701. [CrossRef] [PubMed]
36. Hage, R.; Detrembleur, C.; Dierick, F.; Pitance, L.; Jojczyk, L.; Estievenart, W.; Buisseret, F. DYSKIMOT: An Ultra-Low-Cost Inertial Sensor to Assess Head's Rotational Kinematics in Adults during the Didren-Laser Test. *Sensors* **2020**, *20*, 833. [CrossRef]
37. Kononenko, I. Machine learning for medical diagnosis: History, state of the art and perspective. *Artif. Intell. Med.* **2001**, *23*, 89–109. [CrossRef]
38. Berrar, D. Cross-Validation. *Encycl. Bioinform. Comput. Biol.* **2018**, *1*, 542–545. [CrossRef]
39. Ndiaye, E.; Le, T.; Fercoq, O.; Salmon, J.; Takeuchi, I. Safe grid search with optimal complexity. In Proceedings of the 36th International Conference on Machine Learning, Long Beach, CA, USA, 9–15 June 2019.
40. Kumar, V.M. Sonajharia. Feature Selection: A literature Review. *Smart Comput. Rev.* **2014**, *4*, 211–229. [CrossRef]
41. Franov, E.; Straub, M.; Bauer, C.M.; Ernst, M.J. Head kinematics in patients with neck pain compared to asymptomatic controls: A systematic review. *BMC Musculoskelet. Disord.* **2022**, *23*, 156. [CrossRef]
42. Fukuchi, R.K.; Eskofier, B.M.; Duarte, M.; Ferber, R. Support vector machines for detecting age-related changes in running kinematics. *J. Biomech.* **2011**, *44*, 540–542. [CrossRef]
43. Lai, D.T.; Levinger, P.; Begg, R.K.; Gilleard, W.L.; Palaniswami, M. Automatic recognition of gait patterns exhibiting patellofemoral pain syndrome using a support vector machine approach. *IEEE Trans. Inf. Technol. Biomed.* **2009**, *13*, 810–817. [CrossRef] [PubMed]
44. Suda, E.Y.; Watari, R.; Matias, A.B.; Sacco, I.C.N. Recognition of Foot-Ankle Movement Patterns in Long-Distance Runners With Different Experience Levels Using Support Vector Machines. *Front. Bioeng. Biotechnol.* **2020**, *8*, 576. [CrossRef] [PubMed]
45. Jiang, Y.; Sadeqi, A.; Miller, E.L.; Sonkusale, S. Head motion classification using thread-based sensor and machine learning algorithm. *Sci. Rep.* **2021**, *11*, 2646. [CrossRef] [PubMed]
46. Jairam, V.; Park, H.S. Strengths and limitations of large databases in lung cancer radiation oncology research. *Transl. Lung Cancer Res.* **2019**, *8* (Suppl. 2), S172–S183. [CrossRef] [PubMed]
47. Harper, D.E.; Shah, Y.; Ichesco, E.; Gerstner, G.E.; Peltier, S.J. Multivariate classification of pain-evoked brain activity in temporomandibular disorder. *Pain Rep.* **2016**, *1*, e572. [CrossRef] [PubMed]
48. Guo, R.; Zhou, C.; Wang, C.; Tsai, T.-Y.; Yu, Y.; Wang, W.; Li, G.; Cha, T. In vivo primary and coupled segmental motions of the healthy female head-neck complex during dynamic head axial rotation. *J. Biomech.* **2021**, *123*, 110513. [CrossRef] [PubMed]
49. Moghaddas, D.; de Zoete, R.M.J.; Edwards, S.; Snodgrass, S.J. Differences in the kinematics of the cervical and thoracic spine during functional movement in individuals with or without chronic neck pain: A systematic review. *Physiotherapy* **2019**, *105*, 421–433. [CrossRef]
50. Betsch, M.W.; Blizzard, S.R.; Shinseki, M.S.; Yoo, J.U. Prevalence of degenerative changes of the atlanto-axial joints. *Spine J.* **2015**, *15*, 275–280. [CrossRef]
51. Pan, F.; Arshad, R.; Zander, T.; Reitmaier, S.; Schroll, A.; Schmidt, H. The effect of age and sex on the cervical range of motion—A systematic review and meta-analysis. *J. Biomech.* **2018**, *75*, 13–27. [CrossRef]
52. Liew, B.X.W.; Rugamer, D.; De Nunzio, A.M.; Falla, D. Interpretable machine learning models for classifying low back pain status using functional physiological variables. *Eur. Spine J.* **2020**, *29*, 1845–1859. [CrossRef]

53. Falla, D.; Devecchi, V.; Jiménez-Grande, D.; Rügamer, D.; Liew, B.X.W. Machine learning approaches applied in spinal pain research. *J. Electromyogr. Kinesiol.* **2021**, *61*, 102599. [CrossRef] [PubMed]
54. NOMADe. DidRen VR. Available online: https://www.youtube.com/watch?v=Pqrty4Bj_5A&t=16s (accessed on 12 March 2022).

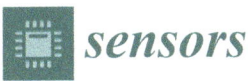

Article

High Specificity of Single Inertial Sensor-Supplemented Timed Up and Go Test for Assessing Fall Risk in Elderly Nursing Home Residents

Frédéric Dierick [1,2,3], Pierre-Loup Stoffel [4], Gaston Schütz [5] and Fabien Buisseret [3,4,6,*]

1. Laboratoire d'Analyse du Mouvement et de la Posture (LAMP), Centre National de Rééducation Fonctionnelle et de Réadaptation—Rehazenter, Rue André Vésale 1, 2674 Luxembourg, Luxembourg; frederic.dierick@rehazenter.lu
2. Faculté des Sciences de la Motricité, Université Catholique de Louvain, Place Pierre de Coubertin 2, 1348 Ottignies-Louvain-la-Neuve, Belgium
3. CeREF-Technique, Chaussée de Binche 159, 7000 Mons, Belgium
4. Forme and Fonctionnement Humain Laboratory, Department of Physical Therapy, Haute Ecole Louvain en Hainaut, Rue Trieu Kaisin 136, 6061 Montignies-sur-Sambre, Belgium; pierreloupstoffel@gmail.com
5. Centre National de Rééducation Fonctionnelle et de Réadaptation—Rehazenter, Rue André Vésale 1, 2674 Luxembourg, Luxembourg; gaston.schuetz@rehazenter.lu
6. Service de Physique Nucléaire et Subnucléaire, UMONS Research Institute for Complex Systems, Université de Mons, Place du Parc 20, 7000 Mons, Belgium
* Correspondence: buisseretf@helha.be

Abstract: The Timed Up and Go test (TUG) is commonly used to estimate the fall risk in the elderly. Several ways to improve the predictive accuracy of TUG (cameras, multiple sensors, other clinical tests) have already been proposed. Here, we added a single wearable inertial measurement unit (IMU) to capture the residents' body center-of-mass kinematics in view of improving TUG's predictive accuracy. The aim is to find out which kinematic variables and residents' characteristics are relevant for distinguishing faller from non-faller patients. Data were collected in 73 nursing home residents with the IMU placed on the lower back. Acceleration and angular velocity time series were analyzed during different subtasks of the TUG. Multiple logistic regressions showed that total time required, maximum angular velocity at the first half-turn, gender, and use of a walking aid were the parameters leading to the best predictive abilities of fall risk. The predictive accuracy of the proposed new test, called i + TUG, reached a value of 74.0%, with a specificity of 95.9% and a sensitivity of 29.2%. By adding a single wearable IMU to TUG, an accurate and highly specific test is therefore obtained. This method is quick, easy to perform and inexpensive. We recommend to integrate it into daily clinical practice in nursing homes.

Keywords: TUG; kinematics; fall risk; logistic regression; elderly; inertial sensor

1. Introduction

The proportion of elderly people is steadily increasing. According to the World Health Organization (WHO) estimates, it will account for 22% of the world's population by 2050. Physiological changes caused by ageing result in deterioration of balance, coordination, and strength, leading to an increased incidence of falls in people over 65 years. Falls are one of the top five causes of death in this age group and their incidence is particularly increasing in people living in nursing homes, with an average of 1.7 falls per bed per year compared to 0.65 in people living independently [1]. In addition, falls lead to more complications in people living in nursing homes, with 10 to 25% of falls resulting in a fracture or open wound [2]. The main risk factors for falls are muscle weakness, balance problems, and gait disturbances [2].

The Timed Up and Go test (TUG) [3] is commonly used in the medical field to predict fall risk in the elderly. Very simply, TUG consists of measuring the time it takes a person to get up from a chair with arms after having heard a "Go", walk forward three meters at a comfortable pace, turn around, walk back to the chair, and sit down again. According to the pioneering study [4], a time greater than 14.0 s indicates a potential fall risk. Obvious advantages of the TUG are the following. It is quick to perform, it requires no equipment other than a chair and a stopwatch, and it involves a sequence of movements common to daily life: getting up, walking, turning, and sitting. In the review [5], it is concluded that the predictive power of the TUG is greater in people living in institutions than in people living independently. This conclusion is shared by [6]. However, this test is limited by the fact that total time is the only parameter measured and that it categorizes fall risk according to a threshold value that is increasingly controversial in the literature. The threshold used to identify fallers in nursing homes actually varies between 13.0 and 32.6 s, depending on the study [5].

Several authors have already proposed ways to improve TUG by adding inertial sensors to measure acceleration or velocity, by combining it with other clinical tests, or by using cameras [7–10]. The corresponding tests are often referred to as instrumented TUG (iTUG). Their predictive performances can be correlated with a gold-standard but more complex functional tests such as Community Balance and Mobility Scale [11]. Among these approaches, we think that the addition of wearable inertial measurement units (IMUs, or inertial sensors) is particularly promising. The information contained in the measured time series (acceleration and angular velocity) goes well beyond the total time measured in TUG, making the iTUG a clinical tool that allows detailed analyses of the TUG's different subtasks. The use of a single IMU is actually adequate to separate the TUG subtasks with sufficient accuracy for clinical applications [10,12,13]. From a methodological point of view, splitting TUG into different subtasks can improve its discriminatory power in various conditions: obese women [14], children with traumatic brain injury [15], and adults with vestibular hypofunction [16].

Using a single IMU placed on a patient's lower back, Buisseret et al. proposed to combine the kinematic data of a 6-min walk test (6MWT) and the result of TUG to improve its predictive accuracy [7]. However, kinematic data of the TUG collected during the latter study were not analysed, despite evidence that a movement such as a trunk rotation is an index of balance measurement that requires special attention [8,11,17–21]. Moreover, among fall-related fractures, hip fractures are the most common. A fall during a turn increases the risk of hip fracture 8-fold compared to a fall in a straight line [18]. Therefore, in this study, we propose a detailed analysis of the two half-turns during TUG from a kinematic point of view by adding to the conventional measures such as duration and maximum angular velocity a parameter called "jerk", which is a measure of movement's smoothness [22].

The aim of this study is to determine: (1) which general characteristics and kinematic parameters are relevant to discriminate fallers (F) from non-fallers (NF) in a population of elderly nursing home residents, based on a dataset previously collected in [7]; (2) which of the relevant variables are best suited to predict a fall within six months using a logistic regression-based model—the model will be called i + TUG in the following to differentiate it from previous attempts called iTUG—and (3) whether i + TUG improves the predictive power of the TUG by assessing its predictive properties (sensitivity, specificity, and overall accuracy). Since our methodology seems to be very similar to the [7] proposal, it is worthwhile to outline here the difference between the present work and the latter. In [7], the duration of TUG was measured and supplemented by kinematic data from a 6MWT. A prediction of fall risk was proposed as a decision process that depends on thresholds for TUG duration and parameters that assess the variability of walk during the 6MWT. Here, fall risk is predicted only from TUG (duration and kinematic data) using multiple logistic regressions. Thus, the proposed assessment of fall risk is intended to be much shorter, with a decision criterion that can be systematically improved.

2. Materials and Methods

2.1. Population

All residents who participated in this study were at least 65 years old and lived in four different nursing homes in the Charleroi region (Belgium). All residents or their legal representatives gave their consent to participate in the study after being informed about the modalities of the study and the possible side effects. The experimental protocol is in accordance with the Declaration of Helsinki on Medical Research Involving Human Subjects and was approved by the Academic Bioethics Committee (reference B200-2017-144). The study was longitudinal and included two evaluations 6 months apart: the first one in May 2018 and the second one in November 2018. Here, we analyze data previously collected, part of which has already been analyzed in [7]. No new measurements were taken and the processed data had not been analyzed in previous studies.

The only inclusion criterion was that residents were at least 65 years old. Residents with lower limb movement disorders that prevented them from walking, cognitive disorders that prevented them from understanding the instructions given during the experiment, or cardio-respiratory disorders that prevented them from walking for 6 min were excluded. Some residents who were originally included in the sample could not be reexamined and were therefore also excluded if: they had dropped out of the study or had been hospitalized during the study period; they had one or more medical conditions that occurred between the two measurements; their medication had changed in a way that affected the measurement; and they were no longer alive.

According to all these criteria, 73 residents took part in the study until the end, giving an initial total of 92 residents. A summary of our resident's general characteristics can be found in Table 1. Cognitive status was assessed with Hodkinson Abbreviated Mental test score (AMTS) [23] that is included in Part 1 of the Fall Risk Assessment Tool [24]. An AMTS score (on 10) ≥ 9 was considered as an intact status [24] and <7 as a possibility of dementia [25]. Residents with a possibility of dementia or diagnosed with Alzheimer's disease were not excluded. The number of residents in faller and non-faller groups with these conditions are reported in Table 1.

Table 1. General characteristics of the residents. Fallers were identified according to the fall records between the 6-months interval (t_1 and t_2). Numerical data are written under the form mean ± standard deviation (*t*-test performed) or median [Q1–Q3] (Mann–Whitney test performed). For the age, the minimum and maximum values in each group are given (second line). Exact Fisher tests were performed for the categorical data (M/F or Yes/No). *p*-values for the comparison between fallers (F) and non-fallers (NF) groups are given in the last column. Total TUG time (T_{TUG}) was assessed with a stopwatch. Medications included: psychotrope, antiarrhythmic, and diuretics. Hypertension is defined as a value > 140/90 mmHg.

Parameter	F	NF	p
Residents (*n*)	24	49	
Age (years)	84 ± 9	83 ± 8	0.646
	66–96	65–96	
Medication	4 [2–5]	3 [2–5]	
FRAT	11 [10–14]	10 [8–12]	
T_{TUG} (s)	24.5 ± 8.5	21.5 ± 8.1	0.096
Gender (M/F)	6/18	22/27	0.128
Walking aid required (Yes/No)	15/9	21/28	0.140
Post-stroke hemiparesis (Yes/No)	2/21	4/45	0.677
Possibility of dementia (Yes/No)	3/21	9/40	0.739
Alzheimer disease (Yes/No)	5/19	14/35	0.577
Previous heart surgery (Yes/No)	8/16	9/40	0.238
Diabetic polyneuropathy (Yes/No)	3/21	8/41	1
Hip or knee replacement (Yes/No)	3/21	9/40	0.739

2.2. Protocol

This study was conducted in two phases. An initial measurement, conducted in May 2018 (t_1), included: (1) a collection of information about each resident, such as medications, presence and type of a walking aid, medical history (fracture, prosthesis, disease, ...); (2) the placement of a DYSKIMOT inertial sensor [7] in the back of each subject at the level of the fourth lumbar vertebra; and (3) a TUG and a 6MWT performed by each resident. The latter test is not taken into account in the present study. TUG data recording began when the "Go" instruction was given and stopped when the participant sat again on the chair. Hence, total TUG time (T_{TUG}) was directly measured from the length of the time series. After this initial measurement, nursing home staff were asked to record resident falls over a 6-month period. In November 2018 (t_2), based on data collected by on-site medical staff, a fall survey was conducted on each resident and they were classified as faller (F) or non-faller (NF). Nursing staff were regularly reminded to record residents' falls through several telephone contacts.

The DYSKIMOT sensor and its placement have been discussed in detail in [7], to which we refer the interested reader. Here, we summarize some key points for completeness. The DYSKIMOT sensor (3 cm × 3 cm, 10.44 g) is based on the commercially available IMU (LSM9DS1, SparkFun Electronics, Niwot, CO, USA), which integrates a triaxial accelerometer, a gyroscope, a magnetometer and a thermometer. The IMU was attached to the resident's back at the level of the fourth lumbar vertebra using an elastic strap. The measured time series are the three components of acceleration, $\vec{a}(t)$, and angular velocity, $\vec{\omega}(t)$, in the sensor's frame with a sample frequency of 100 Hz. Time series were recorded on a computer via the DYSKIMOT software (v. 2.1). The sensor was placed such that the three axes of its frame correspond to the anterio-posterior (AP), medio-lateral (ML) and vertical (V) directions when the resident is standing at rest.

Our data analysis was based on a_{AP}, giving the acceleration in the walking direction, and on ω_V, giving rotation velocity during the two half-turns. These two time series contained the clearest signal in all residents and were used to determine the different subtasks of TUG. Typical traces of the AP acceleration (a_{AP}) and of the V angular velocity (ω_V) during TUG are shown in Figure 1.

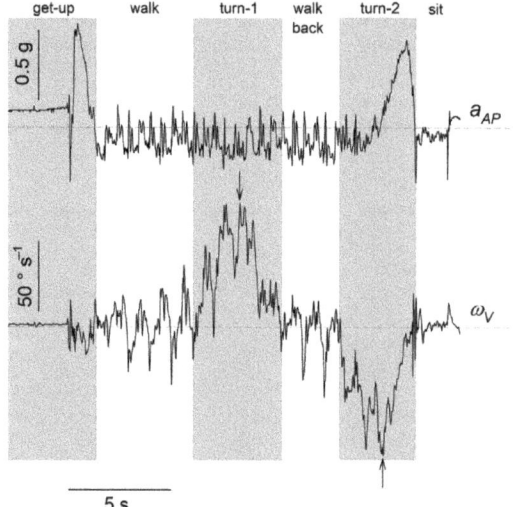

Figure 1. Typical traces of the AP acceleration (a_{AP}) and of the V angular velocity (ω_V) during TUG. Acceleration is expressed in a fraction of $g = 9.81$ m s^{-2}, and angular velocity is expressed in ° s^{-1}. White/gray areas highlight the different subtasks of the TUG. Arrows indicate the peak angular velocity during the two half-turns. Horizontal grey dashed lines show zero value.

2.3. Division of the TUG into Subtasks and Selected Kinematic Parameters

For each resident, we divided the TUG into 6 subtasks by visual inspection of $a_{AP}(t)$ and $\omega_V(t)$, as illustrated in Figure 1: (1) the get-up phase occurred between the beginning of the TUG and the end of the a_{AP} peak (i.e., when a_{AP} comes back to a 0 value after the peak); (2) the walk phase, where ω_V has an oscillatory behaviour around 0; (3) the first half-turn, corresponding to the first peak in ω_V, i.e., when ω_V stops oscillating around 0 to exhibit a global positive or negative trend; (4) the walk back phase, identified as the first one; (5) the second half-turn, identified as the first one; (6) the sit phase, until the end of the time series. A sharp peak in a_{AP} is observed in this phase when the resident's back hits the chair back.

After identification, the durations of the subtasks were recorded: T_{get-up}, T_{walk}, T_{turn-1}, $T_{walk\ back}$, T_{turn-2} and T_{sit}. Then, a more detailed assessment of half-turns was realised, since it is known to be strongly related to participant's stability [18]. Maximal angular velocities (in absolute values) were recorded during the first, ω_{V1}^{max}, and second half-turns, ω_{V2}^{max} (Figure 1). Finally, dimensionless jerks were calculated during the first, J_1, and second, J_2, half-turns as follows [22]:

$$J_i = \ln\left(\frac{T_{turn-i}^3}{\omega_{Vi}^{max\,2}} \int_{a_i}^{b_i} j^2(t)\,dt\right), \quad (1)$$

where $j = \frac{d\omega_V}{dt}$, $i = 1, 2$, and where a_i, b_i are the time values giving the beginning and end of half-turn i, respectively. The derivative was computed by finite differentiation. We recall that dimensionless jerk is a measure of motion's smoothness. The smaller the J_i, the smoother the motion. We hypothesized that NF would reach smaller durations and jerks, and larger maximal angular velocities than F.

2.4. Statistical Analysis

First, we evaluated the differences between the F and the NF groups, with significance level α of 0.05. For this purpose, t-tests were used for continuous variables, Mann–Whitney tests were used for ordinal variables (scores), and exact Fisher tests were used for categorical variables.

Second, based on the results of the above analyses, models predicting falls in our population were designed by resorting to multiple logistic regression. The logistic regression model is given by the following equation:

$$\ln\left(\frac{P}{1-P}\right) = \beta_0 + \sum_{j=1}^{n} \beta_j X_j, \quad (2)$$

where X_j are the n selected parameters, and where β_0, β_j are fitted on the collected data via multiple logistic regression. Once the β_j are fitted on the data, Equation (2) becomes a classification tool: given a set of parameters X_i, measured on one participant, the output P leads either to the value 0 (no predicted fall) or 1 (predicted fall). The model prediction, i.e., fall or no fall, were then compared with the actual falls of the participants. Note that several models were actually used, differing in the number of selected parameters, n, see below. Model performance was measured by computing sensitivity, $Se = \frac{\text{True positive}}{\text{False negative + True positive}}$, specificity, $Sp = \frac{\text{True negative}}{\text{False positive + True negative}}$ and accuracy, $Acc = \frac{\text{True positive + True negative}}{\text{Total}}$. Five models (Mi with i between 0 to 4) were built for different parameter selections:

- (M0) only $X_1 = T_{TUG}$ parameter used when comparing F and NF groups (TUG in Table 2);
- (M1) all parameters with $p < 0.05$ used when comparing F and NF groups (kinTUG in Table 2): $X_1 = \omega_{V1}^{max}$;
- (M2) all parameters with $p < 0.1$ used when comparing F and NF groups (iTUG in Table 2): $X_1 = \omega_{V1}^{max}$ and $X_2 = T_{TUG}$;

- (M3) all parameters with $p < 0.2$ used when comparing F and NF groups (i + TUG in Table 2): $X_1 = \omega_{V1}^{max}$, $X_2 = T_{TUG}$, X_3 = Walking aid required (Yes = 1, No = 0) and X_4 = Gender (M = 1, F = 0);
- (M4) all parameters with $p < 0.3$ when comparing F and NF groups (i + TUG2 in Table 2): $X_1 = \omega_{V1}^{max}$, $X_2 = T_{TUG}$, X_3 = Walking aid required, X_4 = Gender, $X_5 = T_{turn-1}$ and $X_6 = J_1$.

Age was not included in our models because of its large p-value. It therefore has no ability to discriminate between F and NF in our sample, although a positive correlation between age and T_{TUG} has been found in recent works [26,27].

Table 2. First seven rows: β_i coefficients fitted from model (2). The first row gives β_0. Last three rows: performance indicators of the models (*Se*: sensitivity, *Sp*: specificity, *Acc*: accuracy).

Parameters X_i	M0 (TUG)	M1 (kinTUG)	M2 (iTUG)	M3 (i + TUG)	M4 (i + TUG2)
β_0	−1.709	1.423	0.822	1.207	1.553
ω_{V1}^{max}		−0.0245	−0.0213	−0.0208	−0.0231
T_{TUG}	0.0434		0.0139	−0.0046	0.0197
Walking aid required				0.403	0.333
Gender				−0.637	−0.649
J_1					−0.0027
T_{turn-1}					−0.124
Performance Indicators					
Se (%)	8.3	8.3	12.5	29.2	20.8
Sp (%)	95.9	91.8	91.8	95.9	91.8
Acc (%)	67.1	64.4	65.7	74.0	68.5

t-tests, Mann–Whitney tests, exact Fisher tests and multiple logistic regressions were performed using SigmaPlot software (v. 14.0, Systat Software, San Jose, CA, USA).

3. Results

3.1. Population

The general characteristics of the residents are presented in Table 1. The ratio of females to males is 3 to 1 in the F group, compared with 1.2 to 1 in the NF group. The two groups did not differ significantly in any of the recorded parameters. T_{TUG} is higher in F than NF as expected, with a p-value under the M2-threshold (Table 2). Walking aid and gender reached p-values below the M3-threshold (Table 2).

3.2. F versus NF Comparison

The comparison results for kinematic parameters are presented in Table 3. ω_{V1}^{max} was significantly different in both groups, with a higher mean value in NF. The same trend is observed for ω_{V2}^{max} but with a non-significant p-value. Only ω_{V1}^{max} has a p-value below the M1-threshold (Table 2). J_2 and T_{turn-1} can be included in M4 (Table 2), while the other parameters will not be further considered.

3.3. Multiple Logistic Regressions

Results from the multiple logistic regressions are shown in Table 2. It is readily observed that M3 (i + TUG) reaches the best performances (grey area), and that adding extra parameters (M4) does not improve M3.

Table 3. Comparison of kinematic parameters between fallers (F) and non-fallers (NF) groups. Data are written under the form mean ± standard deviation. p-values for the comparison between F and NF groups are given in the last column; parameters are ordered by increasing p-values, with significant values in bold font.

Parameters X_i	F	NF	p
ω_{V1}^{max} (° s^{-1})	82.0 ± 19.0	92.9 ± 23.4	**0.031**
J_1	12.0 ± 2.3	11.6 ± 2.8	0.203
T_{turn-1} (s)	5.2 ± 2.2	4.9 ± 2.5	0.293
J_2	12.0 ± 3.2	11.4 ± 3.9	0.304
ω_{V2}^{max} (° s^{-1})	96.3 ± 24.5	106.2 ± 35.0	0.315
T_{get-up} (s)	4.8 ± 3.5	4.0 ± 2.2	0.338
T_{sit} (s)	3.7 ± 3.4	3.1 ± 1.9	0.545
T_{turn-2} (s)	4.3 ± 2.3	3.8 ± 2.0	0.569
T_{walk} (s)	4.2 ± 2.2	4.0 ± 3.0	0.634
$T_{walk\ back}$ (s)	3.9 ± 2.7	4.0 ± 4.1	0.773

4. Discussion

Our clinical challenge was to improve the predictive ability of the well-known TUG in two ways: (1) by instrumenting it to assess multiple quantitative kinematic parameters specific to the different subtasks of the TUG and (2) by including qualitative features of the residents. Our multiple logistic regressions led to the development of an i + TUG (M3-model in Table 2) for predicting fall risk in our sample that included the parameters of: a TUG with T_{TUG}, an iTUG with ω_{V1}^{max}, and walking aid and gender characteristics.

Thirty-six residents used walking aids to compensate for postural instability and/or mobility decline (F = 11 and NF = 26). In our sample, the postural instability and/or mobility decline typically have several causes, which include diabetic polyneuropathy (F = 3 and NF = 8), Alzheimer's disease (F = 5 and NF = 14), and post-stroke hemiparesis (F = 2 and NF = 4). No residents with Parkinson's disease were included, but this condition was not an exclusion criteria.

The predictive ability of a fall risk test is a critical component of evidence-based patient care, especially among elderly nursing home residents. The indicators of predictive performance we obtained for i + TUG are better than those for TUG, which shows how interesting it is to add additional information to TUG. Our model can be compared with previously proposed models. In [28], the limited predictive ability of TUG for identifying F in a sample of community-dwelling older adults was already pointed out. They showed a sensitivity of 32% (versus 29.2% with our i + TUG) and a specificity of 73% (95.9%).

In a preliminary study conducted with the same sample of residents [7], we improved the discriminative and predictive qualities of TUG by adding kinematic data collected during a 6MWT. The addition of kinematic factors increased the accuracy of the test from 65.7% to 73.9%, with a sensitivity of 85% and a specificity of 50%. Here, we have shown that, based on data collected with the same sensor in the same sample, it is possible to achieve the same predictive accuracy using only data collected during i + TUG. Combining the results of our previous study [7] and the findings obtained here, it appears that an instrumented 6MWT (i6MWT) and the i + TUG developed here are highly complementary, with one test having a high sensitivity and the other high specificity. Because sensitivity refers to the test's potential to identify F residents and specificity refers to the test's potential to identify NF residents, we recommend that, in daily clinical practice and long-term monitoring of nursing home residents, each resident should undergo an i + TUG in the first instance to rule out that he/she is at risk for falls. If the i + TUG can not rule out that he/she is at risk for falls, an i6MWT must also be performed to confirm that he/she is indeed at risk.

The mean T_{TUG} was 24.5 s for F and 21.5 s for NF, both values that are close to the 22.5 s found in [4] and the 22.1 s found in [29]. Furthermore, the inclusion of kinematic data from a single wearable IMU sensor allowed for computing TUG's subtask durations. It appears that our mean T_{get-up} (4.3 ± 2.7 s) is higher than the value reported in [9] (2.1 ± 0.3 s). This discrepancy can be explained by the fact that the get-up movement is first initiated by a trunk tilt (ω_{ML}, not studied here) and terminated by a hip extension (a_{AP}). We chose the latter way of identifying the get-up phase, while, in [9], they chose the former. Our larger value can also be explained by the age of our sample. As shown in [30], there is indeed a relationship between sarcopenia in the elderly and the long time it takes them to get up.

A clear finding in our study is that ω_{V1}^{max} is significantly higher in NF. This result is consistent with previous findings. In the study [18] that led to the development of the "Dite Turn test", it was shown that elderly people who are more prone to fall turn more slowly and unsteadily. They highlighted four characteristics of the turn performed in the TUG that distinguish F from NF: the time required to turn, i.e., T_{turn-i} that we found to be higher in F, but also indirectly ω_{Vi}^{max}; the number of steps to complete the turn; the stable appearance of the subject during the turn and the fact that the subject makes a smooth transition between the turning and walking subtasks. The number of steps was not measured in this work. However, the smoothness/stable appearance of the movement was evaluated using J_i. We found that J_i is decreased in NF, i.e., their motion is smoother in agreement with the observation of [18], although the difference is not significant. In [19,20], it is also highlighted that the duration and velocity of rotation measured by an inertial sensor during a 7-day period were increased in F. The i + TUG is able to reach the same conclusion within a much shorter time period. Same conclusions about ω_{Vi}^{max} have been found in [19]. As for our results, the jerk was measured during the first and second half-turns. It would have been interesting to extend the measurement to the end and the beginning of walking in the case of the first half-turn, and to the end of walking and the beginning of the transition to the sitting position in the case of the second half-turn. Indeed, it was shown in [13] that the strategies for approaching the half-turn differ between young and old participants regarding velocity. Interestingly, ω_{V2}^{max} is not significantly different between F and NF. This could be due to greater variability in our sample. As pointed out in [31], the second half-turn requires more cognitive skills, different motor planning, and greater visual skills because of the need to anticipate the sitting phase.

We acknowledge that our sample size may be considered small for a geriatric population, which is a limitation of our study. In addition, our measurements were performed in nursing homes and may not be representative of the majority of the elderly population. TUG assesses only the person's global mobility; other risk factors such as visual or cognitive impairment, or polymedication [5] need to be considered to capture the entire clinical picture. To address this limitation, it would be interesting to combine the results of the i + TUG with other tests, such as the Falls Risk Assessment Tool (FRAT), which takes into account the other risk factors mentioned above. Our sample was not designed to examine age effects on fall risk because both F and NF have similar means and a large range of ages. However, age increases T_{TUG} [27], and presumably the fall risk. A review paper [32] found that people aged 85 years or older in the United States are four times more likely to be injured in falls than a population aged 65 to 74 years. Lower limb weakness and, more generally, sarcopenia may be partly responsible for this [33,34]. Knee extensor muscle strength was not assessed. Since knee extensor muscle strength could identify the elderly at risk of falling [35], these missing data are also a limitation of our study. Note that the threshold of 85-years in the review [32] is close to the mean age of our sample, illustrating the importance of predicting fall risk in very old people. A wider spread of age would be required, which is an interesting perspective. Finally, we excluded residents with cognitive disorders that prevented them from understanding the instructions given during the experiment. However, even a mild cognitive impairment could affect the iTUG subtasks [31]. Our protocol does not allow us to determine the impact of mild cognitive impairment on our findings.

5. Conclusions

We have shown that integrating kinematic data collected with a single low-cost IMU during TUG and general resident characteristics can improve the accuracy of fall risk prediction. The new i + TUG achieves 74% versus 67% for the TUG. The i + TUG is highly specific (95.9%) and quick to perform; it may be implemented on a smartphone. We recommend integrating the i + TUG into the test battery commonly performed in nursing homes to rule out residents at risk for falls with a high degree of confidence.

It should be kept in mind that the management of an elderly resident in a nursing home must be multifactorial. The i + TUG must therefore be integrated to optimize a care and diagnostic approach that does not neglect the psychosocial and behavioural aspects and always focuses on the resident/caregiver duo.

Author Contributions: Conceptualization, F.B. and F.D.; methodology, F.B. and F.D.; software, P.-L.S.; validation, P.-L.S. and F.B.; data curation, P.-L.S.; writing—original draft preparation, F.D., F.B., P.-L.S. and G.S.; writing—review and editing, F.D., F.B., P.-L.S. and G.S. All authors have read and agreed to the published version of the manuscript.

Funding: This research received no external funding.

Institutional Review Board Statement: The study was conducted according to the guidelines of the Declaration of Helsinki and was approved by the Academic Bioethics Committee (reference B200-2017-144).

Informed Consent Statement: Informed consent was obtained from all subjects involved in the study or from their legal representatives.

Data Availability Statement: Data are available here: https://osf.io/q45ny/ (accessed on 18 January 2022). In particular, the file Analysed_Data.xlsx contains the parameters X_i needed to fit the β_i coefficients according to Equation (2).

Acknowledgments: The authors thank Louis Catinus and Remi Grenard for data collection, and the following Belgian nursing homes for their support to the project: l'Adret (Gosselies), le Centenaire (Châtelet), le home Notre-Dame De Bonne Espérance (Châtelet) and Au Temps des Cerises (Châtelet). The authors also thank CeREF's technical department for having allowed the use of DYSKIMOT sensor and Anne Genette for discussion about logistic regression in early stages of the project.

Conflicts of Interest: The authors declare no conflict of interest.

References

1. WHO. Falls. 2021. Available online: https://www.who.int/news-room/fact-sheets/detail/falls (accessed on 2 January 2022).
2. Rubenstein, L.Z. Falls in older people: Epidemiology, risk factors and strategies for prevention. *Age Ageing* **2006**, *35*, ii37–ii41. [CrossRef] [PubMed]
3. Podsiadlo, D.; Richardson, S. The Timed "Up & Go": A Test of Basic Functional Mobility for Frail Elderly Persons. *J. Am. Geriatr. Soc.* **1991**, *39*, 142–148. [CrossRef] [PubMed]
4. Shumway-Cook, A.; Brauer, S.; Woollacott, M. Predicting the probability for falls in community-dwelling older adults using the Timed Up & Go Test. *Phys. Ther.* **2000**, *80*, 896–903. [PubMed]
5. Schoene, D.; Wu, S.M.S.; Mikolaizak, A.S.; Menant, J.C.; Smith, S.T.; Delbaere, K.; Lord, S.R. Discriminative Ability and Predictive Validity of the Timed Up and Go Test in Identifying Older People Who Fall: Systematic Review and Meta-Analysis. *J. Am. Geriatr. Soc.* **2013**, *61*, 202–208. [CrossRef]
6. Pettersson, B.; Nordin, E.; Ramnemark, A.; Lundin-Olsson, L. Neither Timed Up and Go test nor Short Physical Performance Battery predict future falls among independent adults aged ≥75 years living in the community. *J. Frailty Sarcopenia Falls* **2020**, *5*, 24–30. [CrossRef]
7. Buisseret, F.; Catinus, L.; Grenard, R.; Jojczyk, L.; Fievez, D.; Barvaux, V.; Dierick, F. Timed Up and Go and Six-Minute Walking Tests with Wearable Inertial Sensor: One Step Further for the Prediction of the Risk of Fall in Elderly Nursing Home People. *Sensors* **2020**, *20*, 3207. [CrossRef]
8. Kurosawa, C.; Shimadu, N.; Yamamoto, S. Where do healthy older adults take more time during the Timed Up and Go test? *J. Phys. Ther. Sci.* **2020**, *32*, 663–668. [CrossRef]
9. Salarian, A.; Horak, F.B.; Zampieri, C.; Carlson-Kuhta, P.; Nutt, J.G.; Aminian, K. iTUG, a Sensitive and Reliable Measure of Mobility. *IEEE Trans. Neural Syst. Rehabil. Eng.* **2010**, *18*, 303–310. [CrossRef]
10. Vervoort, D.; Vuillerme, N.; Kosse, N.; Hortobágyi, T.; Lamoth, C.J.C. Multivariate Analyses and Classification of Inertial Sensor Data to Identify Aging Effects on the Timed-Up-and-Go Test. *PLoS ONE* **2016**, *11*, e0155984. [CrossRef]
11. Bergquist, R.; Nerz, C.; Taraldsen, K.; Mellone, S.; Ihlen, E.A.; Vereijken, B.; Helbostad, J.L.; Becker, C.; Mikolaizak, A.S. Predicting Advanced Balance Ability and Mobility with an Instrumented Timed Up and Go Test. *Sensors* **2020**, *20*, 4987. [CrossRef]

12. Beyea, J.; McGibbon, C.A.; Sexton, A.; Noble, J.; O'Connell, C. Convergent Validity of a Wearable Sensor System for Measuring Sub-Task Performance during the Timed Up-and-Go Test. *Sensors* **2017**, *17*, 934. [CrossRef]
13. Mangano, G.R.; Valle, M.S.; Casabona, A.; Vagnini, A.; Cioni, M. Age-Related Changes in Mobility Evaluated by the Timed Up and Go Test Instrumented through a Single Sensor. *Sensors* **2020**, *20*, 719. [CrossRef]
14. Cimolin, V.; Cau, N.; Malchiodi Albedi, G.; Aspesi, V.; Merenda, V.; Galli, M.; Capodaglio, P. Do wearable sensors add meaningful information to the Timed Up and Go test? A study on obese women. *J. Electromyogr. Kinesiol.* **2019**, *44*, 78–85. [CrossRef]
15. Newman, M.A.; Hirsch, M.A.; Peindl, R.D.; Habet, N.A.; Tsai, T.J.; Runyon, M.S.; Huynh, T.; Phillips, C.; Zheng, N. Use of an instrumented dual-task timed up and go test in children with traumatic brain injury. *Gait Posture* **2020**, *76*, 193–197. [CrossRef]
16. Kim, K.J.; Gimmon, Y.; Millar, J.; Brewer, K.; Serrador, J.; Schubert, M.C. The Instrumented Timed "Up and Go" Test Distinguishes Turning Characteristics in Vestibular Hypofunction. *Phys. Ther.* **2021**, *101*, pzab103. [CrossRef]
17. Caronni, A.; Sterpi, I.; Antoniotti, P.; Aristidou, E.; Nicolaci, F.; Picardi, M.; Pintavalle, G.; Redaelli, V.; Achille, G.; Sciumè, L.; et al. Criterion validity of the instrumented Timed Up and Go test: A partial least square regression study. *Gait Posture* **2018**, *61*, 287–293. [CrossRef]
18. Dite, W.; Temple, V.A. Development of a Clinical Measure of Turning for Older Adults. *Am. J. Phys. Med. Rehabil.* **2002**, *81*, 857–866. [CrossRef]
19. Leach, J.M.; Mellone, S.; Palumbo, P.; Bandinelli, S.; Chiari, L. Natural turn measures predict recurrent falls in community-dwelling older adults: A longitudinal cohort study. *Sci. Rep.* **2018**, *8*, 4316. [CrossRef]
20. Mancini, M.; Schlueter, H.; El-Gohary, M.; Mattek, N.; Duncan, C.; Kaye, J.; Horak, F.B. Continuous Monitoring of Turning Mobility and Its Association to Falls and Cognitive Function: A Pilot Study. *J. Gerontol. Ser. A Biol. Sci. Med. Sci.* **2016**, *71*, 1102–1108. [CrossRef]
21. Skrba, Z.; O'Mullane, B.; Greene, B.; Scanaill, C.; Fan, C.W.; Quigley, A.; Nixon, P. Objective real-time assessment of walking and turning in elderly adults. In Proceedings of the 2009 Annual International Conference of the IEEE Engineering in Medicine and Biology Society, Berlin, Germany, 23–27 July 2009. [CrossRef]
22. Balasubramanian, S.; Melendez-Calderon, A.; Burdet, E. A Robust and Sensitive Metric for Quantifying Movement Smoothness. *IEEE Trans. Biomed. Eng.* **2012**, *59*, 2126–2136. [CrossRef]
23. Hodkinson, H.M. Evaluation of a mental test score for assessment of mental impairment in the elderly. *Age Ageing* **1972**, *1*, 233–238. [CrossRef]
24. Stapleton, C.; Hough, P.; Oldmeadow, L.; Bull, K.; Hill, K.; Greenwood, K. Four-item fall risk screening tool for subacute and residential aged care: The first step in fall prevention. *Australas. J. Ageing* **2009**, *28*, 139–143. [CrossRef] [PubMed]
25. Incalzi, R.A.; Cesari, M.; Pedone, C.; Carosella, L.; Carbonin, P. Construct Validity of the Abbreviated Mental Test in Older Medical Inpatients. *Dement. Geriatr. Cogn. Disord.* **2003**, *15*, 199–206. [CrossRef]
26. Steffen, T.M.; Hacker, T.A.; Mollinger, L. Age- and Gender-Related Test Performance in Community-Dwelling Elderly People: Six-Minute Walk Test, Berg Balance Scale, Timed Up & Go Test, and Gait Speeds. *Phys. Ther.* **2002**, *82*, 128–137. [CrossRef]
27. Zarzeczny, R.; Nawrat-Szołtysik, A.; Polak, A.; Maliszewski, J.; Kiełtyka, A.; Matyja, B.; Dudek, M.; Zborowska, J.; Wajdman, A. Aging effect on the instrumented Timed-Up-and-Go test variables in nursing home women aged 80–93 years. *Biogerontology* **2017**, *18*, 651–663. [CrossRef] [PubMed]
28. Barry, E.; Galvin, R.; Keogh, C.; Horgan, F.; Fahey, T. Is the Timed Up and Go test a useful predictor of risk of falls in community dwelling older adults: A systematic review and meta- analysis. *BMC Geriatr.* **2014**, *14*, 14. [CrossRef] [PubMed]
29. Soto-Varela, A.; Rossi-Izquierdo, M.; del Río-Valeiras, M.; Faraldo-García, A.; Vaamonde-Sánchez-Andrade, I.; Lirola-Delgado, A.; Santos-Pérez, S. Modified Timed Up and Go Test for Tendency to Fall and Balance Assessment in Elderly Patients with Gait Instability. *Front. Neurol.* **2020**, *11*, 543. [CrossRef] [PubMed]
30. Chen, T.; Chou, L.S. Effects of Muscle Strength and Balance Control on Sit-to-Walk and Turn Durations in the Timed Up and Go Test. *Arch. Phys. Med. Rehabil.* **2017**, *98*, 2471–2476. [CrossRef] [PubMed]
31. Mirelman, A.; Weiss, A.; Buchman, A.S.; Bennett, D.A.; Giladi, N.; Hausdorff, J.M. Association Between Performance on Timed Up and Go Subtasks and Mild Cognitive Impairment: Further Insights into the Links Between Cognitive and Motor Function. *J. Am. Geriatr. Soc.* **2014**, *62*, 673–678. [CrossRef]
32. Ambrose, A.F.; Paul, G.; Hausdorff, J.M. Risk factors for falls among older adults: A review of the literature. *Maturitas* **2013**, *75*, 51–61. [CrossRef]
33. Oliver, D. Risk factors and risk assessment tools for falls in hospital in-patients: A systematic review. *Age Ageing* **2004**, *33*, 122–130. [CrossRef]
34. Martinez, B.; Gomes, I.; Oliveira, C.; Ramos, I.; Rocha, M.; Forgiarini, L.A., Jr.; Camelier, F.; Camelier, A. Accuracy of the Timed Up and Go test for predicting sarcopenia in elderly hospitalized patients. *Clinics* **2015**, *70*, 369–372. [CrossRef]
35. Pijnappels, M.; van der Burg, P.J.C.E.; Reeves, N.D.; van Dieën, J.H. Identification of elderly fallers by muscle strength measures. *Eur. J. Appl. Physiol.* **2007**, *102*, 585–592. [CrossRef]

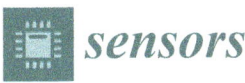

Article

Supervised Exercise Training Improves 6 min Walking Distance and Modifies Gait Pattern during Pain-Free Walking Condition in Patients with Symptomatic Lower Extremity Peripheral Artery Disease

Stefano Lanzi [1,*], Joël Boichat [1], Luca Calanca [1], Lucia Mazzolai [1] and Davide Malatesta [2]

[1] Heart and Vessel Department, Division of Angiology, Lausanne University Hospital, 1011 Lausanne, Switzerland; joel.boichat@unisante.ch (J.B.); luca.calanca@chuv.ch (L.C.); lucia.mazzolai@chuv.ch (L.M.)
[2] Institute of Sport Sciences, University of Lausanne, 1015 Lausanne, Switzerland; Davide.Malatesta@unil.ch
* Correspondence: stefano.lanzi@chuv.ch; Tel.: +41-079-556-49-11

Abstract: This study aimed to investigate the effects of supervised exercise training (SET) on spatiotemporal gait and foot kinematics parameters in patients with symptomatic lower extremity peripheral artery disease (PAD) during a 6 min walk test. Symptomatic patients with chronic PAD (Fontaine stage II) following a 3 month SET program were included. Prior to and following SET, a 6 min walk test was performed to assess the 6 min walking distance (6MWD) of each patient. During this test, spatiotemporal gait and foot kinematics parameters were assessed during pain-free and painful walking conditions. Twenty-nine patients with PAD (65.4 ± 9.9 years.) were included. The 6MWD was significantly increased following SET (+10%; $p \leq 0.001$). The walking speed (+8%) and stride frequency (+5%) were significantly increased after SET ($p \leq 0.026$). The stride length was only significantly increased during the pain-free walking condition (+4%, $p = 0.001$), whereas no significant differences were observed during the condition of painful walking. Similarly, following SET, the relative duration of the loading response increased (+12%), the relative duration of the foot-flat phase decreased (-3%), and the toe-off pitch angle significantly increased (+3%) during the pain-free walking condition alone ($p \leq 0.05$). A significant positive correlation was found between changes in the stride length ($r = 0.497$, $p = 0.007$) and stride frequency ($r = 0.786$, $p \leq 0.001$) during pain-free walking condition and changes in the 6MWD. A significant negative correlation was found between changes in the foot-flat phase during pain-free walking condition and changes in the 6MWD ($r = -0.567$, $p = 0.002$). SET was found to modify the gait pattern of patients with symptomatic PAD, and many of these changes were found to occur during pain-free walking. The improvement in individuals' functional 6 min walk test was related to changes in their gait pattern.

Keywords: intermittent claudication; vascular rehabilitation; 6 min walking test; functional walking

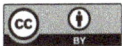

1. Introduction

Lower extremity peripheral artery disease (PAD) is a chronic atherosclerotic vascular morbidity that leads to the narrowing and/or occlusion of lower-limb arteries [1]. PAD affects more than 200 million people worldwide [2]. Intermittent claudication—a pain occurring in the lower limbs during exercise and resolving with rest—is one of the typical manifestations of PAD [1]. Intermittent claudication has a huge impact on patients' daily life activities, leading to reduced quality of life for these individuals [3,4].

Beyond the well-known manifestations of reduced walking capacities, physical function, altered muscular characteristics, and impaired balance [5–9], gait abnormalities have also been documented in patients with PAD [10–17]. Previous investigations reported a reduction in walking speed and cadence, smaller step length, and greater stance phase duration in patients with PAD compared to age-matched non-PAD individuals [13,17,18].

These changes were also observed during pain-free walking conditions [13,15,18]. The attributes of slower gait speed and stride frequency and shorter stride length were recently associated with higher levels of circulating biomarkers of inflammation and endothelial cell oxidative stress [19].

Cardiovascular risk management, pharmacological treatment, and exercise therapy are the main pillars of the treatment of PAD [1]. Following supervised exercise training (SET), greater treadmill walking performance has been well documented, with an improvement of ~82 m and ~120 m in treadmill pain-free and maximal walking distance, respectively [20]. Although less investigated, the 6 min walk test (6MWT)—an overground submaximal functional walking test—is also an effective tool that had been used to assess walking performance following interventions in patients with PAD [21,22]. A meta-analysis showed a mean improvement of ~35 m in 6 min walking distance (6MWD) following SET in individuals with PAD [23].

The question of whether SET induces gait changes, and whether the latter are related to treadmill performance in symptomatic patients with PAD, remains controversial [24–30]. To the best of our knowledge, the recent study by Lanzi et al. [29] is the only study to have assessed this relationship. Their study [29] showed that SET reduced the duration of the push-off and extended the duration of the foot-flat during a constant-speed treadmill exercise. Interestingly, in treadmill tests, gait changes were found to be significantly related to the delayed onset claudication distance [29]. However, the question of whether gait changes following SET are also related to functional walking improvements assessed by the 6MWT remains to be investigated. The investigation of this issue would be clinically relevant, as the 6MWT is representative of the type of walking one commonly partakes in daily life [21]. Following SET, a greater distance covered during the 6MWT is observed alongside an obvious increase in average walking speed. As spatiotemporal gait parameters (such as stride frequency and length) are influenced by walking speed [31], it is expected that gait pattern changes should be observed following SET during the 6MWT.

Previous investigations showed that the durations of the inner-stance phases (e.g., foot-flat and push-off) were altered during an acute treadmill exercise performed at a constant speed in patients with symptomatic PAD [29,32]. These findings showed that, compared to the pain-free walking condition, the duration of foot-flat phase increased and the duration of the push-off phase decreased with the onset of claudication pain [29,32]. The extended duration of the foot-flat phase during exertion may ameliorate the balance between oxygen supply and demand in the active ischemic calf musculature [13,29]. On the other hand, the reduced duration of the push-off phase during the transition from pain-free to painful walking may be related to exercise-induce ischemia, which may lead to calf muscle strength deficit and affect forward propulsion [8]. Notably, even if the onset of the claudication distance was delayed following SET, similar evolutions were observed during a constant-speed treadmill test regarding temporal gait parameters [29]. This suggests that once claudication is established and it worsens to moderate-to-maximal levels, similar gait adaptations occur during an acute bout of exercise before and following SET [29]. However, the evolution of spatiotemporal gait parameters during acute exercise in the form of the 6 min walk test following SET remain to be investigated in these individuals.

The primary aim of this study was to determine the spatiotemporal gait and foot kinematics parameters during an acute bout of 6MWT (acute adaptations) and in response to 3 month SET (chronic adaptations) in patients with symptomatic PAD. It was hypothesized that (1) SET would improve the 6 min walking distance (chronic adaptations); (2) SET would increase walking speed, and as well stride frequency and length (chronic adaptations); and (3) during the transition from pain-free to painful walking, similar acute gait adaptations would be observed during the 6MWT before and after SET.

2. Methods

2.1. Participants

Symptomatic patients with chronic lower extremity PAD were recruited from the Division of Angiology of the University Hospital of Lausanne, Switzerland. As described elsewhere, all the participants were enrolled in the Angiofit study and took part in the SET program [29,33]. For the purpose of this study, we included data regarding all the patients' spatiotemporal gait and foot kinematics parameters during the 6MWT before and following SET. This study was approved by the local ethics committee (study number: 2016-01135) and was conducted in accordance with the Declaration of Helsinki. Before participation, the patients provided written, voluntary, informed consent.

2.2. Experimental Design

Each participant underwent (i) a pre-SET vascular medicine examination; (ii) a pre-SET 6MWT with gait assessment; (iii) a 3-month SET program; (iv) a post-SET 6MWT with gait assessment; and (v) a post-SET vascular medicine examination.

2.2.1. Vascular Medicine Examination

The medical history of each individual was assessed, and physical and vascular evaluations were performed. The ankle–brachial index (ABI) and toe–brachial index (TBI) were measured in accordance with the guidelines [1]. ABI and TBI values related to the most symptomatic leg were considered for the analyses.

2.2.2. Six Min Walk Test

In an indoor 50 m corridor, the patients were asked to walk as far as possible within 6 min to determine their 6MWD [34]. The patients were told that they were allowed to stop during the test and/or lean against the wall. If they did so, they were instructed to resume walking as soon as they could. During the test, standard phrases of encouragement were used in accordance with the guidelines [34]. The pain-free walking time ($PFWT_{6min}$) and distance ($PFWD_{6min}$) during the 6MWT was recorded during the test. These values correspond to the time or distance covered by the patients until the onset of pain. At the end of the test, the rate of perceived exertion on Borg's scale (6: "very very light"; 20: "maximal effort") [35] and the claudication pain severity on the visual analogue scale (VAS; 0: "no pain"; 10: "maximal pain") were also recorded. In the post-SET condition, the 6MWT was performed at least 48 h following the last training session.

2.2.3. Multimodal SET

The patients participated in the clinical multimodal SET program, as previously described [29,33,36,37]. Briefly, the patients performed Nordic walking twice weekly and exercises to strengthen the lower limbs once a week. Each exercise session's duration was 60 min. However, this was the total time available for each training session and does not represent the actual exercising time performed by the patients. Indeed, depending on the exercise tolerance and the baseline functional status of the patient, the actual exercising time at the beginning of the program was around 15–25 min, which increased progressively up to 30–45 min at the end of the program. Each training session started with a 5–10 min warm-up and ended with a 5 min cool down. A clinical exercise physiologist supervised all of the training sessions.

During the outdoor Nordic walking sessions, the patients were asked to walk until they experienced moderate-to-severe claudication leg pain. Subsequently, the patients were asked to rest until they experienced complete (or almost complete) resolution of the pain. To enable complete supervision over the training sessions, patients were asked to walk back and forth over a 100–200 m section of level ground. In addition, the training intensity of the exercise sessions was also monitored using Borg's scale [35]. During the first few weeks of training, patients were asked to exercise at a low intensity (9–11 on Borg's scale). Subsequently, if feasible and safe, the exercise intensity was increased to a moderate or moderate-to-vigorous intensity (12–16 on Borg's scale). The duration of each walking bout depended on the exercise intensity and the induced claudication pain. In general, walking bouts 5–10 min in duration were performed when the exercise intensity (assessed by Borg) was set at a low-to-moderate intensity. On the other hand, walking bouts 1 to 4 min in duration were performed when the exercise intensity was set at a moderate-to-vigorous intensity. The latter, despite inducing a higher cardiovascular stimulation, usually elicits a rapid increase in, and high levels of, claudication pain in these individuals.

The strengthening of the lower limbs was performed indoors with circuit training composed of 5–6 stations. Each station consisted of (1) a different type of walking, such as toe/heel, high knees, side-to-side, or backward walking, or (2) lower-limb resistance exercises (calf/heel raise, lunges, or squats) using body weight, dumbbells, or elastic bands. During the first few weeks of training, the patients were asked to perform 5–15 repetitions of each exercise using their body weight, interspersed with 30 to 60 s of recovery. The exercise training intensity was mainly set at a low level. In the following weeks, the patients were encouraged to exercise at a moderate intensity (12–14 on Borg's scale). To that end, the patients were asked to increase the number of repetitions (20–30 repetitions using their body weight) or to exercise using dumbbells or elastic bands (10–20 repetitions).

During the program, the patients received 6 h of therapeutic workshops on cardiovascular risk factors and a healthy lifestyle (regarding nutrition, physical activity, and tobacco). Compliance with the SET program was defined by the percentage of attended sessions out of the total number of sessions [29].

2.3. Spatiotemporal Gait and Foot Kinematics Parameters

During the 6MWT, the patients wore two Physilog® (GaitUp, Lausanne, Switzerland) inertial sensor units (dimensions: 50 mm × 40 mm × 16 mm, weight: 36 g) [38,39]. These sensors were used to evaluate spatiotemporal gait and foot kinematics parameters [38,39]. Physilog® units integrate a microcontroller, a memory unit, a three-axial accelerometer (range ±3 g), a 3-axial gyroscope (range ±800° s^{-1}), and a battery [38,39]. The inertial sensors displayed good accuracy and precision parameters and showed excellent test–retest reliability [39]. Physilog® units have been validated in young [39] and older adults [38,39]. In addition, these sensors were also validated in individuals affected by stroke [40] and in children with cerebral palsy [41]. Finally, these sensors were previously used in other clinical populations, such as patients with Parkinson's disease [42] and in patients with PAD [29].

The spatiotemporal gait and foot kinematics parameters were recorded during the whole 6MWT. For the analyses, ten consecutive strides were selected 1 min after the beginning of the test (pain-free walking: pain-free) and before the end of the 6 min walk test during the painful walking condition (pain).

During the 6MWT, walking speed, spatiotemporal gait, and foot kinematics parameters were assessed. Stride length was the only spatial parameter. The temporal parameters were stride duration and frequency (i.e., cadence) and the relative duration of the swing, stance, and double support phases (% of gait cycle duration). In addition, the relative duration of the inner-stance phases (i.e., loading response, foot-flat and push-off) were also reported [38,39]. The foot kinematics parameters were the heel-strike pitch angle (the positive angle formed between the level ground and the foot during heel-strike), the toe-off pitch angle (the negative angle formed between the level ground and the foot during toe-off), and the foot clearance (the foot's height during the swing phase). Details regarding the estimation of the spatiotemporal gait and foot kinematics parameters are presented in the supplementary materials.

The symmetry between the legs was assessed by dividing the values of the most symptomatic leg by those of the less or non-symptomatic leg [29].

2.4. Statistical Analysis

The sample size was estimated using our previous data [36], showing that 23 patients were necessary (power 80%; $\alpha = 5\%$). The Kolmogorov–Smirnov test was used to assess the normality of the distribution. First, a two-way repeated measures analysis of variance (ANOVA) (time (before SET vs. after SET) × duration (pain-free vs. pain)) was used to evaluate the symmetry of the spatiotemporal gait and foot kinematics parameters between legs. Second, a two-way ANOVA was also used to compare the gait pattern in the most symptomatic leg alone. If the ANOVAs showed a significant main effect (time or duration) or interaction effect (time × duration), multiple comparison analyses with Bonferroni adjustments were performed to detect the differences. Paired t-tests were used to compare the 6MWT and vascular parameters before and following the multimodal SET program. To determine the relationship between the spatiotemporal gait and foot kinematics changes (i.e., delta; post- minus pre-training values) and changes in 6MWD following SET, partial correlations, controlled for gait baseline values, were performed. The data are expressed as the mean ± SD. The level of significance was set at $p \leq 0.05$. SPSS 27 software (IBM Corporation, Armonk, NY, USA) was used for the statistical analyses.

3. Results

3.1. Participants

Twenty-nine symptomatic patients with chronic PAD were included. All the patients completed the 3 month SET program. Their general characteristics are reported in Table 1. A similar pharmacological therapy was observed before and after SET, except that one patient started antidiabetic therapy during SET. The compliance of the participants with the SET program was 98 ± 4%.

Table 1. Characteristics of the participants.

Variables	Mean ± SD or *n* (%)
Number of included patients	29
Men	15 (52)
Women	14 (48)
Age—years	65.4 ± 9.9
BMI—kg·m^{-2}	28.7 ± 6.2
Cardiovascular risk factors	
Hypercholesterolemia	23 (79)
Hypertension	24 (83)
Smoking (current)	12 (41)
Smoking (former)	13 (45)
Smoking (never)	4 (14)
Family history of CVD	13 (45)
Type 2 diabetes mellitus	8 (28)
Type 1 diabetes	1 (3)
Prior history of CVD	
Cardiac	8 (28)
Cerebrovascular	2 (7)
Prior arterial revascularisation	13 (45)
Ongoing treatment	
Antiplatelet	28 (97)
Antihypertensive	24 (83)
Lipid lowering	23 (79)
Antidiabetic	9 (31)

BMI: body mass index; CVD: cardiovascular disease.

3.2. Vascular Parameters

The values regarding the ABI (before SET: 0.79 ± 0.14 after SET: 0.78 ± 0.14; $p = 0.829$) and TBI (before SET: 0.60 ± 0.15, after SET: 0.60 ± 0.18; $p = 0.971$) were unchanged following SET.

3.3. Six Min Walk Test

Following SET, a significant increase was observed in the 6MWD values (+10%; Table 2). The values regarding $PFWT_{6min}$ and $PFWD_{6min}$ did not change significantly (Table 2). The RPE at the end of the 6MWT was significantly higher after SET (Table 2). Values relating to claudication pain at the end of the 6MWT were unchanged (Table 2).

Table 2. 6 min walk test before and after supervised exercise training.

Variable	Before	After	p Value
6MWD—m	425.5 ± 70.3	468.7 ± 84.3	**≤0.001**
$PFWT_{6min}$—s	125.1 ± 55.4	123.3 ± 54.0	0.869
$PFWD_{6min}$—m	162.5 ± 67.4	179.2 ± 77.6	0.245
$6MWT_{RPE}$	12.3 ± 2.5	13.2 ± 2.2	**0.043**
$6MWT_{VAS}$	6.8 ± 2.2	7.1 ± 1.8	0.432

6MWD: 6 min walking distance; $PFWT_{6min}$: pain-free walking time during the 6 min walk test; $PFWD_{6min}$: pain-free walking distance during the 6 min walk test; $6MWT_{RPE}$: rate of perceived exertion at the end of the 6 min walk test; $6MWT_{VAS}$: claudication pain at the end of the 6 min walk test. Bold p value is statistically significant ($p \leq 0.05$).

3.4. Spatiotemporal Gait and Foot Kinematics Parameters: Acute and Chronic Adaptations

The symmetry of the spatiotemporal gait and foot kinematics parameters between legs showed no significant time, duration, or time × duration interaction effect (data not shown). This suggests that similar acute and chronic adaptations were present in both legs of the participants. Therefore, for sake of clarity, only the results regarding the most symptomatic leg were presented.

3.4.1. Spatiotemporal Gait Parameters (Acute Adaptations)

During the 6MWT, a significant duration effect was observed for all the spatiotemporal gait parameters (Table 3). Multiple comparison analyses demonstrated that walking speed, stride duration, stride frequency, stride length, duration of swing, loading response duration, and push-off phase duration significantly decreased during the transition from the pain-free to painful walking condition, whereas the duration of the stance, foot-flat, and double support phases significantly increased during the 6MWT (Table 3).

3.4.2. Spatiotemporal Gait Parameters (Chronic Adaptations)
Walking Speed

A significant time and time × duration interaction effect was found with regard to the walking speed (Table 3). Multiple comparison analyses revealed that walking speed was significantly increased following SET during the pain-free and painful walking conditions ($p \leq 0.026$, Table 3).

Stride Length

A significant time and time × duration interaction effect was found regarding the stride length (Table 3). Multiple comparison analyses showed that stride length was significantly increased following SET (time effect: $p = 0.013$). Compared to the values recorded before SET, stride length was significantly increased following SET during the pain-free walking condition alone ($p = 0.001$), whereas no significant differences were observed during the painful walking condition ($p = 0.569$).

Stride Duration and Frequency

Following SET, stride duration and frequency significantly increased (time effect: $p \leq 0.001$) with no significant time × duration interaction effect (Table 3).

Table 3. Spatiotemporal gait parameters in the most symptomatic leg during the 6 min walk test before and after supervised exercise training (SET).

Variable	Before SET		After SET		Two-Way ANOVA p-Values		
	Pain-Free	Pain	Pain-Free	Pain	Time Effect	Duration Effect	Time × Duration
Walking speed—m·s^{-1}	1.3 ± 0.2	1.2 ± 0.2 *	1.5 ± 0.2 #	1.3 ± 0.2 *,#	≤0.001	≤0.001	0.031
Spatial Parameter							
Stride length—m	1.4 ± 0.2	1.3 ± 0.2 *	1.4 ± 0.2 #	1.3 ± 0.2 *	0.013	≤0.001	0.020
Temporal Parameters							
Stride duration—s	1.0 ± 0.1	1.1 ± 0.1	1.0 ± 0.1	1.0 ± 0.1	≤0.001	≤0.001	0.502
Stride frequency—Hz	1.0 ± 0.1	0.9 ± 0.1	1.0 ± 0.1	1.0 ± 0.1	≤0.001	≤0.001	0.297
Stance duration—%	60.1 ± 2.0	60.5 ± 1.9	59.6 ± 2.3	60.5 ± 2.4 £	0.431	0.017	0.033
Swing duration—%	39.9 ± 2.0	39.5 ± 1.9	40.4 ± 2.3	39.5 ± 2.4 £	0.431	0.017	0.033
Loading response—%	12.5 ± 3.1	11.0 ± 2.7 *	14.0 ± 3.2 #	11.3 ± 3.0 *	0.013	≤0.001	0.019
Foot-flat—%	55.2 ± 6.3	59.8 ± 6.3 *	53.2 ± 6.4 #	60.4 ± 6.3 *	0.139	≤0.001	0.011
Push-off—%	32.3 ± 4.9	29.2 ± 4.8	32.7 ± 5.5	28.3 ± 5.0	0.706	≤0.001	0.098
Double support—%	20.9 ± 3.5	22.9 ± 3.7	19.5 ± 4.0	21.9 ± 3.9	0.057	≤0.001	0.413

Ten consecutive strides were analyzed during pain-free walking (pain-free) and during painful walking at the end of the 6 min walk test (pain). Bold p value is statistically significant. * $p \leq 0.05$ for significant difference compared to pain-free. # $p \leq 0.05$ for significant difference compared to before SET. £ $p \leq 0.05$ for significant difference to pain-free within after SET condition.

Stance and Swing Phase

After SET, the relative duration of the stance and swing phase was unchanged (time effect: $p = 0.431$); however, a significant time × duration interaction effect was observed (Table 3). Multiple comparison analyses revealed a significant increase in the relative duration of the stance phase during the painful condition compared to the pain-free condition following SET alone ($p = 0.008$). Similarly, a significant decrease in the relative duration of the swing phase was observed during the painful condition compared to the pain-free walking condition following SET alone ($p = 0.008$).

Inner-Stance Phases

A significant time and time × duration interaction effect was observed regarding the relative duration of the loading response (Table 3). Multiple comparison analyses revealed a significant increase in this parameter following SET (time effect: $p = 0.013$). After SET, there was a significant increase in the relative duration of the loading response during the pain-free walking condition alone ($p = 0.001$), whereas no significant differences were observed during the painful walking condition ($p = 0.523$).

The relative duration of the foot-flat phase was unchanged after SET (time effect: $p = 0.139$); however, a significant time × duration interaction effect was observed (Table 3). Multiple comparison analyses revealed a significant decrease following SET during the pain-free walking condition alone ($p = 0.002$), whereas no significant differences were observed during the painful walking condition ($p = 0.420$).

No significant time and time × duration interaction effect was observed for the relative duration of the push-off or for the double support phases (Table 3).

3.5. Foot Kinematics Parameters (Acute Adaptations)

During the 6MWT, all the foot kinematics parameters showed a significant duration effect, except for the first maximal toe clearance (Table 4). Multiple comparison analyses showed that the heel-strike pitch angle, toe-off pitch angle, maximal heel clearance, second maximal toe clearance, and minimal toe clearance significantly decreased during the transition from the pain-free to the painful walking condition during the 6MWT (Table 4).

Table 4. Foot kinematics in the most symptomatic leg during the 6 min walk test before and after supervised exercise training (SET).

Variable	Before SET		After SET		Two-Way ANOVA p-Values		
	Pain-Free	Pain	Pain-Free	Pain	Time Effect	Duration Effect	Time × Duration
Heel-strike pitch angle—°	26.9 ± 6.8	24.4 ± 6.2	27.8 ± 5.9	24.2 ± 5.0	0.463	**≤0.001**	0.080
Toe-off pitch angle—°	−68.8 ± 6.4	−65.2 ± 8.1 *	−70.5 ± 6.3 #	−65.1 ± 7.2 *	0.356	**≤0.001**	**0.047**
Max heel clearance—cm	30.1 ± 5.4	28.9 ± 5.6	30.5 ± 4.5	29.2 ± 5.1	0.517	**0.003**	0.476
First max toe clearance—cm	7.8 ± 4.1	7.6 ± 4.2	7.9 ± 3.2	7.7 ± 3.5	0.837	0.252	0.895
Second max toe clearance—cm	18.1 ± 4.1	16.7 ± 3.4	17.5 ± 4.2	15.6 ± 3.6	0.082	**≤0.001**	0.210
Min toe clearance—cm	2.4 ± 0.9	2.1 ± 0.8	2.4 ± 1.1	2.2 ± 1.1	0.800	**0.013**	0.933

Ten consecutive strides were analyzed during pain-free walking (pain-free) and during painful walking at the end of the 6 min walk test (pain). Bold p value is statistically significant. * $p \leq 0.05$ for significant difference compared to pain-free. # $p \leq 0.05$ for significant difference compared to before SET.

3.6. Foot Kinematics Parameters (Chronic Adaptations)

The toe-off pitch angle was unchanged after SET (time effect: $p = 0.356$); however, a significant time × duration interaction effect was observed (Table 4). Multiple comparison analyses revealed that, compared to before SET, the toe-off pitch angle significantly increased following SET during the pain-free walking condition alone ($p = 0.05$), whereas no significant differences were observed during the painful walking condition ($p = 0.938$). No significant time and time × duration interaction effect was observed regarding the heel-strike pitch angle, maximal heel clearance, second maximal toe clearance, or minimal toe clearance (Table 4).

4. Correlations

The relationships between gait pattern changes during the pain-free walking condition and changes in 6MWD following SET are displayed in Table 5. A significant positive correlation was found between changes in stride length, stride frequency, and second max toe clearance during the pain-free walking condition and changes in 6MWD (Table 5). On the other hand, a significant negative correlation was found between changes in the duration of the foot-flat phase during the pain-free walking condition and changes in 6MWD (Table 5).

Table 5. Relationship between spatiotemporal gait and foot kinematics changes during pain-free walking condition and changes in 6 min walking distance following supervised exercise training.

Gait Pattern Changes	Relationship with the 6 min Walking Distance Changes	p Value
Stride length—m	$r = 0.497$	**0.007**
Stride frequency—Hz	$r = 0.786$	**≤0.001**
Stance duration—%	$r = -0.261$	0.180
Swing duration—%	$r = 0.261$	0.180
Loading response—%	$r = 0.320$	0.097
Foot-flat—%	$r = -0.567$	**0.002**
Push-off—%	$r = 0.303$	0.116
Double support—%	$r = -0.356$	0.060
Heel-strike pitch angle—°	$r = 0.313$	0.105
Toe-off pitch angle—°	$r = -0.100$	0.614
Max heel clearance—cm	$r = -0.112$	0.570
First max toe clearance—cm	$r = 0.035$	0.858
Second max toe clearance—cm	$r = 0.424$	**0.025**
Min toe clearance—cm	$r = -0.117$	0.553

Bold p value is statistically significant ($p \leq 0.05$). All correlations were controlled for gait baseline values.

5. Discussion

The results of this study partially confirm our hypotheses: (1) SET improved the 6MWD in patients with symptomatic PAD; (2) following SET, walking speed, stride frequency and stride length were significantly greater during the 6MWT. However, stride length was significantly increased following SET during the pain-free walking condition alone, whereas no significant differences were observed during the painful walking condition. Similarly, changes in the relative duration of the inner-stance phases (loading response and foot-flat) and the toe-off pitch angle following SET were observed during the pain-free walking condition alone; (3) during the transition from the pain-free to the painful walking condition, the spatiotemporal gait and foot kinematics parameters were shown to undergo a similar evolution before and after SET during the 6MWT. Finally, our results showed that changes in stride length and frequency and in the relative duration of the foot-flat phase during the pain-free walking condition were related to changes in functional walking performance during the 6MWT following SET.

The results of the present investigation confirm previous findings, which showed that SET improves 6MWD in symptomatic patients with PAD [9,23]. We observed a ~43 m improvement in 6MWD, which was greater than the substantial meaningful change of +20 m [43] or +35 m [44] previously observed in these individuals. The greater improvement in 6MWD observed in the present investigation may have been related to the training characteristics of the multimodal SET program. Indeed, the patients combined the strengthening of the lower limbs with Nordic walking, which are both functional training modalities. This type of training likely led to better improvements in functional walking performance. The greater improvement in 6MWD could also be related to the 50 m course length, as previous studies showed that longer course lengths were associated with greater walking distances [45]. By contrast, this improvement was similar to the minimal detectable change of >46 m recently observed in patients with claudication [46]. Taken together, these results suggest that multimodal SET is effective at improving functional walking performance in patients with symptomatic PAD [33,36,37].

During the transition from the pain-free to painful walking conditions, similar acute adaptations were observed for the spatiotemporal gait and foot kinematics parameters during the 6MWT before and after SET. These results extend previous findings observed during constant-speed treadmill exercises in patients with symptomatic PAD [13,29] and highlight that similar acute gait adaptions also occur during the 6MWT, which is a more functional form of walking that represents daily life more accurately [21]. Previous studies have shown that, when compared to aged-matched individuals, gait abnormalities exist from the first step taken (pain-free), suggesting muscle metabolic myopathy in patients with PAD [15,47,48]. Gait worsening was also documented once leg claudication pain was established, highlighting the role of muscle ischemia on gait pattern changes during exertion in these individuals [15]. Our results are in line with these findings. We observed that the walking speed, stride duration, stride frequency, stride length, relative duration of swing, loading response duration, and push-off phase duration decreased (pain-free > end), whereas the duration of the stance, foot-flat and double support phases significantly increased (pain-free < end) during the transition from the pain-free to the painful walking condition during the 6MWT. The extended duration of the stance and the foot-flat phases during exertion may ameliorate the balance between oxygen supply and demand in the active ischemic calf musculature [13,29]. It is also possible that patients adopt this pattern to improve their stability during painful walking [13,29]. The reduced duration of the push-off phase during the transition from the pain-free to the painful walking condition may be related to exercise-induced ischemia, which may lead to calf muscle strength deficit and affect forward propulsion [8]. Consequently, this may also affect walking speed, stride frequency and stride length, and foot kinematics, especially during the 6MWT, where patients are allowed to choose their own walking pace.

In current research, there are a limited number of studies regarding gait pattern changes following exercise interventions in patients with symptomatic PAD, and the findings are inconsistent. Indeed, some studies [27,29,30,49], but not others [24,25,28], observed significant gait changes following SET. The results of the present investigation showed that gait pattern was modified in patients with symptomatic PAD during the 6MWT following multimodal SET. It is, however, interesting to note that many of these changes occurred during the pain-free walking condition alone. Indeed, although walking speed and stride frequency increased following SET, stride length was significantly increased following SET during the pain-free walking condition alone, whereas no significant differences were observed during the painful walking condition. These findings indicate that the increased walking speed observed during the painful walking condition following SET is mainly related to an increased stride frequency rather than increased stride length. Similarly, the relative duration of the loading response phase increased, and the relative duration of the foot-flat phase decreased following SET during the pain-free walking condition alone. The toe-off pitch angle was also increased following SET, but again, during the pain-free walking condition alone. These observations are in contrast to previous findings that show the relative duration of the foot-flat phase was increased during constant-speed maximal treadmill exercises following SET in patients with symptomatic PAD [29]. A possible explanation is that this may have been due to the testing protocol used to assess gait changes following SET. Indeed, compared to the constant-speed treadmill test, walking speed during 6MWT exhibited different values before and after SET. Following SET, the patients demonstrated an improved dynamic balance, which allowed them to walk faster during the 6MWT, causing a reorganization of the durations of the loading response (increased) and foot-flat (decreased) phases during the pain-free walking condition. This is in line with previous observations, which showed that the duration of the foot-flat phase was negatively correlated to walking speed in both PAD and non-PAD individuals [13]. Once claudication pain began and worsened to moderate-to-maximal levels, the walking speed decreased during the 6MWT. Interestingly, the relative durations of the loading response and the foot-flat phases returned to the pre-SET values despite the greater walking speed in the post-SET condition. This suggests that factors other than the walking speed are related to gait pattern changes. These findings indicate the potential role of exercise-induced ischemia and claudication pain on gait adaptations during exertion in patients with symptomatic PAD.

The use of non-invasive inertial sensors with the aim to investigate gait pattern during physical assessment has potential applications with regard to the optimization of the prescription of training in patients with PAD. Indeed, these inertial sensors may easily assess gait pattern evolutions during functional acute exercise performed before and following an exercise training program. This technology allows one to evaluate the gait changes in the transition from the pain-free to painful walking condition, and therefore produces a valid description of daily-life walking pattern in these individuals. In addition, by evaluating the potential correlation between gait pattern and functional performance changes following rehabilitation, specific training approaches could be conceived to optimize patients' benefits. Interestingly, our results showed that the changes in stride length and frequency during the pain-free walking condition were positively correlated to changes in 6MWD. In addition, the changes in the relative duration of the foot-flat phase during the pain-free walking condition were negatively correlated with changes in 6MWD. These findings suggest a link between changes in gait pattern during the pain-free walking condition and improved functional walking performance in patients with symptomatic PAD. These results feature important clinical implications and indicate the need for further investigations regarding the effects of specific gait training modalities on gait pattern and its relation to functional walking performance in these individuals. A previous meta-analysis showed that walking training with cueing of cadence improves spatiotemporal gait parameters more than walking training alone in older patients with cardiovascular disease [50]. Walking training with cueing of cadence, which was usually 5–10% greater than comfortable cadence, improves walking speed, stride length and frequency, and walking symmetry in patients who have experienced a stroke [50]. Based on the gait abnormalities previously observed in patients with PAD [13,15,17,18], these specific gait training modalities could be promising with regard to improving gait pattern and (functional) walking performance in these individuals.

This study featured some limitations. First, the present investigation lacked a control group that did not participate in the 3 month SET. Even though previous findings showed no difference in gait pattern over time in patients with PAD who did not participate in a vascular rehabilitation program [24], future randomized controlled trials are needed to better investigate gait changes following training interventions in these individuals. Second, because of the descriptive nature of our results, it was not possible to elucidate the mechanisms related to our observations. More detailed kinetics and kinematics gait analyses are needed to better describe gait pattern before and after SET. Third, even though it was used in previous works, the inertial system used in the present investigation has never been validated in patients with PAD.

In conclusion, these results show that multimodal SET modifies gait pattern during the 6 min walk test in patients with symptomatic PAD. However, many of these changes (stride length, the relative duration of the loading response and foot-flat phases, and toe-off pitch angle) only occurred during the pain-free walking condition, highlighting the role of claudication pain in gait pattern in this population. In addition, changes in stride length and frequency and in the relative duration of the foot-flat phase during the pain-free walking condition were correlated with changes in 6 min walking distance. These findings suggest that new rehabilitation strategies, including specific gait training modalities, should be further investigated in this population.

Supplementary Materials: The following are available online at https://www.mdpi.com/article/10.3390/s21237989/s1.

Author Contributions: Conceptualization, S.L., D.M.; methodology, S.L., J.B., L.C., L.M. and D.M.; software, S.L., J.B. and D.M.; validation, S.L., J.B., L.C., L.M. and D.M.; formal analysis, S.L., J.B. and D.M.; investigation, S.L., J.B. and L.C.; resources, S.L., J.B., L.C., L.M. and D.M.; data curation, S.L., J.B. and D.M.; writing—original draft preparation, S.L. and D.M.; writing—review and editing, S.L., J.B., L.C., L.M. and D.M.; visualization, S.L., J.B., L.C., L.M. and D.M.; supervision, S.L., L.M. and D.M.; project administration, S.L. and D.M.; funding acquisition, none. All authors have read and agreed to the published version of the manuscript.

Funding: This research received no external funding.

Institutional Review Board Statement: This study was conducted in accordance with the guidelines of the Declaration of Helsinki and approved by the local ethics committee (study number: 2016-01135).

Informed Consent Statement: The subjects provided written, voluntary, informed consent.

Data Availability Statement: The data presented in this study are available on request from the corresponding author.

Conflicts of Interest: The authors declare no conflict of interest.

References

1. Aboyans, V.; Ricco, J.B.; Bartelink, M.E.L.; Bjorck, M.; Brodmann, M.; Cohnert, T. 2017 ESC Guidelines on the Diagnosis and Treatment of Peripheral Arterial Diseases, in collaboration with the European Society for Vascular Surgery (ESVS): Document covering atherosclerotic disease of extracranial carotid and vertebral, mesenteric, renal, upper and lower extremity arteriesEndorsed by: The European Stroke Organization (ESO) The Task Force for the Diagnosis and Treatment of Peripheral Arterial Diseases of the European Society of Cardiology (ESC) and of the European Society for Vascular Surgery (ESVS). *Eur. Heart J.* **2018**, *39*, 763–816.
2. Song, P.; Rudan, D.; Zhu, Y.; Fowkes, F.J.I.; Rahimi, K.; Fowkes, F.G.R.; Rudan, I. Global, regional, and national prevalence and risk factors for peripheral artery disease in 2015: An updated systematic review and analysis. *Lancet Glob. Health* **2019**, *7*, e1020–e1030. [CrossRef]
3. Liles, D.R.; Kallen, M.A.; Petersen, L.A.; Bush, R.L. Quality of Life and Peripheral Arterial Disease. *J. Surg. Res.* **2006**, *136*, 294–301. [CrossRef]
4. Regensteiner, J.G.; Hiatt, W.R.; Coll, J.R.; Criqui, M.H.; Treat-Jacobson, D.; McDermott, M.M. The impact of peripheral arterial disease on health-related quality of life in the Peripheral Arterial Disease Awareness, Risk, and Treatment: New Resources for Survival (PARTNERS). *Program. Vasc. Med.* **2008**, *13*, 15–24. [CrossRef]
5. Gardner, A.W.; Montgomery, P.S. Impaired Balance and Higher Prevalence of Falls in Subjects with Intermittent Claudication. *J. Gerontol. Ser. A Boil. Sci. Med. Sci.* **2001**, *56*, M454–M458. [CrossRef]
6. McDermott, M.M.; Liu, K.; Greenland, P.; Guralnik, J.M.; Criqui, M.H.; Chan, C. Functional decline in peripheral arterial disease: Associations with the ankle brachial index and leg symptoms. *JAMA* **2004**, *292*, 453–461. [CrossRef]
7. Mockford, K.A.; Mazari, F.A.; Jordan, A.R.; Vanicek, N.; Chetter, I.C.; Coughlin, P.A. Computerized Dynamic Posturography in the Objective Assessment of Balance in Patients with Intermittent Claudication. *Ann. Vasc. Surg.* **2011**, *25*, 182–190. [CrossRef] [PubMed]
8. Schieber, M.N.; Hasenkamp, R.M.; Pipinos, I.I.; Johanning, J.M.; Stergiou, N.; DeSpiegelaere, H.K. Muscle strength and control characteristics are altered by peripheral artery disease. *J. Vasc. Surg.* **2017**, *66*, 178–186.e12. [CrossRef] [PubMed]
9. Treat-Jacobson, D.; McDermott, M.M.; Bronas, U.G.; Campia, U.; Collins, T.C.; Criqui, M.H.; Gardner, A.W.; Hiatt, W.R.; Regensteiner, J.G.; Rich, K.; et al. Optimal Exercise Programs for Patients with Peripheral Artery Disease: A Scientific Statement From the American Heart Association. *Circulation* **2019**, *139*, e10–e33. [CrossRef] [PubMed]
10. Celis, R.; Pipinos, I.I.; Scott-Pandorf, M.M.; Myers, S.A.; Stergiou, N.; Johanning, J.M. Peripheral arterial disease affects kinematics during walking. *J. Vasc. Surg.* **2009**, *49*, 127–132. [CrossRef]
11. Chen, S.-J.; Pipinos, I.; Johanning, J.; Radovic, M.; Huisinga, J.M.; Myers, S.A.; Stergiou, N. Bilateral claudication results in alterations in the gait biomechanics at the hip and ankle joints. *J. Biomech.* **2008**, *41*, 2506–2514. [CrossRef] [PubMed]
12. Crowther, R.G.; Spinks, W.L.; Leicht, A.S.; Quigley, F.; Golledge, J. Relationship between temporal-spatial gait parameters, gait kinematics, walking performance, exercise capacity, and physical activity level in peripheral arterial disease. *J. Vasc. Surg.* **2007**, *45*, 1172–1178. [CrossRef]
13. Gommans, L.N.; Smid, A.T.; Scheltinga, M.R.; Cancrinus, E.; Brooijmans, F.A.; Meijer, K.; Teijink, J.A. Prolonged stance phase during walking in intermittent claudication. *J. Vasc. Surg.* **2017**, *66*, 515–522. [CrossRef] [PubMed]
14. Guilleron, C.; Beaune, B.; Durand, S.; Pouliquen, C.; Henni, S.; Abraham, P. Gait alterations in patient with intermittent claudication: Effect of unilateral vs bilateral ischemia. *Clin. Physiol. Funct. Imaging* **2021**, *41*, 292–301. [CrossRef] [PubMed]
15. Koutakis, P.; Johanning, J.M.; Haynatzki, G.R.; Myers, S.; Stergiou, N.; Longo, G.M.; Pipinos, I.I. Abnormal joint powers before and after the onset of claudication symptoms. *J. Vasc. Surg.* **2010**, *52*, 340–347. [CrossRef] [PubMed]
16. Myers, S.A.; Huben, N.B.; Yentes, J.; McCamley, J.; Lyden, E.R.; Pipinos, I.I.; Johanning, J.M. Spatiotemporal Changes Posttreatment in Peripheral Arterial Disease. *Rehabilitation Res. Pract.* **2015**, *2015*, 124023. [CrossRef]
17. Szymczak, M.; Krupa, P.; Oszkinis, G.; Majchrzycki, M. Gait pattern in patients with peripheral artery disease. *BMC Geriatr.* **2018**, *18*, 52. [CrossRef]
18. Gardner, A.W.; Forrester, L.; Smith, G.V. Altered gait profile in subjects with peripheral arterial disease. *Vasc. Med.* **2001**, *6*, 31–34. [CrossRef]
19. Gardner, A.W.; Montgomery, P.S.; Casanegra, A.I.; Silva-Palacios, F.; Ungvari, Z.; Csiszar, A. Association between gait characteristics and endothelial oxidative stress and inflammation in patients with symptomatic peripheral artery disease. *AGE* **2016**, *38*, 64. [CrossRef]
20. Lane, R.; Ellis, B.; Watson, L.; Leng, G.C. Exercise for intermittent claudication. *Cochrane Database Syst. Rev.* **2014**, *12*, CD000990. [CrossRef]
21. McDermott, M.M.; Guralnik, J.M.; Criqui, M.H.; Liu, K.; Kibbe, M.R.; Ferrucci, L. Six-Minute Walk Is a Better Outcome Measure Than Treadmill Walking Tests in Therapeutic Trials of Patients with Peripheral Artery Disease. *Circulation* **2014**, *130*, 61–68. [CrossRef]
22. McDermott, M.M.; Guralnik, J.M.; Tian, L.; Zhao, L.; Polonsky, T.S.; Kibbe, M.R.; Criqui, M.H.; Zhang, D.; Conte, M.S.; Domanchuk, K.; et al. Comparing 6-minute walk versus treadmill walking distance as outcomes in randomized trials of peripheral artery disease. *J. Vasc. Surg.* **2020**, *71*, 988–1001. [CrossRef] [PubMed]
23. Parmenter, B.; Dieberg, G.; Smart, N.A. Exercise Training for Management of Peripheral Arterial Disease: A Systematic Review and Meta-Analysis. *Sports Med.* **2015**, *45*, 231–244. [CrossRef] [PubMed]

24. Crowther, R.G.; Spinks, W.L.; Leicht, A.S.; Sangla, K.; Quigley, F.; Golledge, J. Effects of a long-term exercise program on lower limb mobility, physiological responses, walking performance, and physical activity levels in patients with peripheral arterial disease. *J. Vasc. Surg.* **2008**, *47*, 303–309. [CrossRef] [PubMed]
25. Crowther, R.G.; Spinks, W.L.; Leicht, A.S.; Sangla, K.; Quigley, F.; Golledge, J. The influence of a long term exercise program on lower limb movement variability and walking performance in patients with peripheral arterial disease. *Hum. Mov. Sci.* **2009**, *28*, 494–503. [CrossRef] [PubMed]
26. Dziubek, W.; Bulińska, K.; Stefańska, M.; Woźniewski, M.; Kropielnicka, K.; Jasiński, T.; Jasiński, R.; Pilch, U.; Dąbrowska, G.; Skórkowska-Telichowska, K.; et al. Peripheral arterial disease decreases muscle torque and functional walking capacity in elderly. *Maturitas* **2015**, *81*, 480–486. [CrossRef]
27. Haga, M.; Hoshina, K.; Koyama, H.; Miyata, T.; Ikegami, Y.; Murai, A.; Nakamura, Y. Bicycle exercise training improves ambulation in patients with peripheral artery disease. *J. Vasc. Surg.* **2020**, *71*, 979–987. [CrossRef]
28. King, S.; Vanicek, N.; Mockford, K.A.; Coughlin, P.A. The effect of a 3-month supervised exercise programme on gait parameters of patients with peripheral arterial disease and intermittent claudication. *Clin. Biomech.* **2012**, *27*, 845–851. [CrossRef]
29. Lanzi, S.; Boichat, J.; Calanca, L.; Aubertin, P.; Malatesta, D.; Mazzolai, L. Gait changes after supervised exercise training in patients with symptomatic lower extremity peripheral artery disease. *Vasc. Med.* **2021**, *26*, 259–266. [CrossRef]
30. Schieber, M.N.; Pipinos, I.I.; Johanning, J.M.; Casale, G.P.; Williams, M.A.; DeSpiegelaere, H.K. Supervised walking exercise therapy improves gait biomechanics in patients with peripheral artery disease. *J. Vasc. Surg.* **2019**, *71*, 575–583. [CrossRef]
31. Cavagna, G.A.; Willems, P.A.; Heglund, N.C. The role of gravity in human walking: Pendular energy exchange, external work and optimal speed. *J. Physiol.* **2000**, *528*, 657–668. [CrossRef]
32. Gommans, L.N.; Fokkenrood, H.J.; van Dalen, H.C.; Scheltinga, M.R.; Teijink, J.A.; Peters, R.J. Safety of supervised exercise therapy in patients with intermittent claudication. *J. Vasc. Surg.* **2015**, *61*, 512–518.e2. [CrossRef]
33. Lanzi, S.; Calanca, L.; Berchtold, A.; Mazzolai, L. Improvement in 6-Minute Walking Distance after Supervised Exercise Training Is Related to Changes in Quality of Life in Patients with Lower Extremity Peripheral Artery Disease. *J. Clin. Med.* **2021**, *10*, 3330. [CrossRef]
34. ATS Committee on Proficiency Standards for Clinical Pulmonary Function Laboratories. ATS statement: Guidelines for the six-minute walk test. *Am. J. Respir. Crit. Care. Med.* **2002**, *166*, 111–117. [CrossRef] [PubMed]
35. Borg, G.A. Psychophysical bases of perceived exertion. *Med. Sci. Sports Exerc.* **1982**, *14*, 377–381. [CrossRef]
36. Calanca, L.; Lanzi, S.; Ney, B.; Berchtold, A.; Mazzolai, L. Multimodal Supervised Exercise Significantly Improves Walking Performances Without Changing Hemodynamic Parameters in Patients with Symptomatic Lower Extremity Peripheral Artery Disease. *Vasc. Endovasc. Surg.* **2020**, *54*, 605–611. [CrossRef]
37. Ney, B.; Lanzi, S.; Calanca, L.; Mazzolai, L. Multimodal Supervised Exercise Training Is Effective in Improving Long Term Walking Performance in Patients with Symptomatic Lower Extremity Peripheral Artery Disease. *J. Clin. Med.* **2021**, *10*, 2057. [CrossRef] [PubMed]
38. Dadashi, F.; Mariani, B.; Rochat, S.; Büla, C.J.; Santos-Eggimann, B.; Aminian, K. Gait and Foot Clearance Parameters Obtained Using Shoe-Worn Inertial Sensors in a Large-Population Sample of Older Adults. *Sensors* **2013**, *14*, 443–457. [CrossRef] [PubMed]
39. Mariani, B.; Hoskovec, C.; Rochat, S.; Büla, C.; Penders, J.; Aminian, K. 3D gait assessment in young and elderly subjects using foot-worn inertial sensors. *J. Biomech.* **2010**, *43*, 2999–3006. [CrossRef]
40. Wüest, S.; Massé, F.; Aminian, K.; Gonzenbach, R.; De Bruin, E.D. Reliability and validity of the inertial sensor-based Timed "Up and Go" test in individuals affected by stroke. *J. Rehabil. Res. Dev.* **2016**, *53*, 599–610. [CrossRef]
41. Bregou Bourgeois, A.; Mariani, B.; Aminian, K.; Zambelli, P.Y.; Newman, C.J. Spatiotemporal gait analysis in children with cerebral palsy using foot-worn inertial sensors. *Gait Posture* **2014**, *39*, 436–442. [CrossRef]
42. Mariani, B.; Jimenez, M.C.; Vingerhoets, F.J.; Aminian, K. On-shoe wearable sensors for gait and turning assessment of patients with Parkinson's disease. *IEEE Trans. Biomed. Eng.* **2013**, *60*, 155–158. [CrossRef] [PubMed]
43. McDermott, M.M.; Tian, L.; Criqui, M.H.; Ferrucci, L.; Conte, M.S.; Zhao, L.; Li, L.; Sufit, R.; Polonsky, T.S.; Kibbe, M.R.; et al. Meaningful change in 6-minute walk in people with peripheral artery disease. *J. Vasc. Surg.* **2021**, *73*, 267–276.e1. [CrossRef] [PubMed]
44. Gardner, A.W.; Montgomery, P.S.; Wang, M. Minimal clinically important differences in treadmill, 6-minute walk, and patient-based outcomes following supervised and home-based exercise in peripheral artery disease. *Vasc. Med.* **2018**, *23*, 349–357. [CrossRef]
45. Beekman, E.; Mesters, I.; Hendriks, E.J.; Klaassen, M.P.; Gosselink, R.; Van Schayck, O.C.; De Bie, R.A. Course length of 30 metres versus 10 metres has a significant influence on six-minute walk distance in patients with COPD: An experimental crossover study. *J. Physiother.* **2013**, *59*, 169–176. [CrossRef]
46. Sandberg, A.; Cider, Å.; Jivegård, L.; Nordanstig, J.; Wittboldt, S.; Bäck, M. Test-retest reliability, agreement, and minimal detectable change in the 6-minute walk test in patients with intermittent claudication. *J. Vasc. Surg.* **2020**, *71*, 197–203. [CrossRef]
47. Pipinos, I.I.; Judge, A.R.; Selsby, J.T.; Zhu, Z.; Swanson, S.A.; Nella, A.A. The myopathy of peripheral arterial occlusive disease: Part 1. Functional and histomorphological changes and evidence for mitochondrial dysfunction. *Vasc. Endovasc. Surg.* **2007**, *41*, 481–489. [CrossRef]
48. Pipinos, I.I.; Judge, A.R.; Selsby, J.T.; Zhu, Z.; Swanson, S.A.; Nella, A.A. The myopathy of peripheral arterial occlusive disease: Part 2. Oxidative stress, neuropathy, and shift in muscle fiber type. *Vasc. Endovasc. Surg.* **2008**, *42*, 101–112. [CrossRef] [PubMed]

49. Dziubek, W.; Stefańska, M.; Bulińska, K.; Barska, K.; Paszkowski, R.; Kropielnicka, K.; Jasiński, R.; Rachwalik, A.; Woźniewski, M.; Szuba, A. Effects of Physical Rehabilitation on Spatiotemporal Gait Parameters and Ground Reaction Forces of Patients with Intermittent Claudication. *J. Clin. Med.* **2020**, *9*, 2826. [CrossRef]
50. Nascimento, L.R.; de Oliveira, C.Q.; Ada, L.; Michaelsen, S.M.; Teixeira-Salmela, L.F. Walking training with cueing of cadence improves walking speed and stride length after stroke more than walking training alone: A systematic review. *J. Physiother.* **2015**, *61*, 10–15. [CrossRef]

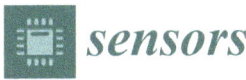

Article

Wearable IMU-Based Human Activity Recognition Algorithm for Clinical Balance Assessment Using 1D-CNN and GRU Ensemble Model

Yeon-Wook Kim [1], Kyung-Lim Joa [2], Han-Young Jeong [2] and Sangmin Lee [1,3,*]

1. Department of Smart Engineering Program in Biomedical Science & Engineering, Inha University, Incheon 22212, Korea; kimywih1@naver.com
2. Department of Physical and Rehabilitation Medicine, Inha University Hospital, Incheon 22332, Korea; drjoakl@gmail.com (K.-L.J.); rmjung@inha.ac.kr (H.-Y.J.)
3. Department of Electronic Engineering, Inha University, Incheon 22212, Korea
* Correspondence: sanglee@inha.ac.kr; Tel.: +82-32-860-7420

Citation: Kim, Y.-W.; Joa, K.-L.; Jeong, H.-Y.; Lee, S. Wearable IMU-Based Human Activity Recognition Algorithm for Clinical Balance Assessment Using 1D-CNN and GRU Ensemble Model. *Sensors* **2021**, *21*, 7628. https://doi.org/10.3390/s21227628

Academic Editors: Fabien Buisseret, Frédéric Dierick and Liesbet Van der Perre

Received: 29 September 2021
Accepted: 15 November 2021
Published: 17 November 2021

Publisher's Note: MDPI stays neutral with regard to jurisdictional claims in published maps and institutional affiliations.

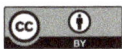

Copyright: © 2021 by the authors. Licensee MDPI, Basel, Switzerland. This article is an open access article distributed under the terms and conditions of the Creative Commons Attribution (CC BY) license (https://creativecommons.org/licenses/by/4.0/).

Abstract: In this study, a wearable inertial measurement unit system was introduced to assess patients via the Berg balance scale (BBS), a clinical test for balance assessment. For this purpose, an automatic scoring algorithm was developed. The principal aim of this study is to improve the performance of the machine-learning-based method by introducing a deep-learning algorithm. A one-dimensional (1D) convolutional neural network (CNN) and a gated recurrent unit (GRU) that shows good performance in multivariate time-series data were used as model components to find the optimal ensemble model. Various structures were tested, and a stacking ensemble model with a simple meta-learner after two 1D-CNN heads and one GRU head showed the best performance. Additionally, model performance was enhanced by improving the dataset via preprocessing. The data were down sampled, an appropriate sampling rate was found, and the training and evaluation times of the model were improved. Using an augmentation process, the data imbalance problem was solved, and model accuracy was improved. The maximum accuracy of 14 BBS tasks using the model was 98.4%, which is superior to the results of previous studies.

Keywords: balance assessment; data augmentation; gated recurrent unit; human activity recognition; inertial measurement unit; one-dimensional convolutional neural network

1. Introduction

Elderly, brain-damaged, and rehabilitation patients often have poor balance. If this and related conditions are not diagnosed promptly, the patients are more likely to suffer further injury by falling [1,2]. Recently, human activity recognition (HAR) was introduced to monitor the motion of a subject in daily life using healthcare devices to determine measures to prevent such accidents [3–5].

In HAR research, various sensors are used, such as an inertial measurement unit (IMU), vision sensors, electrocardiograms (ECGs), and electromyography (EMG) devices [6]. For example, a recent HAR study used a textile stretch sensor attached to patients' clothing [7]. The IMU-based HAR is among the most popular research targets. Even if a non-invasive method is used, such as EMG and ECG, the connections are often unreliable, and they must be changed often, creating fallacious artifact signals [8]. Although cameras are an option, there are limitations to camera installation, owing to bulkiness and obstruction, not to mention privacy issues. Furthermore, lighting and spacing are often problematic [9]. On the other hand, IMUs avoid these problems. Microelectromechanical IMU systems have small size, low cost, and low operational power requirements. Hence, they can be implemented as wearable devices (e.g., smartwatches, fitness bands, and smart clothing [9,10]). Because human health problems are most often expressed as measurable behaviors [11], IMUs are more suitable for daily activity data collection than other sensors. Hence, many IMU-based HAR studies have been accomplished [3–5,9]. Digo's study [12] was conducted to effectively recognize the working condition by wearing only one IMU in the trunk position. This may allow users to wear fewer IMUs, making it easier to use IMUs in daily life. Studies on user motion recognition using an IMU in a smartphone were also performed to recognize motion for daily life [13–15].

Machine-learning models have been widely used [16] for sensor-based HAR measurement, allowing manual and heuristic features to be extracted. Jianchao's study [17] attempted to classify daily patient behaviors with an IMU using global and local features. Global features (e.g., mean and variance) are typically captured using sliding-window techniques, whereas local features typically contain correlation information, such as similarity and error rates. A final feature vector can be determined by using a feature selection algorithm, which shows better classification performance than other methods. In studies using machine learning, the feature selection method often determines the model's performance. In order to extract good manual and heuristic features, sufficient understanding of data and signal processing algorithms is required. Hence, it takes a great deal of time and effort to obtain the desired results because selections and combinations of features must be manually verified [18]. By comparison, deep learning uses raw data as input, and all feature extraction and classification procedures are mathematically combined automatically. Therefore, the process is not only fast and convenient, but it also has the advantage that human error is far less likely. Even features that cannot be recognized by humans can be mathematically extracted. Hence, recently, deep-learning algorithms have been employed more often than machine learning methods, and they have performed well [19]. In a paper by Nathanial Pickle [20], an algorithm was used to estimate whole-body angular momentum and directly determined imbalances by learning wearable IMU data with a one-layer artificial neural network, achieving good performance. In Chung's HAR study [21], data from a multimodal nine degrees-of-freedom IMU was used, and an ensemble model comprising a long short-term memory (LSTM) for each head modality was proposed. Among the many deep-learning studies, the mixed-model convolutional neural network (CNN)/recurrent neural network (RNN) showed better performance than machine-learning models, CNNs, and RNNs alone in many studies [22]. Mekruksa Vanich et al. [23] studied an HAR algorithm using a built-in smartphone IMU. They proposed a four-layer CNN–LSTM model that outperformed the stand-alone LSTM machine-learning model. Mekruksa-Vanich's study [24] demonstrated a CNN-bidirectional gated recurrent unit (GRU) model that showed better classification performance than a machine-learning model, including a CNN with a GRU, against several IMU-based HAR open datasets.

In this work, an HAR algorithm is examined by introducing an IMU system to assess patients via the Berg balance scale (BBS), a clinical test for balance assessment. The BBS is a highly reliable balance test for elderly and stroke patients [25,26]. It consists of 14 static and dynamic motion tasks performed in daily life. Each motion is scored, and the total score is used to assess the patient's probability of falling. A previous study [27] used a machine-learning model for the scoring algorithm. Sensor data with high-scoring contributions were selected for each task. The sum of the energy in the front and rear sections of the motion data was used as a feature, and the amplitudes of frequency components up to 15 Hz were also used. The features were selected by kernel principal component analysis (a feature extraction algorithm), and the data were classified using a support vector machine (SVM). The results showed excellent performance, which improved the performance of Badura's study [3]. However, because these studies used machine-learning models, a great deal of time and effort was required to extract and verify the manual and heuristic features. Hence, in this study, the final feature vector is extracted and classified using a deep-learning algorithm, thus reducing the time and effort requirements of the feature extraction process. It also improves the scoring accuracy. Furthermore, the dataset of the previous study is improved using a signal-processing algorithm, and the performance and computational efficiency of the model are improved. The dataset of the previous paper

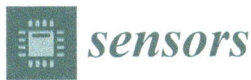

Article

Wearable IMU-Based Human Activity Recognition Algorithm for Clinical Balance Assessment Using 1D-CNN and GRU Ensemble Model

Yeon-Wook Kim [1], Kyung-Lim Joa [2], Han-Young Jeong [2] and Sangmin Lee [1,3,*]

1. Department of Smart Engineering Program in Biomedical Science & Engineering, Inha University, Incheon 22212, Korea; kimywih1@naver.com
2. Department of Physical and Rehabilitation Medicine, Inha University Hospital, Incheon 22332, Korea; drjoakl@gmail.com (K.-L.J.); rmjung@inha.ac.kr (H.-Y.J.)
3. Department of Electronic Engineering, Inha University, Incheon 22212, Korea
* Correspondence: sanglee@inha.ac.kr; Tel.: +82-32-860-7420

Abstract: In this study, a wearable inertial measurement unit system was introduced to assess patients via the Berg balance scale (BBS), a clinical test for balance assessment. For this purpose, an automatic scoring algorithm was developed. The principal aim of this study is to improve the performance of the machine-learning-based method by introducing a deep-learning algorithm. A one-dimensional (1D) convolutional neural network (CNN) and a gated recurrent unit (GRU) that shows good performance in multivariate time-series data were used as model components to find the optimal ensemble model. Various structures were tested, and a stacking ensemble model with a simple meta-learner after two 1D-CNN heads and one GRU head showed the best performance. Additionally, model performance was enhanced by improving the dataset via preprocessing. The data were down sampled, an appropriate sampling rate was found, and the training and evaluation times of the model were improved. Using an augmentation process, the data imbalance problem was solved, and model accuracy was improved. The maximum accuracy of 14 BBS tasks using the model was 98.4%, which is superior to the results of previous studies.

Keywords: balance assessment; data augmentation; gated recurrent unit; human activity recognition; inertial measurement unit; one-dimensional convolutional neural network

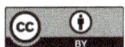

1. Introduction

Elderly, brain-damaged, and rehabilitation patients often have poor balance. If this and related conditions are not diagnosed promptly, the patients are more likely to suffer further injury by falling [1,2]. Recently, human activity recognition (HAR) was introduced to monitor the motion of a subject in daily life using healthcare devices to determine measures to prevent such accidents [3–5].

In HAR research, various sensors are used, such as an inertial measurement unit (IMU), vision sensors, electrocardiograms (ECGs), and electromyography (EMG) devices [6]. For example, a recent HAR study used a textile stretch sensor attached to patients' clothing [7]. The IMU-based HAR is among the most popular research targets. Even if a non-invasive method is used, such as EMG and ECG, the connections are often unreliable, and they must be changed often, creating fallacious artifact signals [8]. Although cameras are an option, there are limitations to camera installation, owing to bulkiness and obstruction, not to mention privacy issues. Furthermore, lighting and spacing are often problematic [9]. On the other hand, IMUs avoid these problems. Microelectromechanical IMU systems have small size, low cost, and low operational power requirements. Hence, they can be implemented as wearable devices (e.g., smartwatches, fitness bands, and smart clothing [9,10]). Because human health problems are most often expressed as measurable behaviors [11], IMUs are more suitable for daily activity data collection than other sensors. Hence, many IMU-based HAR studies have been accomplished [3–5,9]. Digo's study [12] was conducted to effectively recognize the working condition by wearing only one IMU in the trunk position. This may allow users to wear fewer IMUs, making it easier to use IMUs in daily life. Studies on user motion recognition using an IMU in a smartphone were also performed to recognize motion for daily life [13–15].

Machine-learning models have been widely used [16] for sensor-based HAR measurement, allowing manual and heuristic features to be extracted. Jianchao's study [17] attempted to classify daily patient behaviors with an IMU using global and local features. Global features (e.g., mean and variance) are typically captured using sliding-window techniques, whereas local features typically contain correlation information, such as similarity and error rates. A final feature vector can be determined by using a feature selection algorithm, which shows better classification performance than other methods. In studies using machine learning, the feature selection method often determines the model's performance. In order to extract good manual and heuristic features, sufficient understanding of data and signal processing algorithms is required. Hence, it takes a great deal of time and effort to obtain the desired results because selections and combinations of features must be manually verified [18]. By comparison, deep learning uses raw data as input, and all feature extraction and classification procedures are mathematically combined automatically. Therefore, the process is not only fast and convenient, but it also has the advantage that human error is far less likely. Even features that cannot be recognized by humans can be mathematically extracted. Hence, recently, deep-learning algorithms have been employed more often than machine learning methods, and they have performed well [19]. In a paper by Nathanial Pickle [20], an algorithm was used to estimate whole-body angular momentum and directly determined imbalances by learning wearable IMU data with a one-layer artificial neural network, achieving good performance. In Chung's HAR study [21], data from a multimodal nine degrees-of-freedom IMU was used, and an ensemble model comprising a long short-term memory (LSTM) for each head modality was proposed. Among the many deep-learning studies, the mixed-model convolutional neural network (CNN)/recurrent neural network (RNN) showed better performance than machine-learning models, CNNs, and RNNs alone in many studies [22]. Mekruksa Vanich et al. [23] studied an HAR algorithm using a built-in smartphone IMU. They proposed a four-layer CNN–LSTM model that outperformed the stand-alone LSTM machine-learning model. Mekruksa-Vanich's study [24] demonstrated a CNN-bidirectional gated recurrent unit (GRU) model that showed better classification performance than a machine-learning model, including a CNN with a GRU, against several IMU-based HAR open datasets.

In this work, an HAR algorithm is examined by introducing an IMU system to assess patients via the Berg balance scale (BBS), a clinical test for balance assessment. The BBS is a highly reliable balance test for elderly and stroke patients [25,26]. It consists of 14 static and dynamic motion tasks performed in daily life. Each motion is scored, and the total score is used to assess the patient's probability of falling. A previous study [27] used a machine-learning model for the scoring algorithm. Sensor data with high-scoring contributions were selected for each task. The sum of the energy in the front and rear sections of the motion data was used as a feature, and the amplitudes of frequency components up to 15 Hz were also used. The features were selected by kernel principal component analysis (a feature extraction algorithm), and the data were classified using a support vector machine (SVM). The results showed excellent performance, which improved the performance of Badura's study [3]. However, because these studies used machine-learning models, a great deal of time and effort was required to extract and verify the manual and heuristic features. Hence, in this study, the final feature vector is extracted and classified using a deep-learning algorithm, thus reducing the time and effort requirements of the feature extraction process. It also improves the scoring accuracy. Furthermore, the dataset of the previous study is improved using a signal-processing algorithm, and the performance and computational efficiency of the model are improved. The dataset of the previous paper had a data imbalance problem. To resolve this, an oversampling-based data augmentation process was performed to equalize the amount of data for each class and to increase the total amount of data. These efforts led to an increase in the accuracy of the model. Additionally, the previous data suffered oversampling of participants' movement data. This was resolved by finding an optimal sampling rate of data. The sampling rate of the data was reduced. Hence, it is now possible to reduce the computational complexity while preserving classification accuracy. This also lowers the data-sampling rate of the IMU module, which contributes to reducing the power consumption of the wearable device. Furthermore, we further improve the deep-learning model by optimizing the GRU and one-dimensional (1D) CNN models with a shallow structure in consideration of our small dataset. Additionally, performance improvement was achieved by using an ensemble of the two models. As with previous papers, we attempted to create a single model that can cover all BBS tasks. As a result of our experiments, the model comprising two 1D-CNN heads and one GRU head stacking ensemble model had the highest average accuracy on all 14 tasks. This result was superior to previous results [3,27].

2. Materials and Methods

2.1. Experiment

2.1.1. Motion and Experimental Protocol

The BBS was devised to assess the balance of elderly and stroke patients [25,26]. For this exam, subjects are asked to perform 14 functional tasks, and a rehabilitation therapist assigns a score from 0 to 4 for each task. Combined scores of 0 to 20, 21 to 40, and 41 to 56 represent balance impairment, acceptable balance, and good balance, respectively. Table 1 presents a description of the 14 BBS tasks.

Table 1. Berg balance scale tasks.

No.	Task Description
1	Sitting to standing
2	Standing unsupported
3	Sitting unsupported
4	Standing to sitting
5	Transfers
6	Standing with eyes closed
7	Standing with feet together
8	Reaching forward with outstretched arms
9	Retrieving object from floor
10	Turning to look behind
11	Turning 360°
12	Placing alternate foot on stool
13	Standing with one foot in front
14	Standing on one foot

The experiment was performed at the Stroke (brain injury) rehabilitation clinic of the Department of Rehabilitation, Inha University Hospital. The patient wore a wearable IMUs and performed BBS with a rehabilitation therapist in the same manner as the usual BBS assessment. Some patients could not do all tasks, and they perform only tasks that they could do. Patient data had a data imbalance problem in which the amount of data for each score was different and some scores had no data. Therefore, a healthy participant experiment was conducted to complement the lack of data. Healthy participant experiments were advised by rehabilitation specialists and experimented under the coach of rehabilitation therapists. The healthy participants conducted experiments that imitated the patient's movements. The healthy participants performed all the motions with a score of 0 to 4 in the 14 tasks of the BBS assessment. Therefore, in the experiment with healthy participants, it was possible to obtain the same as five times of experiment data per person.

2.1.2. Participants

This study was approved by the Institutional Review Board of Inha University Hospital. Among hospitalized brain disease patients, those expected to be at risk of falling due to poor balance participated. The diseases of each patient differed slightly, but each had either cerebral infarction, cerebral hemorrhage, brain atrophy, or brain embolism. A total of 53 patients (31 male and 22 female) participated, and their ages ranged from 50 to 80 years. The mean age was 64.9, and the standard deviation was 12.6. The healthy experimental participants included three males in their 20s. The average age of healthy participants was 28.7, and the standard deviation of age was 0.6. Figure 1 shows scenes of the BBS experiment conducted with a healthy participant.

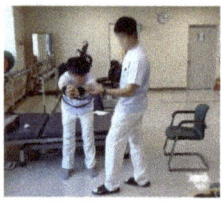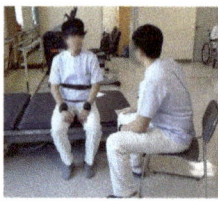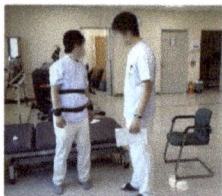

Figure 1. Scenes of BBS experiment conducted with a healthy participant.

2.1.3. Equipment and Data

Noraxon's myoMotion was used for the experiment. This equipment is a multichannel wireless IMU system certified as an ISO 13485 compliant (Registration # MED-0037b) and an FDA 510 K compliant (Registration number #2098416) medical device. The system consists of a multi-channel IMU module capable of wireless data transmission, a receiver, and a Velcro band for attaching the IMU to the human body. The receiver was connected to a computer via USB and records the received data using the provided software. By adding a USB webcam to the configuration, it can record video time-synchronized with IMU data. Because the recorded video and IMU data can be checked simultaneously, the video can be used as the golden state of the IMU data. Figure 2 shows the configuration of the Noraxon myoMotion.

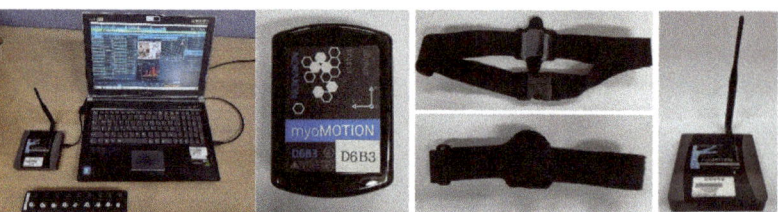

Figure 2. Configuration of the Noraxon myoMotion.

IMU sensors were attached at eight locations: the forehead (FH), back (B), both wrists (RtW: right wrist, LtW: left wrist), both ankles (RtA: right ankle, LtA: left ankle), and both hips (right and left hips). Each IMU sensor yielded nine types of sensor data: three-dimensional (3D) acceleration data (Ac_x, Ac_y, Ac_z); and data that excluded gravity and pitch (P), roll (R), yaw (Y), and 3D rotation data (Ro_x, Ro_y, Ro_z). The rotation data contained the number of accumulated rotations for each 3D axis. The sampling rate of the data was 100 Hz. Figure 3 shows the position of wearable IMU and the types of IMU sensor data.

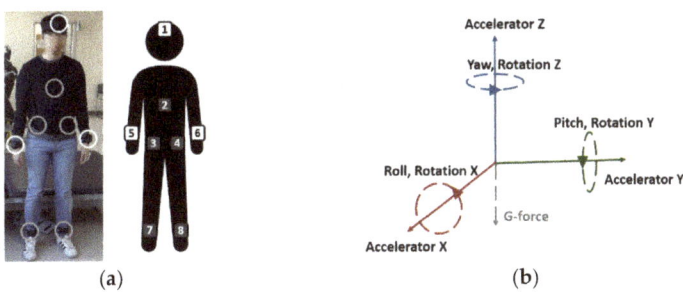

Figure 3. (**a**) Position of wearable IMU sensor; (**b**) the types of IMU sensor data.

2.1.4. Output Data Description

Each IMU outputs nine data types, owing to the eight IMUs used. This provides a total of 72-dimensional time series data items output in real time. Additionally, video was recorded for use as a golden state of IMU data. The duration of the experiment for patient participants was approximately 10–15 min. Some patients could not perform all 14 tasks, resulting in shorter performance times. Fifty-three experimental data were recorded from the patients. Three healthy participants performed all the motions from score 0 to score 4, and 15 experimental data were obtained from the healthy participants. Therefore, the equivalent of 78 experimental data were recorded.

2.2. Methodology of the Proposed Method

Figure 4 presents the methodology of the proposed method. Before training the deep-learning model with the data, the dataset was improved, and 14 models were evaluated by 10-fold cross-validation.

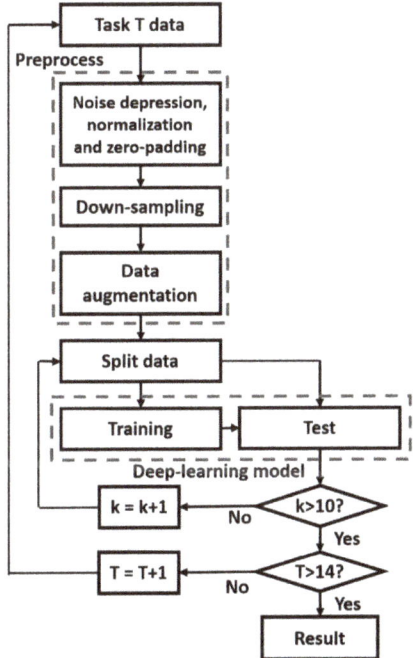

Figure 4. Methodology of the proposed method.

2.2.1. Preprocess

Noise Depression, Normalization, and Zero-Padding

The high-frequency noise of an inertial sensor can be removed using an empirical mode decomposition algorithm [28]. As in a previous study [27], the signal was decomposed into 10 intrinsic mode function (IMF) components and resynthesized from the first to the seventh IMF (low-frequency components) to remove the high-frequency component considered to be noise. Min–max feature scaling normalization was performed on the data to prevent the model from being biased to large values caused by unit differences. Multivariate time-series motion data output from the eight wearable IMUs were continuously recorded from the start to the end of the assessment. Therefore, it was necessary to extract only the section in which the assessment was performed from the data. Using the video, each task execution section was identified, and the IMU data of this section was used as task data. The data length for each task was set to the longest data item in the task, and zero paddings were performed at the end of the data having short lengths.

Data Down-Sampling

According to a previous IMU-based HAR study, even when the sampling rate for 100–250 Hz data was decreased to 12–42 Hz [29], the performance reduction was small, and even the sampling rate of 10 Hz was sufficiently recognizable [21]. Likewise, because the sampling rate of the BBS motion data was 100 Hz, adequate down-sampling was expected to improve the efficiency of the model. To select an appropriate sampling rate, the accumulated information with respect to the frequency was observed, and the accuracy, training time, and evaluation time before and after down-sampling were compared with a classification model. The process is described in detail in Steps 1–5.

1. From the first person in Task 1, an n-point fixed Fourier transform was applied to each of the 72 sensor data outputs from the eight IMUs, and amplitudes from first to the n/2th were extracted.
2. For each person, the amplitude values of all sensors were summed for each frequency component. The accumulated amplitude value for each N Hz frequency was calculated, where N = {1, 2, 3 . . . 50}. The accumulated amplitude for each frequency was divided by the sum of the amplitudes up to 50 Hz, which is the sum of all frequency components, and multiplied by 100 to obtain the percentage (%). Thereafter, the average percentage of the accumulated data for each frequency for all the subjects were calculated.
3. Processes 1–2 were repeated until Task 14, and the average of all tasks in terms of the percentage of accumulated data/information were calculated for each frequency.
4. The trend of the accumulated information was observed for each frequency, and a frequency having a small increase was selected. To restore up to the corresponding frequency component, the sampling rate was set to twice the frequency component based on the Nyquist sampling theory [30].

The accuracy, training time, and evaluation time of the model were compared before and after the data down-sampling.

Data Augmentation Using the Over-Sampling Technique

A medical dataset can easily become unbalanced because it is difficult to obtain negative class data [31]. Therefore, the amount of BBS motion data for each score was unequal. If the model is trained on an unbalanced dataset, the model may be biased toward the majority class, leading to poor performance [32,33]. One way of solving this problem is to balance the dataset by generating new data similar to the original [34–36]. Similarly, BBS motion data can be improved using an oversampling technique [37]. As in Khorshidi's study [38], an over-sampling technique was applied to both the majority and minority classes to equalize the amount of data in each and to increase the total number. Steps 1–3 below describe the data augmentation process:

1. The class set of the scores was A_s. The number of k samples with the closest Euclidean distance to a random sample, x ($x \in A_n$), is x_k ($x_k \in A_n$). x_k can be obtained using the k-nearest neighbor algorithm.
2. The number of n ($n \leq k$) new samples between x and x_k is x_n, and the rule for generating x_n is given by Equation (1):

$$x_n = x + rand(0,1) * |x - x_k| \tag{1}$$

3. Steps 1 and 2 are repeated, so that the amount of class data in each class ($A_0 \sim A_4$) becomes N.

To evaluate the model performance, k = 2 and N = 60 were applied using the augmentation process.

2.2.2. Classification Model

In this study, 1D-CNN and GRU ensemble classification models were introduced for the BBS scoring algorithm. The 1D-CNN and LSTM models often show good performance on multivariate time-series data [39–41]. Because the amount of BBS data is small, each 1D-CNN and GRU model was constructed with a shallow structure, which is advantageous for small amounts of data [42,43]. The following describes the 1D-CNN and GRU structures used in the experiment and the ensemble model that showed the best performance.

1D-CNN Head and GRU Head

The 1D-CNN head has one convolution layer followed by a max-pooling layer with a size of two, followed by a flattening layer. The kernel size of the convolution layer was three, the number of filters was 64, and the rectified linear unit was used as the activation function. The padding option was the same, and stride was set to one.

The GRU head had a one-time-distributed GRU layer, and its output was flattened. The input size of the GRU unit was 64, and the output size was 64. When using a non-time-distributed GRU layer, the information of all units in the layer was compressed into one vector having a fixed size. Therefore, if the input is long, information may be lost, leading to low model performance [44]. However, the time-distributed GRU layer outputs a feature vector for each unit, and this problem can be alleviated.

1D-CNN, GRU Stacking Ensemble Model

The 1D-CNN and GRU stacking ensemble model is composed of three heads. The three heads include two 1D-CNN heads having a kernel size of one and three, and one GRU head is composed of a one-time distributed GRU layer. The outputs of the three heads are then concatenated, followed by a dense layer with 100 perceptrons. In this case, between these two layers, a 50% dropout was applied to prevent overfitting and to generalize the model. The last layer was a softmax with five perceptrons.

The overall structure was a stacking ensemble. The three heads represented each of the models, and the subsequent layers were meta-learners. The meta-learner was equally applied to the proposed model and other experimental models. Figure 5 shows the structure of the 1D-CNN and GRU stacking ensemble model.

Training and Evaluation

The model optimizer was Adam with a learning rate of 0.001. The loss function used was the categorical cross entropy, and the batch size was optimized for each task. Batch $size_{1\sim14}$ = {64, 32, 64, 16, 32, 32, 32, 64, 32, 64, 64, 64, 64, 64}. Early stopping was applied; the training was completed when the loss no longer decreased, the patience number was 20, and the maximum number of epochs was limited to 500.

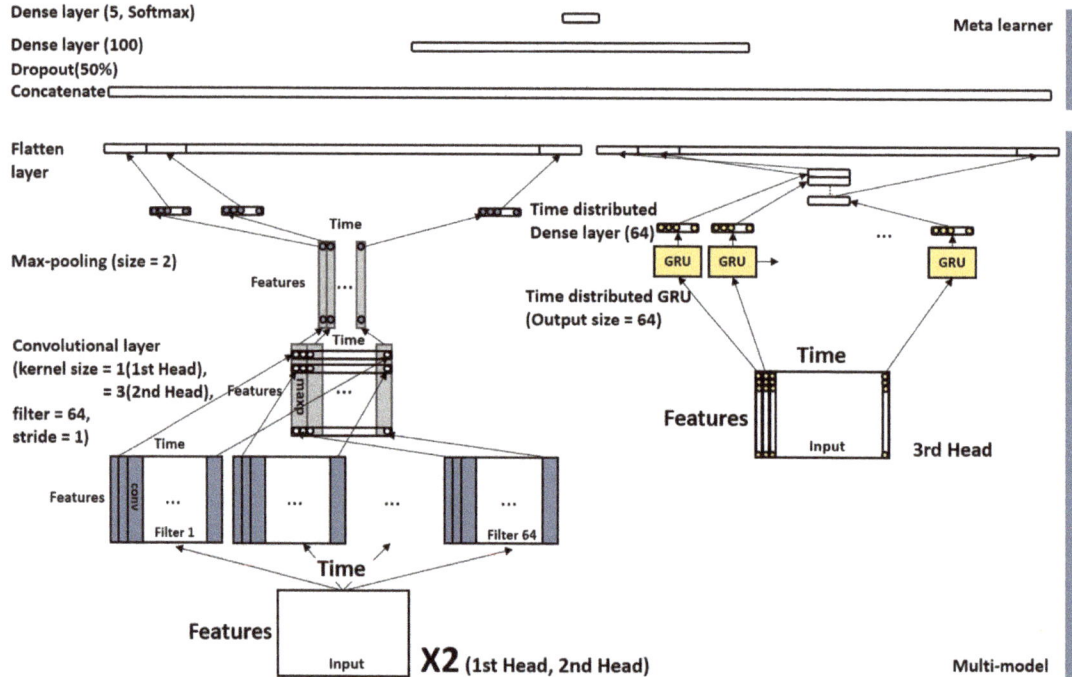

Figure 5. Structure of the 1D-CNN and GRU stacking ensemble model.

When evaluating the accuracy of a model with data randomly split into training and testing, there may be differences in the accuracy, depending on the split data. Therefore, the model performance was evaluated using the average of the Stratified K-fold cross-validation accuracy. Stratified K-fold cross-validation maintains the ratio of the amount of data per class of the original dataset when splitting the training and test data in K-fold cross-validation. Because the amount of data for each class was equalized by improving the dataset, the data for each class for training and testing were also equalized. Only accuracy was used as the evaluation metric because the model was trained on balanced data; hence, it was not necessary to use an evaluation metric such as the F1 score used in the case of imbalanced data [45]. When evaluating the model, the average performance of all BBS tasks was used; this was to make a good model that could cover all BBS tasks, as in previous studies [3,27].

3. Results and Discussion

3.1. Improving Model Efficiency through a Data Down-Sampling Process

To determine an appropriate sampling rate, the accumulated data for each frequency were analyzed. Figure 6 shows the amount of accumulated data with respect to the frequency.

As the frequency increases, the increase in the amount of data tends to decrease. The sum of the frequency components under 10 Hz was more than 90% of the total information, thus confirming that most of the information is in the low-frequency region. In the 5–10 Hz range, the increase in the information rapidly decreases and thereafter remains small. Therefore, the appropriate sampling rate was set such that the frequency component below 10 Hz could be restored. According to the Nyquist sampling theory [30], the sampling rate required to restore a frequency component of n Hz is $2 \times n$ Hz. Therefore, the appropriate sampling rate was set to 20 Hz.

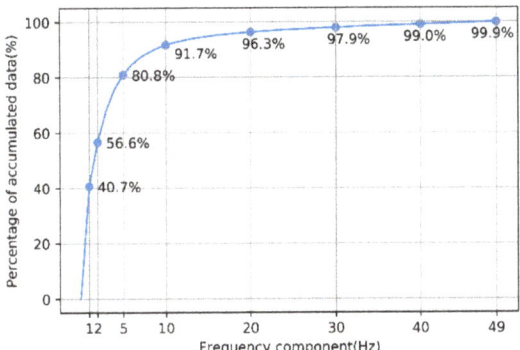

Figure 6. Percentage of accumulated data with respect to the frequency.

When down-sampling data from 100 to 20 Hz, the amount of data was reduced by 80%; however, the amount of information was reduced by 8.3%. The classification performance of the scoring model was compared to the data before and after down-sampling to determine the degree to which this loss of information affects the scoring performance. Figure 7 shows the scoring accuracy of 14 tasks using the 1D-CNN model before and after down-sampling. Input data of the model was preprocessed multidimensional time-series data output from the eight IMUs.

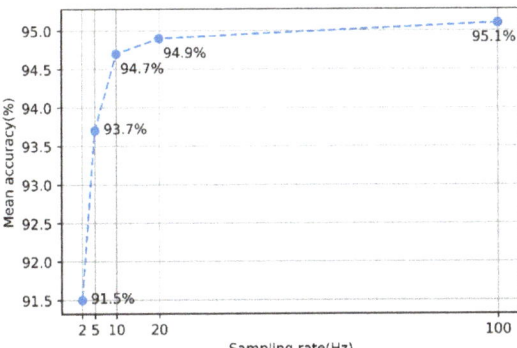

Figure 7. Sampling rate vs. accuracy of the 1D-CNN model.

When the sampling rate was 20 Hz, the average accuracy of the model decreased by 0.2%. When the data sampling rate was 20 Hz, the training time was reduced by 67.7% compared with when the sampling rate was 100 Hz; in addition, the epoch time was reduced by 66.4%, and the evaluation time was reduced by 58.6%. After down-sampling the data, the gain in the computational efficiency of the model was greater than the loss, owing to the performance decrease caused by information loss. As shown in Figure 7, when the sampling rate was below 20 Hz, the decrease in accuracy was greater; therefore, it was not appropriate to further lower the sampling rate. By observing the graph of Figures 6 and 7, given the similarity in the shapes, the correlation between the amount of information and the model performance is considered to be high. Therefore, predicting the decrease in the model performance based on the amount of information is a reasonable method.

3.2. Classification Model

The 1D-CNN and RNN based models, which show good performance on multivariate time-series data, were used as the scoring algorithms. In many studies, the performance could be improved with the 1D-CNN- and RNN-based ensemble models rather than using them alone [23,46–48]. This study also tried to find the model structure with the best performance by combining the 1D-CNN model and the RNN-based model using various model structures. Table 2 presents the average performance of the model in the 14 tasks. The performance on each task is the average performance of 10-fold cross-validation. The model names listed in the table are abbreviated as follows: 1D-CNN: C; GRU: G; Double head 1D-CNN: DC; Triple-head 1D-CNN: TC; 1D-CNN after GRU: C-G; 1D-CNN and GRU parallel: C+G; and double-head 1D CNN and GRU parallel: DC+G.

Table 2. Performance of 1D-CNN, GRU-based model.

Model	C	G	DC	TC	C-G	C+G	DC+G
Mean accuracy (%)	94.9	95.6	95.6	95.3	95.3	95.9	96.1
Standard deviation of accuracy (%)	4.4	4.1	4.0	4.4	4.7	4.1	3.8
Max accuracy (%)	99.8	99.8	100	99.8	100	100	100
Min accuracy (%)	87.1	87.4	87.6	86.4	85.7	87.2	88.8
Mean epoch	64.9	80.6	69.9	63.8	80.1	71.7	78.8
Mean training time (s)	5.172	21.351	8.383	10.270	13.304	21.729	26.551
Epoch time (s)	0.081	0.265	0.120	0.161	0.166	0.303	0.337
Evaluation time (s)	0.099	0.073	0.142	0.153	0.115	0.095	0.129

Before constructing the ensemble model, the parameters of the single 1D-CNN and GRU models were optimized, and their performance was checked. Between the two models, the mean accuracy of the GRU model was 95.6%, which is 0.7% higher than that of the 1D-CNN model. However, the training time of the 1D-CNN model was about 76% shorter than that of the GRU model. Therefore, the 1D-CNN and GRU model were both excellent. After this test, various 1D-CNN and GRU ensemble models were tested to find the optimal model.

First, a double-head 1D-CNN model with kernel sizes of one and three was tested for the scoring algorithm. In previous studies [49,50], the performance of multi-head 1D-CNN was found to be better than that of the single-head 1D-CNN and LSTM. The test results showed that the mean accuracy of the double-head 1D-CNN was 95.6%, which is 0.7% higher than that of the 1D-CNN single model and the same as that of the GRU single model. However, the training time was 60% shorter than that of the GRU single model. Therefore, it could be helpful in improving performance. Additionally, triple-head 1D-CNN models with kernel sizes of one, three, and five were tested. The experimental results showed that the performance of the triple-head 1D-CNN was not better than that of the double-head 1D-CNN because the mean accuracy of the triple-head 1D-CNN model was 0.3% lower than that of the double-head 1D-CNN model, and the training time of the triple-head 1D-CNN model was 23% longer than that of the double-head 1D-CNN model; hence, adding three or more 1D-CNN heads did not improve performance.

Second, a model comprising a GRU layer after the 1D-CNN layer was tested. It is natural for the GRU layer to come after the CNN layer in theory [51]. Therefore, many studies have used this model and have obtained good performance [52,53]. The test results showed that the mean accuracy of the 1D-CNN after the GRU model was 95.3%, which is 0.4% higher than that of the 1D-CNN single model, but it was 0.3% lower than that of the GRU single model. Additionally, the training time of the 1D-CNN after the GRU model was 59% longer, and the mean accuracy was 0.3% lower than that of the double-head 1D-CNN model.

Third, the 1D-CNN and GRU parallel models were tested. In XU's study [54], the CNN and LSTM parallel models outperformed the 1D-CNN and LSTM single models.

From the test results, the mean accuracy of the 1D-CNN and GRU parallel models was 95.6%, which is 1.0 and 0.3% higher than that of the 1D-CNN and GRU single models, respectively. It was also 0.3% higher than the double-head 1D-CNN model, whose mean accuracy was the highest.

From the previous test results, the performance improved in two cases: double-head 1D-CNN model and 1D-CNN and GRU parallel models. Therefore, a model with two 1D-CNN heads and one GRU head, which is a stacking ensemble model, was tested. The results of the test showed that the mean accuracy of the two 1D-CNN heads and one GRU head model was 96.1%, which was the highest of all tested models. Additionally, the stability of this model was the best because the standard deviation of the accuracy of the model was 0.2–0.9% lower than that of the other models.

3.3. Improvement in Model Performance through Data Augmentation

One of the objectives of this study was to develop a model that shows good performance in all BBS tasks. Therefore, the amount of data for each score in all the tasks was made the same so that the effect of augmentation was equal for each task. The amount of data for each score was set to 60 for the model tests. Because Task 2 "Standing unsupported," which had the most imbalanced data, had 56 participants' motion data with Score 4. The under-sampling technique was not considered because over-sampling showed generally better performance in the data imbalance problem [37]. Many studies have improved the performance of classification models using the oversampling technique [34–36,55]. However, the over-sampling technique also decreases the model performance because new data increases noise or can cause overlapping between classes [56]. Therefore, the amount of data for each score was fixed at 60 to reduce the complexity of the experiment. Subsequently, using the model with the best performance, the test was performed to determine whether the model performance could be improved when the amount of data was increased. Figure 8 shows the model performance with respect to the amount of data for each score.

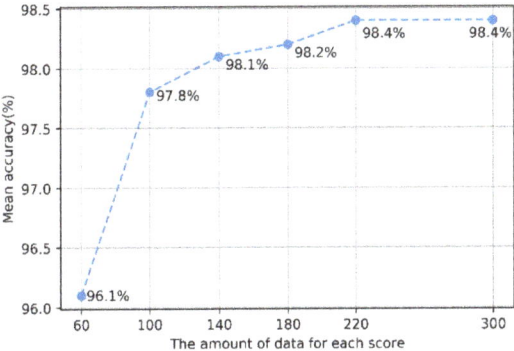

Figure 8. Accuracy of the best model with respect to the amount of data for each score.

The average accuracy increases with the increase in the amount of data for each score. The model performance was saturated when the amount of data for each score was 220. Therefore, it was confirmed that the appropriate amount of data for each score to maximize the model performance was 220. When the amount of data for each score was 220, the average accuracy on the 14 tasks was 98.4%. Figures 9 and 10 show boxplots of the accuracy of the model in the 14 tasks when the amount of data for each score was 60 and 220, respectively. The accuracy increased, and the variance of the accuracy decreased when the amount of data for each score was 220.

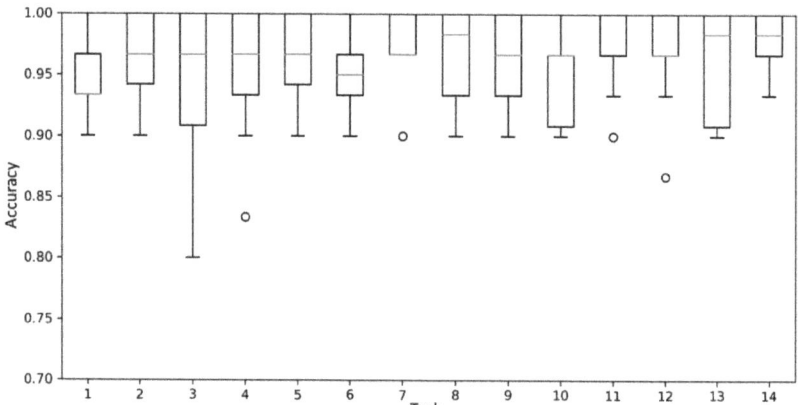

Figure 9. Mean accuracy of the best model when the amount of data for each score was 60.

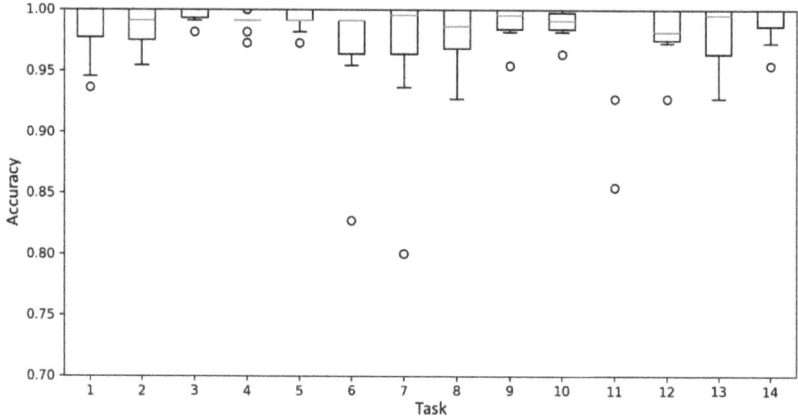

Figure 10. Mean accuracy of the best model when the amount of data for each score was 220.

3.4. Comparison with Previous Study

This study evaluated model excellence by comparing the results of previous studies. Prior studies include those of Badura [3] and Kim [27]. Kim's was a study in which the performance was improved by changing the feature extraction process and machine learning classification model of Badura's study. Unlike previous studies, this study applied a deep-learning algorithm and performed feature extraction using the deep-learning model. The data sampling rate of the previous studies (100 Hz) was down-sampled to 20 Hz, and the computational complexity was improved without reducing model accuracy. Reducing the sampling rate of data is meaningful in that it can contribute to reducing power consumption by lowering the sampling rate of the wearable devices. The dataset of the previous study had a data imbalance problem in which the amount of data for each score was different. In this study, this problem was solved by performing data augmentation based on the oversampling algorithm. As a result, the classification accuracy was increased. Additionally, a healthy participant experiment was performed to compensate for the insufficient amount of data in some classes. Because healthy participants performed all actions from zero to four on all tasks, the amount of data was equal to five times the patient data per healthy participant. The total amount of data was 78, 53 of which were patient data, and 15 were created by three healthy participants. By using the 10-fold cross-validation average accuracy as the evaluation method of the model, the evaluation method of previous studies, which can produce good results only in some splits, was improved overall. Table 3 summarizes the improvement points of this study compared with these previous studies.

Table 3. Improvements in this study compared to previous studies.

Study	Badura's Study	Kim's Study	This Study
Classification model	Multi-layer perceptron (MLP)	Support vector Machine (SVM)	Double head 1D-CNN and single head GRU stacking ensemble
Feature extraction	Manual (Frequency and time domain feature, Feature selection: Fisher's linear discriminant)	Manual (Frequency domain and energy feature, Feature selection: KPCA)	Automatic in deep learning
Sampling rate of data (Hz)	100	100	20 (Introduce data down-sampling)
Data imbalance problem	Yes	Yes	No (Introduce data augmentation)
Amount of experimental data	63	53	78
Evaluation method	Random split Training: Test = 7:3	Random split Training: Test = 7:3	Mean accuracy of 10-fold cross validation

The main achievement of this study is the improvement of accuracy. Table 4 shows the scoring accuracy of the model in the previous studies and the model that showed the best performance in this study. The model names listed in the table are abbreviated as follows: double-head 1D CNN and GRU stacking ensemble: DC+G.

Table 4. Comparison of results of previous study with this study.

Task	Badura's MLP Accuracy (%)	Kim's SVM Accuracy (%)	DC+G Accuracy (%)
1	87.5	100	98.5
2	92.2	100	98.5
3	100	100	99.6
4	89.1	87.5	99.0
5	70.3	76.5	96.7
6	89.1	100	97.9
7	76.6	100	99.0
8	76.6	92.9	98.9
9	89.1	100	97.8
10	70.3	78.6	98.2
11	78.1	100	97.8
12	79.7	80.0	98.2
13	62.5	90.0	98.1
14	67.2	100	99.1
Average	80.6	93.2	98.4
Standard deviation	10.9	9.1	0.7

The average accuracy of the model in this study was about 18% higher than that of the multi-layer perceptron model of Badura's study [3] and about 5% higher than that of the SVM model of Kim's study [27]. It was also confirmed that the standard deviation of the accuracy for the BBS task from 1 to 14 of the models of this study was 0.7%, which was much smaller than 10.9% of the MLP model of Badura's study and 9.1% of Kim's SVM model. This means that the model of this study can cover all BBS tasks well.

4. Conclusions

In this study, a deep learning-based BBS auto-scoring algorithm was developed. The best model was the stacking ensemble model with a meta-learner comprising a simple dense layer behind two 1D-CNN heads and one GRU head. The computational complexity and accuracy of the model were improved by improving the dataset during preprocessing. During the down-sampling process, it was possible to find a reasonable sampling rate by analyzing the accumulated information amount and the trend in the accumulated information amount with respect to the frequency change. After down-sampling, the computational complexity of the model was reduced. During the data augmentation process, the dataset was improved using the over-sampling technique. By creating data similar to the original data, the amount of data for each score was equalized, and that of both minority and majority classes was increased so that the deep-learning model could learn the data more generally. As a result, the scoring performance of the model was improved without a performance decrease caused by noise or class overlapping that occurs otherwise due to the generated data [56]. The accuracy was saturated when the amount of data for each score exceeded a certain threshold. The maximum average accuracy of the model in the 14 tasks was 98.4%, which was superior to previously reported results.

In the previous study [27], the efficiency of the algorithm could be increased by using only sensor data, which is advantageous to score classification for each BBS task. Of course, the deep-learning method performs this process inside the model by adjusting the weights between perceptrons. However, it has a disadvantage in that the amount of computations is large because all sensor data must be entered as an input. Therefore, in a follow-up study, an attention model deep-learning method will be introduced, and weights will be visualized to exclude data having a low contribution to scoring classification. This will not only increase the computational efficiency of the model, but it will also have the advantage that users can wear fewer sensors. Furthermore, we will introduce the latest deep-learning techniques and improve the dataset with signal processing algorithms to increase performance.

The algorithm of this study can be applied to a wearable healthcare device that evaluates the balance ability in the daily life of elderly or brain-disease patients who are at risk of falling. With wearable healthcare devices, users can know their balance ability and probability of falling at any time without having to visit a hospital, and it will be helpful for falling prevention.

Author Contributions: Conceptualization, Y.-W.K., K.-L.J., H.-Y.J. and S.L.; methodology, Y.-W.K. and S.L.; software, Y.-W.K.; validation, Y.-W.K., K.-L.J., H.-Y.J. and S.L.; formal analysis, Y.-W.K. and S.L.; investigation, Y.-W.K., K.-L.J., H.-Y.J. and S.L.; resources, K.-L.J. and H.-Y.J.; data curation, Y.-W.K. and K.-L.J.; writing—original draft preparation, Y.-W.K.; writing—review and editing, Y.-W.K. and S.L.; visualization, Y.-W.K.; supervision, S.L. and H.-Y.J.; project administration, S.L. and H.-Y.J. All authors have read and agreed to the published version of the manuscript.

Funding: This research was funded by INHA UNIVERSITY Research Grant and the National Research Foundation of Korea (NRF-2020R1A2C2004624).

Institutional Review Board Statement: The study was conducted according to the guidelines of the Declaration of Helsinki and approved by the Institutional Review Board of INHA UNIVERSITY HOSPITAL, Incheon, Korea (IRB license number 2016-08-012 and date of approval 2016-10-10).

Informed Consent Statement: Informed consent was obtained from all subjects involved in the study.

Conflicts of Interest: The authors declare no conflict of interest.

References

1. Herdman, S.J.; Blatt, P.; Schubert, M.C.; Tusa, R.J. Falls in patients with vestibular deficits. *Otol. Neurotol.* **2000**, *21*, 847–851.
2. Wolfson, L.I.; Whipple, R.; Amerman, P.; Kaplan, J.; Kleinberg, A. Gait and balance in the elderly: Two functional capacities that link sensory and motor ability to falls. *Clin. Geriatr. Med.* **1985**, *1*, 649–659. [CrossRef]

3. Badura, P.; Pietka, E. Automatic berg balance scale assessment system based on accelerometric signals. *Biomed. Signal Process. Control* **2016**, *24*, 114–119. [CrossRef]
4. Mohammadian Rad, N.; Van Laarhoven, T.; Furlanello, C.; Marchiori, E. Novelty detection using deep normative modeling for imu-based abnormal movement monitoring in parkinson's disease and autism spectrum disorders. *Sensors* **2018**, *18*, 3533. [CrossRef] [PubMed]
5. Romijnders, R.; Warmerdam, E.; Hansen, C.; Welzel, J.; Schmidt, G.; Maetzler, W. Validation of IMU-based gait event detection during curved walking and turning in older adults and Parkinson's Disease patients. *J. Neuroeng. Rehabil.* **2021**, *18*, 1–10. [CrossRef]
6. Yu, B.; Liu, Y.; Chan, K. A Survey of Sensor Modalities for Human Activity Recognition. In Proceedings of the 12th International Joint Conference on Knowledge Discovery, Budapest, Hungary, 2–4 November 2020; INSTICC: Rua dos Lusíadas, Portugal, 2020; pp. 282–294.
7. Vu, C.C.; Kim, J.K. Human motion recognition using SWCNT textile sensor and fuzzy inference system based smart wearable. *Sens. Actuators A* **2018**, *283*, 263–272. [CrossRef]
8. Rodrigues, S.M.; Fiedler, P.; Küchler, N.; Domingues, P.R.; Lopes, C.; Borges, J.; Haueisen, J.; Vaz, F. Dry electrodes for surface electromyography based on architectured titanium thin films. *Materials* **2020**, *13*, 2135. [CrossRef]
9. Raeis, H.; Kazemi, M.; Shirmohammadi, S. Human Activity Recognition with Device-Free Sensors for Well-Being Assessment in Smart Homes. *IEEE Instrum. Meas. Mag.* **2021**, *24*, 46–57. [CrossRef]
10. Wang, Y.; Cang, S.; Yu, H. A survey on wearable sensor modality centred human activity recognition in health care. *Expert Syst. Appl.* **2019**, *137*, 167–190. [CrossRef]
11. Ponciano, V.; Pires, I.M.; Ribeiro, F.R.; Marques, G.; Villasana, M.V.; Garcia, N.M.; Zdravevski, E.; Spinsante, S. Identification of Diseases Based on the Use of Inertial Sensors: A Systematic Review. *Electronics* **2020**, *9*, 778. [CrossRef]
12. Digo, E.; Agostini, V.; Pastorelli, S.; Gastaldi, L.; Panero, E. Gait Phases Detection in Elderly using Trunk-MIMU System. In Proceedings of the 14th International Joint Conference on Biomedical Engineering Systems and Technologies (BIOSTEC 2021), Vienna, Austria, 11–13 February 2021; pp. 58–65.
13. Choudhury, N.A.; Moulik, S.; Roy, D.S. Physique-based Human Activity Recognition using Ensemble Learning and Smartphone Sensors. *IEEE Sens. J.* **2021**, *21*, 16852–16860. [CrossRef]
14. Nan, Y.; Lovell, N.H.; Redmond, S.J.; Wang, K.; Delbaere, K.; van Schooten, K.S. Deep Learning for Activity Recognition in Older People Using a Pocket-Worn Smartphone. *Sensors* **2020**, *20*, 7195. [CrossRef]
15. Wu, B.; Ma, C.; Poslad, S.; Selviah, D.R. An Adaptive Human Activity-Aided Hand-Held Smartphone-Based Pedestrian Dead Reckoning Positioning System. *Remote Sens.* **2021**, *13*, 2137. [CrossRef]
16. Lara, O.D.; Labrador, M.A. A survey on human activity recognition using wearable sensors. *IEEE Commun. Surv. Tutor.* **2012**, *15*, 1192–1209. [CrossRef]
17. Lu, J.; Zheng, X.; Sheng, M.; Jin, J.; Yu, S. Efficient Human Activity Recognition Using a Single Wearable Sensor. *IEEE Internet Things J.* **2020**, *7*, 11137–11146. [CrossRef]
18. Vanrell, S.R.; Milone, D.H.; Rufiner, H.L. Assessment of homomorphic analysis for human activity recognition from acceleration signals. *IEEE J. Biomed. Health Inform.* **2017**, *22*, 1001–1010. [CrossRef] [PubMed]
19. Wang, J.; Chen, Y.; Hao, S.; Peng, X.; Hu, L. Deep learning for sensor-based activity recognition: A survey. *Pattern Recognit. Lett.* **2019**, *119*, 3–11. [CrossRef]
20. Pickle, N.T.; Shearin, S.M.; Fey, N.P. Dynamic neural network approach to targeted balance assessment of individuals with and without neurological disease during non-steady-state locomotion. *J. Neuroeng. Rehabil.* **2019**, *16*, 1–9. [CrossRef]
21. Chung, S.; Lim, J.; Noh, K.J.; Kim, G.; Jeong, H. Sensor data acquisition and multimodal sensor fusion for human activity recognition using deep learning. *Sensors* **2019**, *19*, 1716. [CrossRef]
22. Ramanujam, E.; Perumal, T.; Padmavathi, S. Human activity recognition with smartphone and wearable sensors using deep learning techniques: A review. *IEEE Sens. J.* **2021**, *21*, 13029–13040. [CrossRef]
23. Mekruksavanich, S.; Jitpattanakul, A. LSTM networks using smartphone data for sensor-based human activity recognition in smart homes. *Sensors* **2021**, *21*, 1636. [CrossRef]
24. Mekruksavanich, S.; Jitpattanakul, A. Deep Convolutional Neural Network with RNNs for Complex Activity Recognition Using Wrist-Worn Wearable Sensor Data. *Electronics* **2021**, *10*, 1685. [CrossRef]
25. Blum, L.; Korner-Bitensky, N. Usefulness of the Berg Balance Scale in stroke rehabilitation: A systematic review. *Phys. Ther.* **2008**, *88*, 559–566. [CrossRef]
26. Muir, S.W.; Berg, K.; Chesworth, B.; Speechley, M. Use of the Berg Balance Scale for predicting multiple falls in community-dwelling elderly people: A prospective study. *Phys. Ther.* **2008**, *88*, 449–459. [CrossRef] [PubMed]
27. Kim, Y.W.; Cho, W.H.; Joa, K.L.; Jung, H.Y.; Lee, S. A New Auto-Scoring Algorithm for Bance Assessment with Wearable IMU Device Based on Nonlinear Model. *J. Mech. Med. Biol.* **2020**, *20*, 2040011. [CrossRef]
28. Huang, N.E.; Shen, Z.; Long, S.R.; Wu, M.C.; Shih, H.H.; Zheng, Q. The empirical mode decomposition and the Hilbert spectrum for nonlinear and non-stationary time series analysis. *Proc. R. Soc. Lond. Ser. A* **1998**, *454*, 903–995. [CrossRef]
29. Khan, A.; Hammerla, N.; Mellor, S.; Plötz, T. Optimising sampling rates for accelerometer-based human activity recognition. *Pattern Recognit. Lett.* **2016**, *73*, 33–40. [CrossRef]
30. Landau, H.J. Sampling, data transmission, and the Nyquist rate. *Proc. IEEE* **1967**, *55*, 1701–1706. [CrossRef]

31. Khushi, M.; Shaukat, K.; Alam, T.M.; Hameed, I.A.; Uddin, S.; Luo, S.; Reyes, M.C. A Comparative Performance Analysis of Data Resampling Methods on Imbalance Medical Data. *IEEE Access* **2021**, *9*, 109960–109975. [CrossRef]
32. Liu, Z.; Cao, W.; Gao, Z.; Bian, J.; Chen, H.; Chang, Y.; Liu, T.Y. Self-paced ensemble for highly imbalanced massive data classification. In Proceedings of the 2020 IEEE 36th International Conference on Data Engineering (ICDE), Dallas, TX, USA, 20–24 April 2020; IEEE: New York, NY, USA; pp. 841–852.
33. Thabtah, F.; Hammoud, S.; Kamalov, F.; Gonsalves, A. Data imbalance in classification: Experimental evaluation. *Inf. Sci.* **2020**, *513*, 429–441. [CrossRef]
34. Sun, J.; Lang, J.; Fujita, H.; Li, H. Imbalanced enterprise credit evaluation with DTE-SBD: Decision tree ensemble based on SMOTE and bagging with differentiated sampling rates. *Inf. Sci.* **2018**, *425*, 76–91. [CrossRef]
35. Xu, Z.; Shen, D.; Nie, T.; Kou, Y. A hybrid sampling algorithm combining M-SMOTE and ENN based on random forest for medical imbalanced data. *J. Biomed. Inform.* **2020**, *107*, 103465. [CrossRef]
36. Abdoh, S.F.; Rizka, M.A.; Maghraby, F.A. Cervical cancer diagnosis using random forest classifier with SMOTE and feature reduction techniques. *IEEE Access* **2018**, *6*, 59475–59485. [CrossRef]
37. Chawla, N.V.; Bowyer, K.W.; Hall, L.O.; Kegelmeyer, W.P. SMOTE: Synthetic minority over-sampling technique. *J. Artif. Intell. Res.* **2002**, *16*, 321–357. [CrossRef]
38. Khorshidi, H.A.; Aickelin, U. Synthetic Over-sampling with the Minority and Majority classes for imbalance problems. *arXiv* **2020**, arXiv:2011.04170. in preprint.
39. Canizo, M.; Triguero, I.; Conde, A.; Onieva, E. Multi-head CNN–RNN for multi-time series anomaly detection: An industrial case study. *Neurocomputing* **2019**, *363*, 246–260. [CrossRef]
40. Jiang, Z.; Lai, Y.; Zhang, J.; Zhao, H.; Mao, Z. Multi-factor operating condition recognition using 1D convolutional long short-term network. *Sensors* **2019**, *19*, 5488. [CrossRef]
41. Xie, X.; Wang, B.; Wan, T.; Tang, W. Multivariate abnormal detection for industrial control systems using 1D CNN and GRU. *IEEE Access* **2020**, *8*, 88348–88359. [CrossRef]
42. Pasupa, K.; Sunhem, W. A comparison between shallow and deep architecture classifiers on small dataset. In Proceedings of the 2016 8th International Conference on Information Technology and Electrical Engineering (ICITEE), Yogyakarta, Indonesia, 5–6 October 2016; IEEE: New York, NY, USA; pp. 1–6.
43. Brigato, L.; Iocchi, L. A close look at deep learning with small data. In Proceedings of the 2020 25th International Conference on Pattern Recognition (ICPR), Milan, Italy, 10–15 January 2021; IEEE: New York, NY, USA; pp. 2490–2497.
44. Cho, K.; Van Merriënboer, B.; Bahdanau, D.; Bengio, Y. On the properties of neural machine translation: Encoder-decoder approaches. *arXiv* **2014**, arXiv:1409.1259. in preprint.
45. Chen, H.; Ji, M. Experimental Comparison of Classification Methods under Class Imbalance. *EAI Trans. Scalable Inf. Syst.* **2021**, *sis18*, e13. [CrossRef]
46. Ordoñez, F.J.; Roggen, D. Deep convolutional and lstm recurrent neural networks for multimodal wearable activity recognition. *Sensors* **2016**, *16*, 115. [CrossRef] [PubMed]
47. Qian, Y.; Bi, M.; Tan, T.; Yu, K. Very deep convolutional neural networks for noise robust speech recognition. *IEEE/ACM Trans. Audio Speech Lang. Process.* **2016**, *24*, 2263–2276. [CrossRef]
48. Tsironi, E.; Barros, P.; Weber, C.; Wermter, S. An analysis of convolutional long short-term memory recurrent neural networks for gesture recognition. *Neurocomputing* **2017**, *268*, 76–86. [CrossRef]
49. Ahmad, W.; Kazmi, B.M.; Ali, H. Human activity recognition using multi-head CNN followed by LSTM. In Proceedings of the 2019 15th international conference on emerging technologies (ICET), Peshawar, Pakistan, 2–3 December 2019; IEEE: New York, NY, USA; pp. 1–6.
50. Perenda, E.; Rajendran, S.; Pollin, S. Automatic modulation classification using parallel fusion of convolutional neural networks. In Proceedings of the 2019 3rd International Balkan Conference on Communications and Networking (IBCCN) (BalkanCom'19), Skopje, North Macedonia, 10–12 June 2019; IEEE: New York, NY, USA.
51. Lee, K.; Kim, J.K.; Kim, J.; Hur, K.; Kim, H. CNN and GRU combination scheme for bearing anomaly detection in rotating machinery health monitoring. In Proceedings of the 2018 1st IEEE International Conference on Knowledge Innovation and Invention (ICKII), Jeju Island, Korea, 23–27 July 2018; IEEE: New York, NY, USA; pp. 102–105.
52. Hamad, R.A.; Yang, L.; Woo, W.L.; Wei, B. Joint learning of temporal models to handle imbalanced data for human activity recognition. *Appl. Sci.* **2020**, *10*, 5293. [CrossRef]
53. Hamad, R.A.; Hidalgo, A.S.; Bouguelia, M.R.; Estevez, M.E.; Quero, J.M. Efficient activity recognition in smart homes using delayed fuzzy temporal windows on binary sensors. *IEEE J. Biomed. Health Inform.* **2019**, *24*, 387–395. [CrossRef]
54. Xu, M.; Yin, Z.; Wu, M.; Wu, Z.; Zhao, Y.; Gao, Z. Spectrum sensing based on parallel cnn-lstm network. In Proceedings of the 2020 IEEE 91st Vehicular Technology Conference (VTC2020-Spring), Virtual, Antwerp, Begium, 25 May–31 July 2020; IEEE: New York, NY, USA; pp. 1–5.
55. Wang, K.J.; Makond, B.; Chen, K.H.; Wang, K.M. A hybrid classifier combining SMOTE with PSO to estimate 5-year survivability of breast cancer patients. *Appl. Soft Comput.* **2014**, *20*, 15–24. [CrossRef]
56. Fernández, A.; Garcia, S.; Herrera, F.; Chawla, N.V. SMOTE for learning from imbalanced data: Progress and challenges, marking the 15-year anniversary. *J. Artif. Intell. Res.* **2018**, *61*, 863–905. [CrossRef]

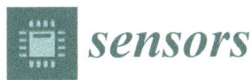

Article

Connected Skiing: Motion Quality Quantification in Alpine Skiing

Cory Snyder [1,2,*], Aaron Martínez [1,2], Rüdiger Jahnel [1], Jason Roe [3] and Thomas Stöggl [1,2]

[1] Department of Sport and Exercise Science, University of Salzburg, Schlossallee 49, 5400 Hallein/Rif, Austria; aaron.martinez@sbg.ac.at (A.M.); ruediger.jahnel@sbg.ac.at (R.J.); Thomas.stoeggl@sbg.ac.at (T.S.)
[2] Athlete Performance Center, Red Bull Sports, Brunnbachweg 71, 5303 Thalgau, Austria
[3] Atomic Austria GmbH, Atomic Strasse 1, 5541 Altenmarkt, Austria; jason.roe@atomic.com
* Correspondence: cory.snyder@sbg.ac.at

Abstract: Recent developments in sensing technology have made wearable computing smaller and cheaper. While many wearable technologies aim to quantify motion, there are few which aim to qualify motion. (2) To develop a wearable system to quantify motion quality during alpine skiing, IMUs were affixed to the ski boots of nineteen expert alpine skiers while they completed a set protocol of skiing styles, included carving and drifting in long, medium, and short radii. The IMU data were processed according to the previously published skiing activity recognition chain algorithms for turn segmentation, enrichment, and turn style classification Principal component models were learned on the time series variables edge angle, symmetry, radial force, and speed to identify the sources of variability in a subset of reference skiers. The remaining data were scored by comparing the PC score distributions of variables to the reference dataset. (3) The algorithm was able to differentiate between an expert and beginner skier, but not between an expert and a ski instructor, or a ski instructor and a beginner. (4) The scoring algorithm is a novel concept to quantify motion quality but is limited by the accuracy and relevance of the input data.

Keywords: IMU; principal component analysis; wearable; scoring; carving

1. Introduction

Recent developments in sensor technology have made sensing units cheaper and easier to implement. These developments have made the application of "wearable technology" or smart sporting equipment appealing to not only scientists and elite athletes, but also recreational athletes. Such users are interested in more than the quantity of a movement performed (e.g., steps, ski turns, or kilometers per run); they are also interested in the quality of motion, or how well they performed the activity [1]. Together, the recent developments and new users of wearable technology have led to a number of recent publications concerning the measurement of motion quality during skiing, especially during in-field experiments [1–4].

A popular sensor choice in the field-based measurements are inertial measurement units (IMUs). These sensors combine accelerometers, gyroscopes, and optionally, magnetometers to record three-dimensional acceleration, angular velocity, and magnetic field signals. IMUs have been used to measure center of mass kinematics [5], skier posture [6], trunk orientation [7], vibration transmission [8], knee joint angles [9], edge angle [10], as well as the estimation of skier kinetics [11]. Despite the variety of approaches to quantify skiing performance, these studies focused exclusively on competitive alpine skiing [12]. Although the results of these studies provide motion quality parameters to scientists and coaches regarding athlete performance or injury risk, the methods used are not "plug-and-play" systems. In general, the methods utilized in the studies above require extensive sensor calibration, bulky measurement equipment, or offline post-processing [13]. While these processes can be quite simple, they can also be quite complex and can significantly

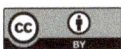

influence data quality [14]. Indeed, this limitation was a key finding in one of the earliest publications regarding wearable systems to measure motion quality during skiing [15]. This study used an extensive sensor setup (tri-axial accelerometer, tri-axial gyroscope, force-sensing resistors, radar, and infrared distance sensors) to estimate a wide variety of parameters related to competitive skiing simulations. The main intent of this system was to provide data to augment feedback normally given by a human coach. The authors of this paper highlighted that although the measurement system was quite comprehensive, it was prohibitively obtrusive for regular everyday use, and future systems should focus on providing an interface that is easy and intuitive to operate and interpret.

More recently, there have been further developments in the area of motion quality assessment in alpine skiing. Yamagiwa and colleagues developed a simple system based on a single IMU mounted on the trunk of a skier to assess skiing quality based on turning tempo (turn frequency) [16]. The algorithm assessed only the variability of tempo during a run in order to differentiate between high- and low-skill skiers. However, this study only presented the development of the algorithm; it did not report any group statistics and included a limited number of participants. Kos and Umek [17,18] proposed a more complex system, integrating bending and load transducers directly into a ski in addition to an IMU placed on the torso of skiers. Although this system was quite comprehensive and provided real-time feedback to users, the hardware requirements (data-logger, backpack, cables) and calibration procedures (static and dynamic requirements) rendered it infeasible for realistic everyday frictionless use.

Recent work addressing the literature gap regarding low-friction systems has developed a wearable-system based on IMUs mounted on the cuffs of both ski boots and a smartphone hub for data recording, storage, and online data processing within a custom application [3]. This provides the platform for the automated detection of turns [4], data processing and extraction of skiing specific metrics [19], and turn classification into carving, drifting, or non-parallel turning styles [2]. Together, these steps fit within the activity recognition chain (ARC, segmentation, enrichment, classification) [20]. Brunauer and colleagues [21] have proposed an extension of the ARC, going beyond answering the question of "What did X do?", to "How well has X performed?" and "What should X do to improve?" In order for this proposed extension to function, it requires an objective quantification of which parameters define motion quality (i.e., edge angle, radial force, CoM speed, turning radius). One approach to answer these types of questions is principal component analysis (PCA). PCA is a common tool in statistics and machine learning used to reduce the dimensionality of large time series datasets, where many variables contain redundancy with respect to the total variability of the dataset [22]. In the context of human movement analysis, PCAs have been utilized to identify unique gait patterns during walking [23], to discriminate between patients with and without knee osteoarthritis [24], and to evaluate motion quality during functional movements and classify athletes as novice or elite [25]. PCAs have also been implemented in other smart sports equipment settings—for example, to detect errors during balance board tasks [26]. In the context of skiing, PCAs have been used to identify the main motions or principal movements related to skiing technique during slalom racing [27]. While PCAs would normally be applied to an entire dataset, in the context of wearables and smart coaching, an alternative approach would be to apply a PCA model to individual time series variables in order to identify the specific components of individual parameters which contribute to overall variability. In this way, a wearable system could be developed which is more sensitive to individual parameter shapes, rather than traditional metrics such as mean, standard deviation, maximum, or minimum.

In order to develop a robust model of skiing movement quality, we develop a principal component analysis (PCA)-based model of motion quality during alpine skiing using a simple sensor system, and we evaluate the performance of the algorithm during in-field skiing conditions compared to expert raters.

2. Materials and Methods

2.1. Participants

Nineteen advanced or expert skiers (8 male/11 female, age 34.6 ± 7.8 years, height 1.73 ± 0.1 m, weight 72.7 ± 11.0 kg) were recruited to participate in this study. All participants were either ski instructors or current or former competitive alpine skiers, including four former FIS Alpine World Cup athletes. Additionally, three separate participants, one beginner, one ski instructor, and one expert skier, were recruited to complete a separate algorithm validation. Participants were informed of the testing procedures in detail, including possible benefits and risks of the investigation, prior to signing the consent form as approved by the local ethics committee (EK-GZ: 11/2018). This experiment was conducted in accordance with the Declaration of Helsinki.

2.2. Overall Design

In order to construct a "systematic" dataset comprising a variety of skiing styles, participants completed seven skiing runs, performing at least ten consecutive turns during each run. Participants performed carving and drifting style turns. In both styles, turns were performed in long, medium, and short radii. Long-radius turns were defined as at least three snow-cat groomed widths (>12 m), medium-radius turns were defined as roughly two snow-cat groomed widths (~8 m), and short-radius turns were defined as less than two snow-cat groomed widths (<8 m). The seventh test run was a "maximum performance" run performed at the participants self-selected turn radius and style. Additionally, participants performed one snowplow steering and one pure snowplow run; however, data from these runs were not included in the analysis. All tests were performed at three Austrian ski resorts between January and March 2019. In order to ensure consistent slope conditions, all tests were performed before 11 am. All tests were completed on freshly groomed blue or red pistes with limited fresh snowfall (<6 cm).

2.3. Data Acquisition

All tests were performed on commercially available recreational race skis. Long- and medium-radius turns, as well as the "maximum performance" runs, were performed on a "giant slalom" model (Atomic Redster G9 171/177/183 cm length, 18.6 m radius). Short-radius and non-parallel turns were performed on "slalom" skis (Atomic Redster S9, 155/165 cm length, 12.7 m radius). Prior to testing sessions, participants completed at least one run to familiarize themselves with the test skis.

The wearable system consisted of two IMUs (configuration: 2.5 × 3 × 0.83 mm ± 16 g and ±1000 dps full-scale resolution, board by Movesense [28]) mounted on the upper posterior cuff of each ski boot using a custom housing and strap. The Y axis of the IMU was aligned with the vertical axis of the boot pointing superiorly, the X axis with the lateral axis pointing to the right, and the Z axis with the roll axis pointing posteriorly (Figure 1). Both the accelerometer and gyroscope sampled at 833 Hz. The raw signals were filtered by an analog anti-aliasing low-pass filter, and again after A/D conversion by a digital low-pass filter (filter cutoff: 416.5 Hz—accelerometer; 245 Hz—gyroscope) The filtered signals were transmitted via Bluetooth at 54 Hz to a smartphone running a custom application, where they were stored for further processing. Additionally, global navigation satellite system (GNSS) signals were recorded at 1 Hz by the same custom application on the mobile phone. A central requirement of the wearable system is its "plug-and-play" character; therefore, after factory calibration, no further IMU calibrations were performed.

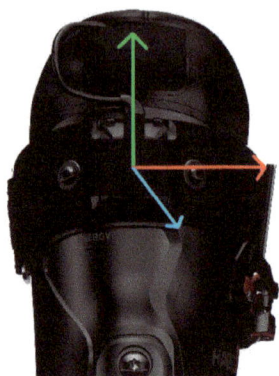

Figure 1. Measurement system and axis orientation. The X axis (red) points to the right, the Y axis (green) points vertically, and the Z axis (blue) points posteriorly.

2.4. Pre-Processing

All collected data were processed according to the process outlined by the ARC proposed by Brunauer and colleagues [21]. Each run was segmented into turns using the algorithm described by Martinez et al. [3,4]. Briefly, this algorithm detects peaks in the roll axis gyroscope signal to segment turns based on the pendulum model of skiing. The first and last detected turn from each run, as well as turns with an average speed one median absolute deviation below the median speed for that run, were excluded from the dataset in order to exclude turns within each sequence where the skier was either accelerating or decelerating (i.e., the beginning and end of a run). Pre-processed data from each turn were enriched with the metrics, speed, radial force, edge angle, and edge angle symmetry (left–right turn differences) according to the algorithms proposed by Snyder and colleagues [19] and speed based on the mobile phone GNSS. Finally, each turn in the segmented, enriched dataset was classified as either carving, drifting, or non-parallel style according to the classification algorithm described by Neuwirth and colleagues [2]. Although this algorithm was able to distinguish among styles with high accuracy (~93%), not all turns within one style are similar, specifically with regard to turn size. Therefore, in order to add a further layer of specificity to the scoring algorithm, each classified turn was further classified according to the assigned turn size (small, medium, and large). Although the turn style for each run was specified, the classified turn styles assigned by the classification algorithm were not always identical to the style intended. Table 1 shows the number of turns from each participant classified in each turning style/radius, as well as the "intended" turn styles included. Due to synchronization errors, specific runs from 10 participants were excluded. These participants were all included in the test dataset, preventing their "lack" of data from influencing the model results.

The processed dataset was split participant-wise into reference (42%) and test (58%) datasets. The reference dataset was used to learn a PCA model and develop a scoring system. The test dataset was then used as "new data" to test the performance of the algorithm. The participants placed into the reference dataset were selected based on their objectively high skiing level. These five "gold-standard" skiers included one male and one female professional instructor and three retired male World Cup athletes (retired after 2006). These skiers had a combined 49 World Cup Victories, 13 World Championship medals, 4 Olympic Medals, and 9 World Cup Overall or discipline crystal globes.

Table 1. Turns classified per participant as carving or drifting in long, medium, and short radii. Although participants were instructed to complete turns of specific styles, some turns were classified as different styles or radii. Experience levels: WC corresponds to retired world cup ski racers, while FIS corresponds to retired FIS level ski racers.

#	Experience Level	Group	Carving			Drifting			Completed Runs
			Long	Medium	Short	Long	Medium	Short	
1	WC	Ref	10	42	29	9	25	1	CL, CM, CS, DL, DM, DS, Max
3	WC	Test	3	4	0	~	~	~	CL
4	Instructor	Test	~	~	~	~	~	34	DS
5	Instructor	Test	~	~	~	~	~	37	DS
6	FIS	Test	~	~	~	~	18	10	DS
7	Instructor	Test	~	~	~	~	1	23	DS
8	Instructor	Test	~	~	12	~	~	22	CS, DS
9	Instructor	Test	~	~	5	~	2	18	DS
11	Instructor	Test	~	~	~	~	2	15	DS
12	Instructor	Test	1	10	7	~	~	17	CM, DS, Max
14	Instructor	Test	15	16	2	8	11	2	CL, CM, CS, DL, DM, DS, Max
15	FIS	Test	4	42	22	5	17	47	CL, CM, CS, DL, DM, DS, Max
16	Instructor	Test	~	33	4	7	43	35	CL, CM, CS, DL, DM, DS, Max
17	Instructor	Ref	2	73	12	14	24	3	CL, CM, CS, DL, DM, DS, Max
19	Instructor	Ref	8	18	30	6	12	5	CL, CM, CS, DM, DS
20	Instructor	Test	5	54	25	12	22	45	CL, CM, CS, DL, DM, DS, Max
21	FIS	Test	13	21	14	6	16	20	CL, CM, CS, DL, DM, DS, Max
23	WC	Ref	10	59	59	20	6	27	CL, CM, CS, DL, DM, DS, Max
24	WC	Ref	11	43	~	21	9	~	CL, CM, DL, DM, Max
Total			82	415	221	108	208	361	84

2.5. Scoring Alogirthm

A PCA model was applied to the reference dataset to learn the signal characteristics (principal components) of the reference skiers. The principal components scores (the linear representations of each sample in the principal component space) of the first three principal components were retained and used as a reference distribution to assess the similarity between the reference and test datasets (scoring).

A centered PCA model was learned separately on each input variable (edge angle, radial force, speed, symmetry) for each skiing style in the reference dataset. Therefore, each variable is represented by an $n \times 101$ dimensional matrix, P_{ref}, where n is the number of samples (turns) and 101 is the number of features—in this case, the signal normalized to 100% turn duration. The PCA yields two results, a matrix of eigenvectors and a matrix of eigenvalues. The eigenvectors represent the direction of the largest sources of variability in P_{ref} and are ordered by the magnitude of variability that they explain. These are termed principal component loading vectors $\vec{PC}_{ref}$. The eigenvalues of each eigenvector are the representations of the original dataset in the principal component space and are termed PC scores, PCS_{ref}, and they represent the amount of variability contributed by each sample to each PC loading vector. In this way, $\vec{PC}_{ref}$ can be thought of as a transformation matrix from the PC space and the original data space. The mean vector response of each variable and $\vec{PC}_{ref}$ were retained as the required data to transform new data to the PC space, where the transformed data can be scored.

While the eigenvectors $\vec{PC}_{ref}$ are used to transform new data into the PC space, the eigenvalues PCS_{ref} are scalars which describe the contribution of each PC to the overall variability of the dataset. Therefore, assuming that the skiers in the reference dataset represent the "gold standard" of skiing performance, within one PC of one variable (ex. PC 1 of edge angle), the distribution of PCS_{ref} describes the optimal weighting of that PC for that variable, where scores close to the middle of the distribution are desirable, and those at each tail are less desirable.

An absolute Z-score for each PC of each variable was calculated and transformed into discrete scoring bins, where Z < 0.75 = 4, Z > 0.75 and Z < 1.5 = 3, Z > 1.5 and Z < 3 = 2, Z > 3 = 1. These Z-scores were normalized by the variance explained by each PC and summed within variables so that PC that contributed most to the variability of the reference dataset carried the most weight in the score. The final score for each turn was calculated as the sum of normalized Z-scores across variables, expressed as a percentage of the maximum score, where higher scores represent higher similarity to the reference dataset. In order to form a single continuous scale for all turns, those turns classified as carving were scaled from 7 to 10, and those classified as drifted turns from 3 to 6. Not addressed in this study were the turns classified as snowplow and snowplow steering [2]. These classes were not scored by this algorithm but assigned scores of 1 (snowplow) and 2 (snowplow steering) in order to complete the 1–10 scale. None of the turns included in this study were classified as snowplow.

The final scoring model consists of a set of vectors representing the mean response of each variable, a set of loading vector means ($\vec{PC}_{ref}$) and loading vector standard deviations for each PC of each variable, in each turn size (small, medium, large) of each turning style (carving and drifting).

The test dataset was processed according to the same pre-processing steps as the reference dataset (segmentation, enrichment, and classification). Rather than learning a new PCA model in the incoming dataset, each variable of each metric was scaled by the mean response of the reference dataset and transformed to the PC space using the matrix $\vec{PC}_{ref}$. The test dataset was then scored according to the scoring algorithm described above.

Finally, three skiers completed a shortened protocol consisting of three runs in set radii (long, short, and self-selected) and self-selected turning style, using the instrumented ski boot, while being observed by three professional ski instructors. The instructors rated the skiing quality using two items, the overall quality ("On a scale of 1–4, how is the overall skiing quality? 1 being not able to ski, 4 being excellent"), the skiing dynamics ("On a scale of 1–4, how dynamic is the skiing? 1 being static, 4 being very dynamic"), and the skiing turn style ("What is the skiing style: carving, drifted, or mixed?"). The scores were scaled using the assigned style (3–6, drifting, 5–8 mixed, 7–10 carving) in order to match the scale of score provided by the wearable system. Data from the instrumented boot were processed according to the algorithm above, and the mean score from each run was compared to the scores assigned by the expert raters using Pearson correlations. Correlations less than 0.3 were interpreted as small, between 0.3 and 0.6 as medium, and greater than or equal to 0.6 as large [29]. Finally, the scores from all turns from each skier were compared using a Kruskal–Wallis test to determine if the algorithm was able to assign different scores to skiers of different skill levels.

3. Results

3.1. Explained Variability

The first three PCs of each variable in each turning condition explained at least 85% of the variability of the reference dataset for all variables in all skiing styles (Figure 2). The first three PCs of speed explained 99.1 ± 1.6%, 0.9 ± 1.6%, and 0.03 ± 0.1% of the total variability across all skiing styles. Similarly, the first three PCs of edge angle explained 95.9 ± 2.9%, 2.7 ± 1.4%, and 1.3 ± 1.5% of the total variability across all skiing styles. For radial force, the first three PCs explained 75.5 ± 9.9%, 4.4 ± 5.2%, and 6.6 ± 3.0% of the total variability. Finally, for symmetry, the first three PCs explained 60.4 ± 10.3%, 26.0 ± 9.1%, and 9.0 ± 3.6% of the total variability.

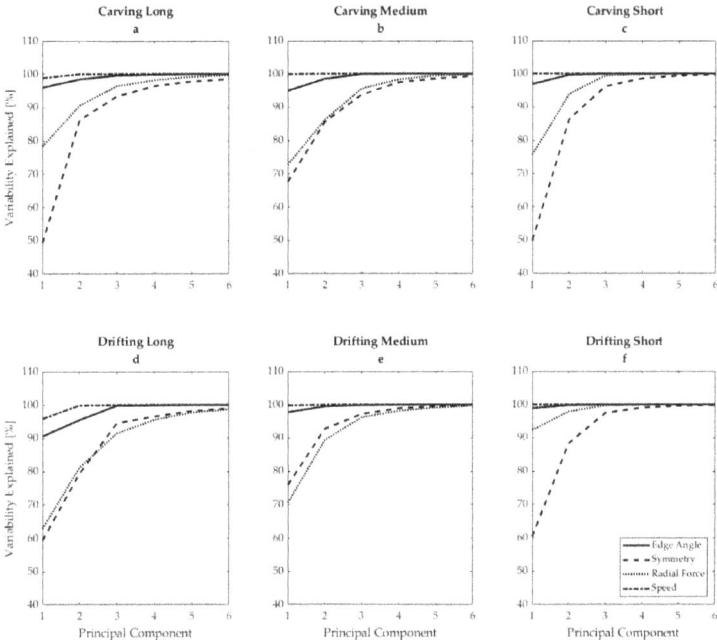

Figure 2. Cumulative explained variability of the first six principal components from the reference dataset for edge angle (solid line), edging symmetry (dashed line), radial force (dotted line), and speed (dot–dash line), in (**a**) carving long radius, (**b**) carving medium radius, (**c**) carving short radius, (**d**) drifting long radius, (**e**) drifting medium radius, and (**f**) drifting short radius.

3.2. PC Response and Score Response

A sample response of each variable in the PC space is shown in Figure 3 for carving short radius. For example, the third row (Figure 3g–i) shows the responses of the first three PCs of radial force. Higher PC 1 scores for radial force indicate lower radial force, while lower scores indicate higher radial force. For PC 2, high scores indicate peak radial forces occurring later in turn duration, while lower PC 2 scores indicate peak radial forces earlier in the turn. Finally, in Figure 3i, higher PC 3 scores indicate single peaks in radial force, with longer transition phases where radial forces are low, while lower PC 3 scores indicate double peaks in radial force.

3.3. Test Score Distribution

The scores assigned by the wearable system to the training dataset are shown in Figure 4. In all styles except carving medium, the scores were moderately skewed towards higher scores (carving long: −0.58, carving medium: 0.01, carving short −0.36, drifting long: −0.82, drifting medium: −0.52, drifting short: −0.38).

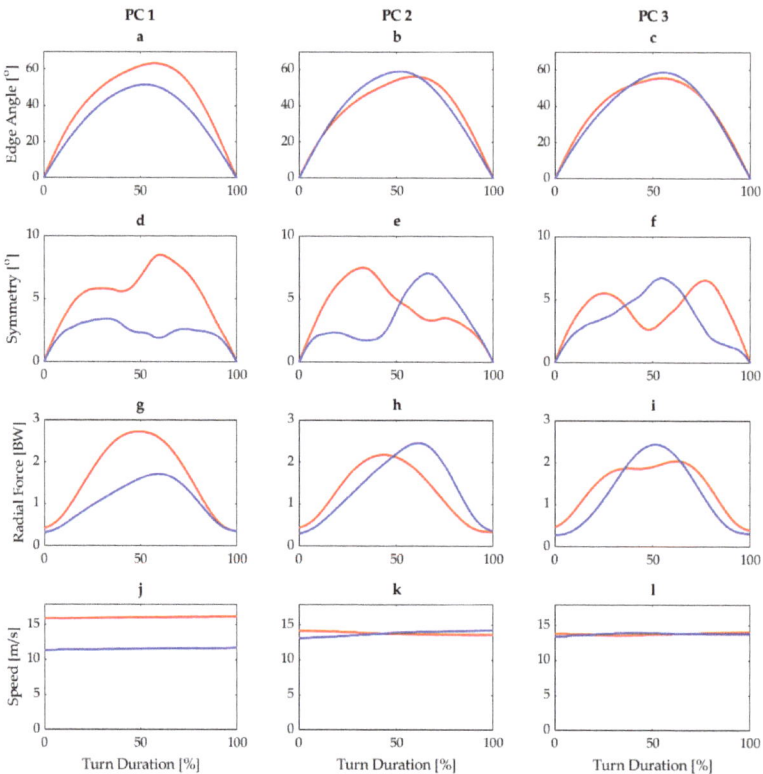

Figure 3. Responses for first three principal components for edge angle (**a**–**c**), edge angle symmetry (**d**–**f**), radial force (**g**–**i**), and speed (**j**–**l**) for carving short from the reference dataset. Blue lines represent the mean load score −1SD and red lines represent mean load score +1SD.

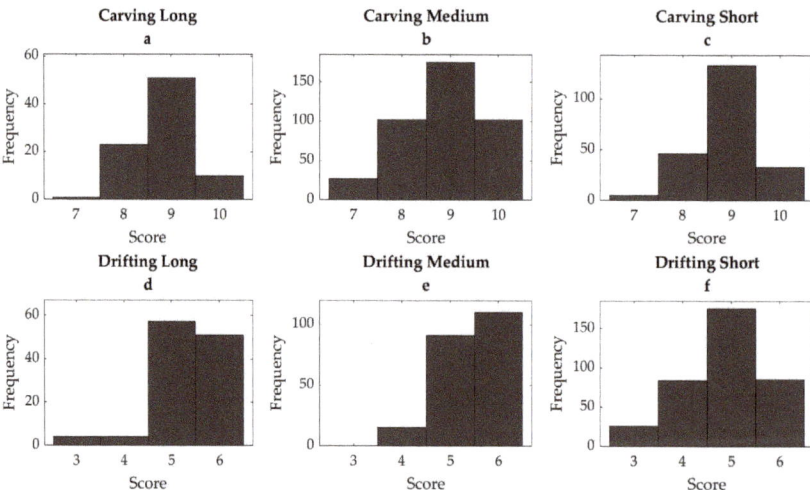

Figure 4. Distribution of algorithm-assigned scores from the test dataset for the skiing styles carving and drifting in long (**a**,**d**), medium (**b**,**e**), and short (**c**,**f**) radius.

3.4. Validation Test

A large correlation was observed between the expert assigned dynamic score and the median score of all turns assigned by the wearable system within each run (r = 0.71, p = 0.048), but not between the overall quality score and the score assigned by the wearable system (r = 0.59, p = 0.120). Additionally, differences were observed between the algorithm-assigned scores for the beginner and expert skiers (p = 0.02), but not between the ski instructor and the expert skier (p = 0.23) and the beginner and the ski instructor (p = 0.44).

4. Discussion

The goal of the study was to develop a wearable sensor system-based scoring algorithm to assess motion quality during skiing. The system proposed in the current study is both well suited for use in a mobile application and is able to discriminate between high- and low-skill skiers, but only when the skiing style is sufficiently different (i.e., carving vs. drifting). Additionally, this scoring system embraces the previous steps proposed by the ARC (segmentation/enrichment/classification) and assesses motion quality relative to the performed technique and turn size [21].

A critical aspect of a scoring system is that it provides outputs which are prepared to feed further motion quality algorithms, such as the extended ARC [21]. For example, an algorithm which only provides a single numeric score is appropriate for comparing athletes or students but does not provide sufficient information to address further questions, such as "What should X do?". As the inputs of the algorithm proposed by this paper are easily interpretable, context-relevant parameters (e.g., edge angle, radial force, speed, and symmetry), the sub-scores calculated for each feature could be used to translate the scores for each PC into concrete coaching steps.

Although a PCA is typically used to address the main sources of variability in a dataset and reduce the number of input variables, in this case, PCAs are applied to each signal separately in order to identify the main variability sources within each signal independently, specifically so that the results could be translated into context-relevant coaching instructions. For example, consider a skier whose lowest sub-score comes from the radial force variable. Their PC 1 score was lower than the target. A low PC 1 score for radial force indicates that they ski with higher radial force than the target so they should aim for a lower radial force turn. Their PC 2 score was higher than the target, which, for radial force, indicates that the radial force peak was later in the turn. Therefore, they should aim to have their peak radial force earlier in the turn. Finally, for PC 3, their score was similar to the target, so the duration of the turn with higher radial force was similar to the reference.

Additionally, the scoring algorithm incorporates signals related to multiple aspects of alpine skiing and is able to assess the motion quality across all of the aspects independently of each other. For example, although skier A achieved a good score for PC 1 of edge angle, they received a low PC 2 score: both of these aspects are related to skiing performance; however, the magnitude of edge angle is more important for the timing of the peak edge angle, as, during carving skiing, the edge angle is directly related to the turn radius [30]. This is also reflected in the PCA results, as the variance explained by PC 1 (related to signal magnitude) in all skiing styles and all variables explained 82 ± 17% of the total variance, while PC 2 and PC 3 (generally related to signal timing and duration) explained 14 ± 15% and 3 ± 4% of the total variance of the dataset, respectively. The algorithm also considers this fact, scaling the contribution of each PC to the total score for each variable by the variance explained for each PC. For example, if a skier were to score a perfect 4 in each PC of radial force, their scores would be 2.78, 0.88, and 0.34, as PC 1–3 explain 70%, 22%, and 5%, respectively, of the total variance in the radial force signal. This prevents poor scores in PCs, which contribute very little to the overall variability from exacting an outsized influence on the overall score—for example, speed, where PC 1 explains ~99% of the variability across all styles. In the case of speed, the 1 Hz GPS signal is linearly interpolated to the 54 Hz IMU sample frequency by the application. Therefore, only the magnitude of the signal and not the shape of the signal is meaningful. In this case, the PCA is also "smart" enough to treat this parameter in the same way that a maximum value only would be scored.

The primary consideration for a scoring algorithm is its ability to distinguish between high- and low-skill skiers. In general, it can be observed that higher scores are associated with higher edge angles, higher symmetry, higher radial force, and higher speed, which generally matches the assumptions of higher performance observed in competitive environments [12]. The simplest proof of concept would be to use the algorithm to compare two skiers, one retired WC athlete and one beginner skier. The beginner skier was able to complete drifting turns with a low motion quality, but not carving turns. Given that the two skiers in this test completed the same test protocol, the mean score from the two skiers should represent their overall skiing quality. The average score for skier A, the retired WC athlete, across all collected turns was ~8.4, reflecting their high motion quality even in "lower-skill" drifted turns. The average score for skier B, the beginner, was 5.9. Although this skier was instructed to perform carving turns, according to the algorithm, this skier was unable to perform carving turns, and thus a majority of their turns were classified as drifting and thus scored below 7.

The results of the in-field validation show that the scoring algorithm was correlated with scores representing skiing dynamics, but not with the overall skiing quality. Therefore, it appears that the algorithm scores movement quality more based on the dynamics of the movement than the subjective motion quality as assessed by expert raters. This is a logical outcome, since the dynamics were the parameters directly measured by the IMU system (acceleration and angular velocities). Although the algorithm was able to correctly rank the skills of the three test skiers (beginner < instructor < expert), and the scores assigned accurately distinguished between the beginner and expert skier, Figure 5 shows that, outside of edge angle and speed, the scores were generally quite similar across all variables. Due to these similarities, the scores assigned by this algorithm are likely only discriminant enough to differentiate between skiers when the skiing style is sufficiently different (higher vs. lower dynamics).

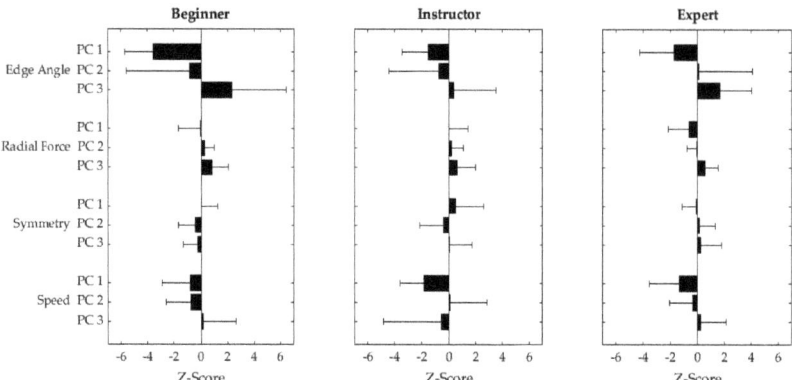

Figure 5. Mean +/− 1 standard deviation Z-transformed PC scores for PC 1–3 (top to bottom) across all runs (long, short, self-selected) for a beginner skier (**left**), a ski instructor (**middle**), and an expert skier (**right**).

The observation that the algorithm scores skiers based on their skiing dynamics highlights the importance of the choice of skiers included in the reference dataset. The scores assigned by the algorithm to the test dataset were generally skewed towards higher scores, which would be expected since the skiers in this dataset were all either instructors or former competitive alpine skiers. Although the reference group in this study contained only elite alpine skiers (retired WC athletes), the algorithm only assesses how similar the variability new data was to the set of reference skiers for each individual skiing style.

Therefore, it is possible to receive a negative score when PC scores are either above or below the reference skiers' values. For example, a skier with extremely high edge angles might receive the same score as a skier with a lower edge angle because they are both equally different from the reference dataset but in opposite directions, even though the case of the extremely high edge angle indicates objectively better skiing quality. Additionally, it is possible that the variability contained in this dataset (containing only expert skiers) might not represent the variability that might be contained by a dataset that includes more intermediate or novice skiers. On the contrary, such a dataset might not generate meaningful targets, as the variability of such a dataset would represent the variability between skill groups rather than the variability of a reference group. This highlights the importance of the selection of an appropriate reference group, which should match the quality of skiing to be evaluated by the algorithm.

In this context, a distinct advantage of this algorithm is its flexibility in adapting to a new reference. A user could simply record a new selected group of reference skiers, and the algorithm could learn a new reference model based on this new dataset, provided that it contained an appropriate volume of turns in all desired skiing styles. This could also be done on an individual level to provide a baseline for competitive skiers to detect subtle changes in skiing technique possibly related to fatigue and increased injury risk during longer training sessions [31].

A limitation of an approach such as the extended ARC is the issue of dependency. The accuracy of each step in the extended ARC is dependent on the accuracy of the previous step. For example, the accuracy of the ski style classification is dependent on the accuracy of the feature extraction step, which is dependent on the accuracy of the segmentation step. Despite this limitation, all of the steps in the extended ARC proposed above have been previously validated. Martinez and colleagues performed in-lab [3] and in-field [4] validations of the turn detection and segmentation algorithm, and the accuracy and precision of the estimated features edge angle and radial force have been shown to be $-0.77 \pm 1.00°$ and $1.50 \pm 1.33°$, respectively, and the classification algorithm proposed by Neuwirth and colleagues was able to distinguish between drifting and carving turns with an accuracy of 95%. This indicates that the error contributed from previous processing steps likely imposes a minimal influence on the accuracy of the scoring system. Additionally, the algorithm was designed based on input data processed via the same input algorithms, and, thus, the error contributed by the system itself is inherently included in the model of skiing motion quality.

5. Conclusions

The scoring algorithm presented in this study is a first step towards developing a wearable system to evaluate skiing motion quality that could be implemented in a stand-alone application for regular use by both recreational and competitive alpine skiers. The proposed system is a novel approach to quantifying motion quality and was able to differentiate between high- and low-skill skier abilities. Additionally, the system is easy to use, flexible, and could be easily adapted to accommodate reference skiers of varying abilities. Future work should focus on validating the algorithm in a wider range of skiing conditions, such as powder or moguls, using a more accurate reference scoring and incorporating further features (e.g., pressure distribution, ski bending, or mechanical energy dissipation) into the algorithm in order to provide a more robust and comprehensive view of motion quality during alpine skiing [12].

Author Contributions: Conceptualization, C.S., A.M., R.J., J.R. and T.S.; Data curation, C.S., A.M. and T.S.; Formal analysis, C.S.; Investigation, C.S.; Methodology, C.S., A.M. and R.J.; Project administration, T.S.; Resources, J.R.; Software, C.S., A.M. and T.S.; Supervision, T.S.; Validation, C.S.; Visualization, C.S.; Writing—original draft, C.S.; Writing—review and editing, C.S., A.M., R.J., J.R. and T.S. All authors have read and agreed to the published version of the manuscript.

Funding: This research was funded by the Austrian Federal Ministry for Transport, Innovation and Technology and the Austrian Federal Ministry for Digital and Economic Affairs and the federal state of Salzburg, (Grant number: 872574).

Institutional Review Board Statement: The study was conducted according to the guidelines of the Declaration of Helsinki, and approved by the Ethics Committee of the Paris Lodron—Universität Salzburg (EK—GZ: 11/2018, 31 July 2018).

Informed Consent Statement: Informed consent was obtained from all subjects involved in the study.

Data Availability Statement: The data presented in this study are available on request from the corresponding author.

Acknowledgments: The authors would like to thank Isabella Fessl and Simon Mayrhofer for their assistance during data collection and instrumentation, as well as Wolfgang Kremser, Richard Brunauer, and Christina Kranzinger for their assistance in algorithm design and data processing. Open Access Funding by the University of Salzburg.

Conflicts of Interest: The authors declare no conflict of interest.

References

1. Camomilla, V.; Bergamini, E.; Fantozzi, S.; Vannozzi, G. Trends supporting the in-field use of wearable inertial sensors for sport performance evaluation: A systematic review. *Sensors* **2018**, *18*, 873. [CrossRef]
2. Neuwirth, C.; Snyder, C.; Kremser, W.; Brunauer, R.; Holzer, H.; Stöggl, T. Classification of alpine skiing styles using gnss and inertial measurement units. *Sensors* **2020**, *20*, 4232. [CrossRef]
3. Martinez, A.; Jahnel, R.; Buchecker, M.; Snyder, C.; Brunauer, R.; Stöggl, T. Development of an automatic alpine skiing turn detection algorithm based on a simple sensor setup. *Sensors* **2019**, *19*, 12. [CrossRef] [PubMed]
4. Martínez, A.; Brunauer, R.; Venek, V.; Snyder, C.; Jahnel, R.; Buchecker, M.; Thorwartl, C.; Stöggl, T. Development and validation of a gyroscope-based turn detection algorithm for alpine skiing in the field. *Front. Sports Act. Living* **2019**, *1*, 18. [CrossRef] [PubMed]
5. Fasel, B.; Spörri, J.; Schutz, P.; Lorenzetti, S.; Aminian, K. An inertial sensor-based method for estimating the athlete's relative joint center positions and center of mass kinematics in alpine ski racing. *Front. Physiol.* **2017**, *8*, 850. [CrossRef] [PubMed]
6. Nemec, B.; Petric, T.; Babic, J.; Supej, M. Estimation of alpine skier posture using machine learning techniques. *Sensors* **2014**, *14*, 18898–18914. [CrossRef] [PubMed]
7. Spörri, J.; Kröll, J.; Fasel, B.; Aminian, K.; Müller, E. Course setting as a prevention measure for overuse injuries of the back in alpine ski racing: A kinematic and kinetic study of giant slalom and slalom. *Orthop. J. Sports Med.* **2016**, *4*. [CrossRef] [PubMed]
8. Sporri, J.; Kroll, J.; Fasel, B.; Aminian, K.; Muller, E. The use of body worn sensors for detecting the vibrations acting on the lower back in alpine ski racing. *Front. Physiol.* **2017**. [CrossRef]
9. Fasel, B.; Spörri, J.; Chardonnens, J.; Kröll, J.; Müller, E.; Aminian, K. Joint inertial sensor orientation drift reduction for highly dynamic movements. *IEEE J. Biomed. Health Inform.* **2018**, *22*, 77–86. [CrossRef]
10. Yu, G.; Jang, Y.J.; Kim, J.; Kim, J.H.; Kim, H.Y.; Kim, K.; Panday, S.B. Potential of imu sensors in performance analysis of professional alpine skiers. *Sensors* **2016**, *16*, 463. [CrossRef]
11. Fasel, B.; Spörri, J.; Gilgien, M.; Boffi, G.; Chardonnens, J.; Müller, E.; Aminian, K. Three-dimensional body and centre of mass kinematics in alpine ski racing using differential gnss and inertial sensors. *Remote Sens.* **2016**, *8*, 13. [CrossRef]
12. Hebert-Losier, K.; Supej, M.; Holmberg, H.-C. Biomechanical factors influencing the performance of elite alpine ski racers. *Sports Med.* **2014**, *44*, 519–533. [CrossRef] [PubMed]
13. Spörri, J.; Schiefermuller, C.; Müller, E. Collecting kinematic data on a ski track with optoelectronic stereophotogrammetry: A methodological study assessing the feasibility of bringing the biomechanics lab to the field. *PLoS ONE* **2016**, *11*, e0161757. [CrossRef]
14. Fasel, B.; Spörri, J.; Schutz, P.; Lorenzetti, S.; Aminian, K. Validation of functional calibration and strap-down joint drift correction for computing 3d joint angles of knee, hip, and trunk in alpine skiing. *PLoS ONE* **2017**, *12*, e0181446. [CrossRef] [PubMed]
15. Michahelles, F.; Schiele, B. Sensing and monitoring professional skiers. *IEEE Pervasive Comput.* **2005**, *4*, 40–45. [CrossRef]
16. Yamagiwa, S.; Ohshima, H.; Shirakawa, K. Skill Scoring System for Ski's Parallel Turns; icSPORTS: Rome, Italy, 2014; pp. 121–128.
17. Umek, A.; Kos, A.; Tomazic, S. Smartski: Application of sensors integrated into sport equipment. In Proceedings of the 2016 International Conference on Identification, Information and Knowledge in the Internet of Things, Beijing, China, 20–21 October 2016; pp. 122–127.
18. Kos, A.; Umek, A. Smart sport equipment: Smartski prototype for biofeedback applications in skiing. *Pers. Ubiquitous Comput.* **2018**, *22*, 535–544. [CrossRef]
19. Snyder, C.; Kremser, W.; Brunauer, R.; Holzer, H.; Stöggl, T. Validation of a wearable system for edge angle estimation during alpine skiing. In *Science and Skiing Viii*; Magdalena Karczewska-Lindinger, A.H., Vesa, L., Stefan, L., Eds.; Vuokatti Sports Technology Unit of the Faculty of Sport and Health Sciences of the University of Jyväskylä: Jyväskylä, Finland, 2020.

20. Roggen, D.; Magnenat, S.; Waibel, M.; Tröster, G. Wearable computing. *IEEE Robot. Autom. Mag.* **2011**, *18*, 83–95. [CrossRef]
21. Brunauer, R.; Kremser, W.; Stöggl, T. *From Sensor Data to Coaching in Alpine Skiing—A Software Design to Facilitate Immediate Feedback in Sports*; Springer International Publishing: Cham, Switzerland, 2020; pp. 86–95.
22. Robertson, G.E.; Caldwell, G.E.; Hamill, J.; Kamen, G.; Whittlesey, S. *Research Methods in Biomechanics*; Human Kinetics: Champaign, IL, USA, 2013.
23. Wu, J.N.; Wang, J.; Liu, L. Feature extraction via kpca for classification of gait patterns. *Hum. Mov. Sci.* **2007**, *26*, 393–411. [CrossRef]
24. Deluzio, K.J.; Astephen, J.L. Biomechanical features of gait waveform data associated with knee osteoarthritis: An application of principal component analysis. *Gait Posture* **2007**, *25*, 86–93. [CrossRef]
25. Ross, G.B.; Dowling, B.; Troje, N.F.; Fischer, S.L.; Graham, R.B. Objectively differentiating movement patterns between elite and novice athletes. *Med. Sci. Sports Exerc.* **2018**, *50*, 1457–1464. [CrossRef]
26. Kranz, M.; Möller, A.; Hammerla, N.; Diewald, S.; Plötz, T.; Olivier, P.; Roalter, L. The mobile fitness coach: Towards individualized skill assessment using personalized mobile devices. *Pervasive Mob. Comput.* **2013**, *9*, 203–215. [CrossRef]
27. Federolf, P.; Reid, R.; Gilgien, M.; Haugen, P.; Smith, G. The application of principal component analysis to quantify technique in sports. *Scand. J. Med. Sci. Sports* **2014**, *24*, 491–499. [CrossRef] [PubMed]
28. Movesense. Available online: https://www.movesense.com/wp-content/uploads/2017/11/Movesense-SensorDatasheet-_-20171109.pdf (accessed on 1 May 2021).
29. Cohen, J. Statistical power analysis. *Curr. Dir. Psychol. Sci.* **1992**, *1*, 98–101. [CrossRef]
30. Jentschura, U.D.; Fahrbach, F. Physics of skiing: The ideal carving equation and its applications. *Can. J. Phys.* **2004**, *82*, 249–261. [CrossRef]
31. Kröll, J.; Mueller, E.; Seifert, J.G.; Wakeling, J.M. Changes in quadriceps muscle activity during sustained recreational alpine skiing. *J. Sport. Sci. Med.* **2011**, *10*, 81–92.

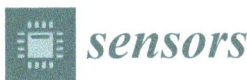

Communication

Detection of Movement Events of Long-Track Speed Skating Using Wearable Inertial Sensors

Yosuke Tomita [1,*], Tomoki Iizuka [1,2], Koichi Irisawa [1] and Shigeyuki Imura [1]

[1] Department of Physical Therapy, Graduate School of Health Care, Takasaki University of Health and Welfare, Takasaki 370-0033, Gunma, Japan; 1930201@takasaki-u.ac.jp (T.I.); irisawa@takasaki-u.ac.jp (K.I.); s-imura@takasaki-u.ac.jp (S.I.)

[2] Department of Rehabilitation, Kurosawa Hospital, Takasaki 370-1203, Gunma, Japan

* Correspondence: tomita-y@takasaki-u.ac.jp; Tel.: +81-27-352-1291 (ext. 285)

Abstract: Inertial measurement units (IMUs) have been used increasingly to characterize long-track speed skating. We aimed to estimate the accuracy of IMUs for use in phase identification of long-track speed skating. Twelve healthy competitive athletes on a university long-track speed skating team participated in this study. Foot pressure, acceleration and knee joint angle were recorded during a 1000-m speed skating trial using the foot pressure system and IMUs. The foot contact and foot-off timing were identified using three methods (kinetic, acceleration and integrated detection) and the stance time was also calculated. Kinetic detection was used as the gold standard measure. Repeated analysis of variance, intra-class coefficients (ICCs) and Bland-Altman plots were used to estimate the extent of agreement between the detection methods. The stance time computed using the acceleration and integrated detection methods did not differ by more than 3.6% from the gold standard measure. The ICCs ranged between 0.657 and 0.927 for the acceleration detection method and 0.700 and 0.948 for the integrated detection method. The limits of agreement were between 90.1% and 96.1% for the average stance time. Phase identification using acceleration and integrated detection methods is valid for evaluating the kinematic characteristics during long-track speed skating.

Keywords: inertial measurement unit; movement analysis; long-track speed skating; validity

1. Introduction

Long-track speed skating is a skillful sport where athletes glide on a 400-m ice rink at a speed of more than 50 km/h. The athletes accelerate their body using the ground reaction force exerted by the ice through an approximately 1 mm wide blade attached to the bottom of the skate shoe. Various studies have identified kinematic features of different movement phases, such as changes in the knee and trunk angles during races [1,2], that may influence the performance of long-track speed skating athletes. Additionally, a smaller push-off angle, which is the angle of the shank with respect to the floor in the frontal plane, has been shown to be associated with a greater power output [3] and skating velocity during a 5000-m race [1,2], although such a relationship was not observed during a 1500-m race [2]. Changes in the blade tilt angle during a 4000-m long-distance skating event have also been reported [4]. Several studies have also demonstrated the benefit of a greater knee flexion angle before the push-off to generate increased kinetic energy [3,5,6].

The majority of the studies that have investigated kinematic features during long-track speed skating has primarily used video analysis [1–6]. However, conventional kinematic measurements using video analysis have several limitations [7]. First, video analysis is largely influenced by the visibility of body landmarks. However, landmark visibility is often interfered by people or objects during long-track speed skating competitions or training sessions. Therefore, researchers need to synchronize measurements with multiple cameras and/or incorporate special environmental conditions to quantify kinematics with good body landmark visibility. Consequently, most kinematic analyses of long-track speed skating only measure an isolated segment of an entire race [1,2]. Although one study showed significant variability in the knee joint angles of athletes with similar performance levels [8], the source of the variability may partly be explained by the limited precision of the measurements.

Second, video analysis requires an enormous amount of time for data processing, which includes the identification of movement phases and digitization of body landmark positions. This limits the use of acquired data for immediate feedback to the athletes. Therefore, feedback regarding skating techniques must be provided predominantly based on visual or qualitative assessments from observers, without the benefit of a quantitative assessment.

In an effort to solve these limitations, inertial measurement units (IMUs) have been used increasingly in recent years as an alternative method to measure kinematics in various sports, such as speed skating, running and skiing. An IMU utilizes three axial accelerometers, gyroscopes and geomagnetometers [7]. The validity of IMUs for gait event detection has been well established [9,10], while evidence is limited for movement phase detection during sports performance. IMUs have several advantages over conventional video analyses. First, IMUs are not restricted by the visibility of body landmarks because the IMU system does not use positional data to compute kinematic outcomes. This allows for a kinematic measurement in a crowd and for a wide range of performance areas. Second, a kinematic analysis with IMUs does not require the digitization of body landmarks, allowing for a real-time display of kinematic features, including the angular velocity, acceleration and joint and segment angles. Therefore, the IMU is a promising tool for use in kinematic data acquisition in various situations, including sporting events and clinical rehabilitation.

The validity of joint angles derived from IMUs during gait and running has been widely examined by comparing them with gold standard measurements (e.g., an optical 3D motion capture system and a magnetic motion capture system) [11–13]. However, the validity of IMUs for the identification of movement phase classifications during long-track speed skating remains unknown. While no standardized movement phase classifications exist for long-track speed skating, foot contact and foot-off of each leg represent the start of the stance and swing, respectively, and both are important features for characterizing skating strokes [4]. Therefore, in this study, we focused on the identification of foot contact and foot-off. The objective of this study was to estimate the accuracy of IMUs for identification of foot contact and foot-off in competitive speed skaters during long-track speed skating by comparing the method with phase identification using the foot pressure sensor system. The validation of IMUs would advance the applicability of the system for use during long-track speed skating competitions and training sessions to allow for comprehensive kinematic analyses in flexible environments and instant feedback to athletes.

2. Materials and Methods

2.1. Participants

Twelve healthy competitive athletes on a university long-track speed skating team participated in the study after signing an informed consent form. All the participants had more than 10 years of speed skating experience. The demographic characteristics of the participants are shown in Table 1. This study was approved by the ethics committee of the Takasaki University of Health and Welfare (approval number: 1904) in accordance with the Declaration of Helsinki. The participants had no musculoskeletal or neurological pathologies that could affect task performance.

Table 1. The demographics of the study participants (n = 12).

Sex (Female:Male)	5:7
Height (mean ± SD), m	165.6 ± 6.12
Body weight (mean ± SD), kg	63.46 ± 5.85
Personal best time for 1000 m (mean ± SD), sec	77.41 ± 11.76

SD: standard deviation.

2.2. Data Acquisition

Data recording was performed during a full-speed 1000-m skating event from a static start position on a 400-m, two-lane indoor oval (Meiji Hokkaido-Tokachi Oval, Obihiro, Hokkaido, Japan).

The kinematic data were acquired using eight IMU sensors at a sampling rate of 100 Hz (myoMOTION, Noraxon, Scottsdale, AZ, USA). A data logger was embedded in each sensor, allowing data recording over a wide area. The IMU sensors were attached with double-sided tape to the skin at standardized locations on the lower thorax and pelvis and bilaterally on the thighs, shanks and feet. The specific sensor locations are shown in Table 2. Subsequently, the subjects wore compressive racing suits designed specifically for the body shape of each of the individual participants, which ensured that displacement of the sensors did not occur while recording was taking place. The foot sensors on the skating shoes were also stabilized with tape. The sensor locations were marked on the skin or skating shoes with a pen, as each sensor was attached, and we verified that there were no changes in the sensor locations before and after the data recordings.

Table 2. Sensor locations.

Lower Thoracic	In line with the spinal column at L1/T12
Pelvic	Body area of the sacrum
Thigh	Frontal and distal half (where there is less muscle displacement during motion)
Shank	Front and slightly medial (along the tibia)
Foot	Upper foot, slightly below the ankle

The kinetic data were acquired using a portable foot pressure measurement system at a sampling rate of 100 Hz (F-Scan System, TeckScan, South Boston, MA, USA). The system consists of two sensor sheets, two cuff units, one data logger unit and two cables connecting the cuff units and the data logger. Two sensor sheets were trimmed to the participant's foot size and a sensor sheet was inserted and attached to the sole of each of the skate shoes using double-sided tape. The cuff units were stabilized at the middle shanks and the data logger was attached to the back waist using Velcro tape. The IMU and foot pressure systems were synchronized using an electrical synch signal.

2.3. Data Analysis

We excluded the data from the first and last straights (first and last 50 m) and the first curve (100-m) from the analysis because the skating technique during these segments differs substantially from the remaining segment. Therefore, we analyzed the data for the remaining 800-m (400-m straight and 400-m curve) segment. The data from each side (left and right) were analyzed separately for both the straight and the curve. We adopted three types of analytical methods to detect foot contact and foot-off (Table 3).

Table 3. Overview of the three analytical methods used to detect foot contact and foot-off.

Name	Type of Sensor	Type of Signal
Kinetic detection	Foot pressure	Force
Acceleration detection	IMU	Foot sagittal acceleration
Integrated detection	IMU	Foot sagittal acceleration + knee flexion angle

IMU: inertial measurement unit.

The first detection (the kinetic detection method) was based on the foot pressure data. Foot contact and foot-off were defined as the moments in which the foot pressure exceeded (foot contact; the vertical solid line in Figure 1A) and diminished below (foot-off; the vertical dotted line in Figure 1A) 20% of the peak foot pressure, which was calculated from all evaluated strokes (the horizontal dashed line in Figure 1A). Based on our empirical observations of the data obtained from all the participants in this study, 20% peak foot pressure was high enough to avoid false detections due to noise, but low enough to detect both the foot contact and foot-off.

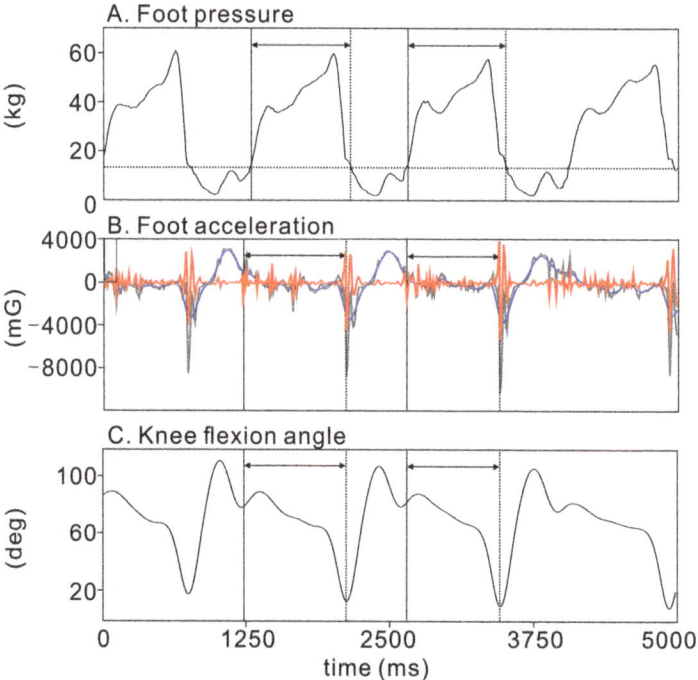

Figure 1. The timing identifications using three different detection methods. The vertical solid and dotted lines in each panel show the foot contact and foot-off timing, respectively. We calculated the stance time by computing the duration of the foot contact and foot-off for each skating stroke (intervals within horizontal arrows). (**A**) **Kinetic detection using the foot pressure**. The horizontal dotted line indicates the threshold level (20% peak) for the identification of foot contact and foot-off. (**B**) **Acceleration detection using the sagittal foot acceleration**. Gray line: raw sagittal acceleration. Red line: high-pass filtered sagittal acceleration. Blue line: low-pass filtered sagittal acceleration. (**C**) **Integrated detection using both the foot sagittal acceleration and the knee flexion angle**.

The second detection (the acceleration detection method) was based on the foot sagittal (anterior-posterior direction of the foot) acceleration data obtained from the IMU sensors on each foot. The sagittal acceleration signal was used because it showed consistent changes at both the foot contact and foot-off throughout the entire 1000-m of skating. The measured sagittal acceleration signals were filtered and decomposed to their high-frequency (Butterworth high-pass filter at a cut-off frequency of 20 Hz; the red line in Figure 1B) and low-frequency (Butterworth low-pass filter at a cut-off frequency of 10 Hz; the blue line in Figure 1B) components. The high-frequency component represents instant acceleration changes and clearly shows foot contact (the vertical solid line in Figure 1B) and foot-off (the vertical dotted line in Figure 1B). The low-frequency component represents slower acceleration changes and shows the swing movement of the leg. We divided the data such that each segment comprised the start and end of the swing movement based on the low-frequency component of the acceleration. We then looked for the moment at which the high-frequency component of the foot sagittal acceleration reached its peak. The first and second peaks were set as the foot contact and foot-off, respectively.

The third detection (the integrated detection method) was based on the combination of the foot acceleration and the knee flexion angle. Raw data were automatically filtered using a robust fusion algorithm (Kalman filter) optimized for IMU data by the IMU software (myoRESEARCH 3.10, Noraxon, Scottsdale, AZ, USA). Four element quaternion values were derived by combining the elemental sensor component axes to estimate the angular offset of each sensor from the calibrated position in the global coordinate [14,15]. The knee flexion angle was automatically calculated using the biomechanical model adopted by the IMU system software. The bias (normalized root mean square) of the knee flexion angle, derived by the present IMU software from the angle based on the model recommended by the International Society of Biomechanics [16], has been reported to be $16.9 \pm 5.1\%$ during gait. The knee flexion angle showed a phasic pattern within each stroke (Figure 1C), allowing for clear segmentation of the strokes. We divided the data such that each segment comprised the start and end of the phasic pattern, which constituted one stroke and swing of each leg. We then looked for the moment at which the high-frequency component of the foot sagittal acceleration reached its peak. The first and second peaks were set as the foot contact (the vertical solid line in Figure 1C) and foot-off (the vertical dotted line in Figure 1C), respectively. All the timing detections were performed by combining the automated and visual identifications.

Based on previous studies that reported the validity of IMU systems to detect gait events [17,18], we calculated the stance time for each stroke (calculated as the time from foot contact to foot-off for each stroke) separately for each leg (right and left), section (straight and curve) and detection method (kinetic, acceleration and integrated detection). The data analysis was performed using custom-made programs (MATLAB 2014a, MathWorks, Natick, MA, USA).

2.4. Statistical Analysis

The stance time as calculated based on the kinetic detection method was considered as the gold standard measure in our study. The difference in the stance times among the three detection methods was examined by a repeated measures analysis of variance (ANOVA). The Tukey honestly significant difference test was performed for the post-hoc pairwise comparisons. We used the intra-class coefficient (ICC) to examine the similarity between the kinetic detection and acceleration/integrated detection methods by computing the ICC (2,1) and their 95% confidence intervals (95% CIs). To assess the validity of the proposed detection method, Bland-Altman plots and limits of agreement were calculated for both the acceleration and integrated detection methods, where we estimated the level of agreement between the proposed methods and the gold standard measure (i.e., the kinetic detection method). The bias between the proposed methods and the gold standard measure was calculated as the mean difference between the measurements from each method. The upper and lower limits of agreement, which defined the margin in which 95% of the differences between the methods were expected to lie, were calculated as a bias of ± 1.96 SD. The precision of the limits of agreement is reported as the 95% confidence interval. SPSS ver. 21 (IBM, Armonk, NY, USA) was used for the statistical analyses. A statistical significance level of $p < 0.05$ was used for all the tests.

3. Results

In total, 1036 strokes (86.3 ± 10.4 strokes per participant) were analyzed in this study. The stance times detected by the three methods are summarized in Table 4. The results of the repeated measures ANOVA showed significant differences of stance time among detection methods on the right side (straight: $F = 15.236$, $p < 0.001$; curve: $F = 92.298$, $p < 0.001$). The post-hoc analysis showed that acceleration and integrated detection methods on the right side significantly overestimated the stance time by 2.4–3.6%, compared to the kinetic detection method ($p < 0.05$; Table 4). No significant difference was found between acceleration and integrated detections.

Table 4. Stance time detected by kinetic, acceleration and integrated detection methods.

Section	Side	Kinetic Detection Mean (SD), ms	Acceleration Detection Mean (SD), ms	Δ%	LOA%	Integrated Detection Mean (SD), ms	Δ%	LOA%	F	p
Straight	Right	713.1 (243.3)	730.5 (252.2) *	2.4	95.4	738.8 (259.4) *	3.6	94.2	15.236	<0.001
	Left	736.7 (261.2)	740.2 (250.1)	0.5	91.8	744.8 (264.6)	1.1	90.1	0.670	0.512
Curve	Right	614.7 (142.6)	629.4 (153.5) *	2.4	96.1	632.3 (150.2) *	2.9	93.4	92.298	<0.001
	Left	587.6 (127.1)	587.8 (108.5)	0.0	93.8	583.3 (102.2)	0.7	95.0	0.479	0.619

The differences between the acceleration and integrated detection methods and the kinetic detection methods are shown as Δ%. The proportion of cases within the limits of agreement is shown as LOA%. The F value and p value were obtained by the repeated measures analysis of variance. * Significantly different from the kinetic detection method in the post-hoc analysis.

The ICC (2,1) results for each detection method are summarized in Table 5. The ICC (2,1) was ≥0.700 for the integrated detection method for all the sections on both sides, while the ICC (2,1) was 0.657 for the acceleration detection method in the curve for the left side.

Table 5. The intra-class coefficient as computed by the acceleration and integrated detection methods.

Section	Detection Method	Right ICC (2,1) [95% CI]	Left ICC (2,1) [95% CI]
Straight	Acceleration	0.927 [0.906−0.943]	0.882 [0.852−0.907]
	Integrated	0.948 [0.925−0.963]	0.868 [0.834−0.895]
Curve	Acceleration	0.904 [0.875−0.926]	0.657 [0.582−0.721]
	Integrated	0.891 [0.529−0.956]	0.700 [0.633−0.757]

ICC: intra-class coefficient; 95% CI: 95% confidence interval.

The Bland-Altman plot is shown separately for each section (straight and curve), side (right and left), and detection method (acceleration and integrated) (Figures 2 and 3).

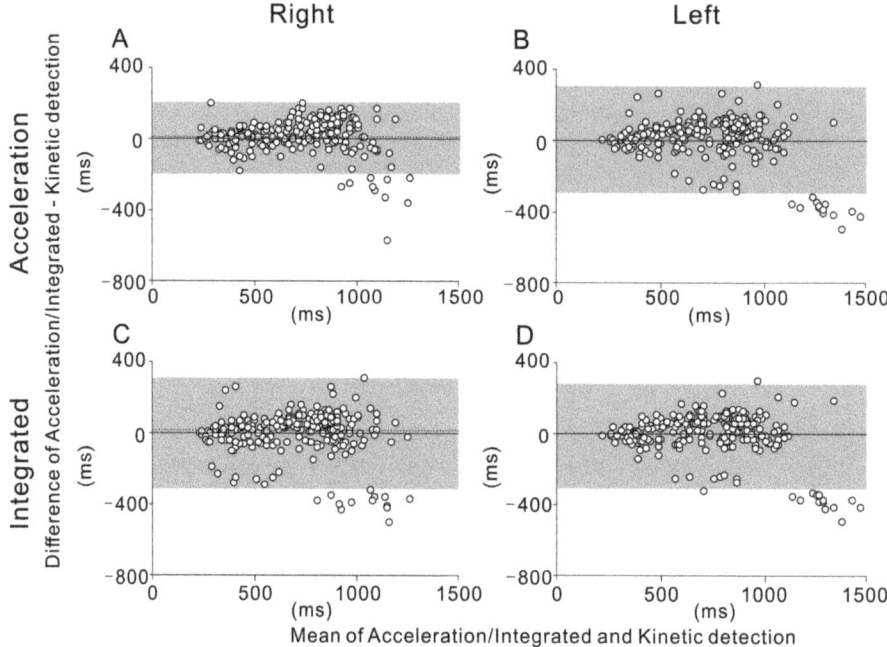

Figure 2. The Bland-Altman plot depicts the differences between the different detection methods in the straight, with 95% limits of agreement. The mean difference is shown by the dotted line. The 95% confidence intervals of the limits of agreement are also depicted (gray-shaded area). (**A**) Acceleration detection on the right side. (**B**) Acceleration detection on the left side. (**C**) Integrated detection on the right side. (**D**) Integrated detection on the left side.

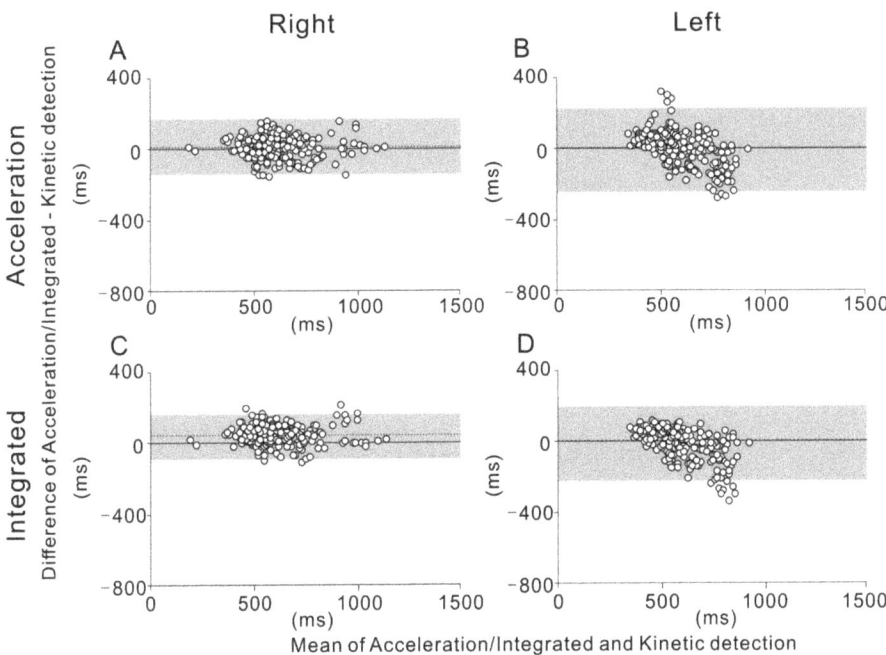

Figure 3. The Bland-Altman plot depicts the differences between the different detection methods in the curve, with 95% limits of agreement. The mean difference is shown by the dotted line. The 95% confidence intervals of the limits of agreement are also depicted (gray-shaded area). (**A**) Acceleration detection on the right side. (**B**) Acceleration detection on the left side. (**C**) Integrated detection on the right side. (**D**) Integrated detection on the left side.

The gray-shaded areas in the figures show the limits of agreement of the two detection methods. The proportion of cases within the limits of agreement was greater than 90% for all the measurements (LOA% in Table 4).

4. Discussion

In this study, we aimed to estimate the accuracy of IMUs for the phase identification of long-track speed skating for competitive speed skaters by comparing it with phase identification using the foot pressure sensor system. We examined the agreements of the acceleration and integrated detection methods with the gold standard measurements (i.e., the kinetic detection method) to calculate the stance time based on the foot contact and foot-off identified by each detection method.

The main finding of this study is the high degree of agreement between the kinetic and acceleration/integrated detection methods measured with the foot pressure sensor and IMU systems, as shown by the moderate to high ICCs. This was true for both sides (left and right) and segments (the straight and the curve). While statistically significant differences between the methods were found for the stroke time on the right side for both the straight and the curve, these differences were within 3.6%. The significant difference may partly be due to the large number of strokes used for the comparison, while the magnitude of the observed errors may not be very meaningful. Our Bland-Altman analysis shows that in the straight, the extent of the bias was proportional to the observed stance time (Figure 2). It is known that, during running, the stance time is prolonged as the running speed decreases [19]. Therefore, it should be noted that both the acceleration and integrated methods may be biased when the stance time is greater and the skating speed is slower (e.g., during long-distance skating). Our results also suggest that during the curve, the ICCs for the left side were substantially lower than those for the right side. This side-specific difference may be related to the asymmetrical skating form during the curve. Further study is needed to investigate the side-specific difference of the skating form during the curve in speed skating.

The acceleration and integrated detection methods were in significant agreement with the gold standard measure for the computation of the stance time, which suggests that the timing of the foot contact and foot-off for each leg and stroke can be accurately detected by these methods. The identification of foot contact and foot-off during skating is crucial for characterizing skating performance. It has been shown that the force measured by the sensor embedded in the skate shoe is greater when the subject stands on one leg (single leg stance), while the force substantially decreases when both legs are on the ice (double leg stance) [20]. The detection methods proposed in this study can be used to characterize skating performance using only IMUs, with minimal interference to the performance of the subject. The accuracy of acceleration and integrated methods was similar in our study, suggesting either method can be used for the detection of foot contact and foot-off. However, the phases of the speed skating motion can be divided into more details than just foot contact and foot-off [21]. IMUs have the potential to be used to identify a more detailed phase classification. In particular, the knee flexion, hip flexion and hip extension angles may potentially be used for a more detailed phase classification, as these angles show phase-dependent changes [22]. Therefore, the combined use of acceleration and the joint angle profiles obtained by IMUs would be ideal for future studies.

This study had several limitations. First, we only included healthy competitive athletes from a university long-track speed skating team. Further studies are necessary to generalize the results to different populations. Second, we used a foot pressure system as the gold standard measure, although the system itself could exhibit a measurement bias. Specifically, we used 20% peak force as the threshold for the foot contact and foot-off timing for the kinetic detection method. The 20% threshold was selected based on the observation of all trials from all participants, assuring no false detection in the kinetic detection, while the threshold may not be generalizable to other datasets. Furthermore, in reality, foot contact and foot-off occurred respectively earlier and later than the timing identified by the kinetic detection. This time lag between the actual and detected events can explain the systematic bias observed between the detection methods (i.e., all the positive Δ% values in Table 4). This time lag can overestimate the bias, while providing conservative results for the objective of this study.

5. Conclusions

In this study, we examined the agreement among the acceleration and integrated detection methods and the gold standard measure (i.e., the kinetic detection method) to calculate the stance time based on the foot contact and foot-off identified by each detection method. Despite the statistically significant differences between the acceleration/integrated detection methods and the gold standard measure on the right side, these differences were within 3.6%. The current data show that phase identification using acceleration and integrated detection is valid for evaluating the kinematic characteristics during long-track speed skating.

Author Contributions: Conceptualization, Y.T., T.I., K.I. and S.I.; methodology, Y.T. and T.I.; data collection, Y.T. and T.I.; formal analysis, Y.T. and T.I.; data curation, Y.T. and T.I.; writing—original draft preparation, Y.T. and T.I.; writing—review and editing, Y.T., T.I., K.I. and S.I.; supervision, Y.T. and S.I.; funding acquisition, Y.T. All authors have read and agreed to the published version of the manuscript.

Funding: This research was supported by Kakenhi (Grant-in-Aid for Early-Career Scientists No. 19K20011).

Institutional Review Board Statement: The study was conducted according to the guidelines of the Declaration of Helsinki and approved by the Ethics Committee of the Takasaki University of Health and Welfare (approval number: 1904, 17 May 2019).

Informed Consent Statement: Informed consent was obtained from all subjects involved in the study.

Data Availability Statement: Data available on request due to ethical restrictions.

Acknowledgments: We thank all participants who volunteered for our study.

Conflicts of Interest: The authors declare no conflict of interest.

References

1. Noordhof, D.A.; Foster, C.; Hoozemans, M.J.; de Koning, J.J. Changes in speed skating velocity in relation to push-off effectiveness. *Int. J. Sports Physiol. Perform.* **2013**, *8*, 188–194. [CrossRef] [PubMed]
2. Noordhof, D.A.; Foster, C.; Hoozemans, M.J.; de Koning, J.J. The association between changes in speed skating technique and changes in skating velocity. *Int. J. Sports Physiol. Perform.* **2014**, *9*, 68–76. [CrossRef]
3. van Ingen Schenau, G.J.; de Groot, G.; de Boer, R.W. The control of speed in elite female speed skaters. *J. Biomech.* **1985**, *18*, 91–96. [CrossRef]
4. Yuda, J.; Yuki, M.; Aoyanagi, T.; Fujii, N.; Ae, M. Changes in Blade Reaction Forces During the Curve Phase Due to Fatigue in Long Distance Speed Skating. *Int. J. Sport Health Sci.* **2004**, *2*, 195–204. [CrossRef]
5. de Koning, J.J.; de Groot, G.; van Ingen Schenau, G.J. Ice friction during speed skating. *J. Biomech.* **1992**, *25*, 565–571. [CrossRef]
6. Upjohn, T.; Turcotte, R.; Pearsall, D.J.; Loh, J. Three-dimensional kinematics of the lower limbs during forward ice hockey skating. *Sports Biomech.* **2008**, *7*, 206–221. [CrossRef] [PubMed]
7. Faisal, A.I.; Majumder, S.; Mondal, T.; Cowan, D.; Naseh, S.; Deen, M.J. Monitoring Methods of Human Body Joints: State-of-the-Art and Research Challenges. *Sensors* **2019**, *19*, 2629. [CrossRef] [PubMed]
8. van Ingen Schenau, G.J. The influence of air friction in speed skating. *J. Biomech.* **1982**, *15*, 449–458. [CrossRef]
9. Simonetti, E.; Villa, C.; Bascou, J.; Vannozzi, G.; Bergamini, E.; Pillet, H. Gait event detection using inertial measurement units in people with transfemoral amputation: A comparative study. *Med. Biol. Eng. Comput.* **2020**, *58*, 461–470. [CrossRef] [PubMed]
10. Romijnders, R.; Warmerdam, E.; Hansen, C.; Welzel, J.; Schmidt, G.; Maetzler, W. Validation of IMU-based gait event detection during curved walking and turning in older adults and Parkinson's Disease patients. *J. Neuroeng. Rehabil.* **2021**, *18*, 28. [CrossRef]
11. Bonnet, V.; Joukov, V.; Kulić, D.; Fraisse, N. Monitoring of Hip and Knee Joint Angles Using a Single Inertial Measurement Unit During Lower Limb Rehabilitation. *IEEE Sens. J.* **2016**, *16*, 1557–1564. [CrossRef]
12. Seel, T.; Raisch, J.; Schauer, T. IMU-based joint angle measurement for gait analysis. *Sensors* **2014**, *14*, 6891–6909. [CrossRef] [PubMed]
13. Reenalda, J.; Maartens, E.; Homan, L.; Buurke, J.H.J. Continuous three dimensional analysis of running mechanics during a marathon by means of inertial magnetic measurement units to objectify changes in running mechanics. *J. Biomech.* **2016**, *49*, 3362–3367. [CrossRef] [PubMed]
14. Berner, K.; Cockcroft, J.; Louw, Q. Kinematics and temporospatial parameters during gait from inertial motion capture in adults with and without HIV: A validity and reliability study. *Biomed. Eng. Online* **2020**, *19*, 57. [CrossRef] [PubMed]
15. Mundt, M.; Thomsen, W.; David, S.; Dupré, T.; Bamer, F.; Potthast, W.; Markert, B. Assessment of the measurement accuracy of inertial sensors during different tasks of daily living. *J. Biomech.* **2019**, *84*, 81–86. [CrossRef] [PubMed]
16. Wu, G.; Siegler, S.; Allard, P.; Kirtley, C.; Leardini, A.; Rosenbaum, D.; Whittle, M.; D'Lima, D.D.; Cristofolini, L.; Witte, H.; et al. Standardization and Terminology Committee of the International Society of Biomechanics. ISB recommendation on definitions of joint coordinate system of various joints for the reporting of human joint motion—part I: Ankle, hip, and spine. International Society of Biomechanics. *J. Biomech.* **2002**, *35*, 543–548. [CrossRef]
17. Mariani, B.; Hoskovec, C.; Rochat, S.; Büla, C.; Penders, J.; Aminian, K. 3D gait assessment in young and elderly subjects using foot-worn inertial sensors. *J. Biomech.* **2010**, *43*, 2999–3006. [CrossRef] [PubMed]
18. Brégou Bourgeois, A.; Mariani, B.; Aminian, K.; Zambelli, P.Y.; Newman, C.J. Spatio-temporal gait analysis in children with cerebral palsy using, foot-worn inertial sensors. *Gait Posture* **2014**, *39*, 436–442. [CrossRef]
19. Clark, K.P.; Weyand, P.G. Are running speeds maximized with simple-spring stance mechanics? *J. Appl. Physiol.* **2014**, *117*, 604–615. [CrossRef] [PubMed]
20. van der Kruk, E.; Veeger, H.E.J.; van der Helm, F.C.T.; Schwab, A.L. Design and verification of a simple 3D dynamic model of speed skating which mimics observed forces and motions. *J. Biomech.* **2017**, *64*, 93–102. [CrossRef] [PubMed]
21. van der Kruk, E.; Schwab, A.L.; van der Helm, F.C.T.; Veeger, H.E.J. Getting in shape: Reconstructing three-dimensional long-track speed skating kinematics by comparing several body pose reconstruction techniques. *J. Biomech.* **2018**, *69*, 103–112. [CrossRef] [PubMed]
22. Khuyagbaatar, B.; Purevsuren, T.; Park, W.M.; Kim, K.; Kim, Y.H. Interjoint coordination of the lower extremities in short-track speed skating. *Proc. Inst. Mech. Eng. H* **2017**, *231*, 987–993. [CrossRef] [PubMed]

MDPI
St. Alban-Anlage 66
4052 Basel
Switzerland
Tel. +41 61 683 77 34
Fax +41 61 302 89 18
www.mdpi.com

Sensors Editorial Office
E-mail: sensors@mdpi.com
www.mdpi.com/journal/sensors

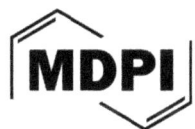

www.ingramcontent.com/pod-product-compliance
Lightning Source LLC
LaVergne TN
LVHW070616100526
838202LV00012B/660